METHODS IN MOLECULAR BIOLOGY

Series Editor
John M. Walker
School of Life and Medical Sciences
University of Hertfordshire
Hatfield, Hertfordshire, AL10 9AB, UK

For further volumes:
http://www.springer.com/series/7651

Marine Genomics

Methods and Protocols

Edited by

Sarah J. Bourlat

Department of Marine Sciences, University of Gothenburg, Gothenburg, Sweden

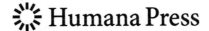 Humana Press

Editor
Sarah J. Bourlat
Department of Marine Sciences
University of Gothenburg
Gothenburg, Sweden

ISSN 1064-3745   ISSN 1940-6029   (electronic)
Methods in Molecular Biology
ISBN 978-1-4939-8135-9   ISBN 978-1-4939-3774-5   (eBook)
DOI 10.1007/978-1-4939-3774-5

Cover caption: Ephyra larva of the barrel jellyfish, *Rhizostoma pulmo* captured in a zooplankton haul off the Swedish west coast. – Photo By: Erik Selander, Department of Marine Sciences, University of Gothenburg, Sweden

Printed on acid-free paper

This Humana Press imprint is published by Springer Nature
The registered company is Springer Science+Business Media LLC New York

Preface

Marine genomics includes all aspects of genes and genomes of marine organisms aimed at understanding their evolution, function, biodiversity and environmental interactions. The field of genomics has been revolutionized by next generation sequencing, providing novel insights into one of the largest biomes on our planet.

In this book, we present the latest protocols for both laboratory and bioinformatics based analyses in the field of marine genomics. The chapters presented here cover a wide range of topics, including the sampling and genomics of bacterial communities, DNA extraction in marine organisms, high-throughput sequencing of whole mitochondrial genomes, phylogenomics, SNP discovery, SNP arrays for species identification, digital PCR-based quantification methods, environmental DNA for invasive species surveillance and monitoring, microarrays for the detection of waterborne pathogens, DNA barcoding of marine biodiversity, metabarcoding protocols for marine eukaryotes, analytical protocols for the visualization of eukaryotic diversity, and applications of genomic data to benthic indices for environmental monitoring.

These trusted protocols provide detailed step-by-step instructions, regents and materials as well as tips and troubleshooting, making this volume a valuable resource for researchers, students, and policy makers in the field of marine biology.

Gothenburg, Sweden   *Sarah J. Bourlat*

Contents

Contributors

HENRIK ARONSSON • *Department of Biological and Environmental Sciences, University of Gothenburg, Gothenburg, Sweden*

EVA AYLAGAS • *AZTI, Marine Research Division, Sukarrieta, Bizkaia, Spain*

ANDERS BLOMBERG • *Department of Marine Sciences, University of Gothenburg, Strömstad, Sweden*

SARAH J. BOURLAT • *Department of Marine Sciences, University of Gothenburg, Gothenburg, Sweden*

ANDREW GEORGE BRISCOE • *Department of Life Sciences, Natural History Museum, London, UK*

R. ANDREW CAMERON • *Division of Biology and Biological Engineering, California Institute of Technology, Pasadena, CA, USA*

JOHANNA TAYLOR CANNON • *Department of Zoology, Naturhistoriska Riksmuseet, Stockholm, Sweden*

YIPING CAO • *Southern California Coastal Water Research Project Authority, Costa Mesa, CA, USA*

PETER DAHL • *Department of Chemistry and Molecular Biology, University of Gothenburg, Gothenburg, Sweden*

AGATA DRYWA • *Institute of Oceanology, Polish Academy of Sciences, Sopot, Poland*

JENNIE FINNMAN • *Sahlgrenska Academy, Gothenburg University Genomics Core Facility, Gothenburg, Sweden*

VERA G. FONSECA • *Zoological Research Museum Alexander Koenig (ZFMK), Centre for Molecular Biodiversity Research, Bonn, Germany*

ANNA GODHE • *Department of Marine Sciences, University of Gothenburg, Gothenburg, Sweden*

MIRIAM GÖTTING • *Department of Biology, University of Turku, Turku, Finland*

JOHN F. GRIFFITH • *Southern California Coastal Water Research Project Authority, Costa Mesa, CA, USA*

QUITERIE HAENEL • *Department of Biology and Environmental Sciences, University of Gothenburg, Gothenburg, Sweden*

PAUL D.N. HEBERT • *Centre for Biodiversity Genomics, Biodiversity Institute of Ontario, University of Guelph, Guelph, ON, Canada*

KEVIN PETER HOPKINS • *Department of Life Sciences, Natural History Museum, London, UK*

CHRISTOPHER L. JERDE • *Department of Biology, Aquatic Ecosystems Analysis Laboratory, University of Nevada, Reno, NV, USA*

KERSTIN JOHANNESSON • *Department of Marine Sciences, University of Gothenburg, Strömstad, Sweden*

MATTHEW KENT • *Centre for Integrative Genetics (CIGENE), Department of Animal and Aquacultural Sciences, IHA, Norwegian University of Life Sciences, NMBU, Ås, Norway*

NANCY KNOWLTON • *National Museum of Natural History, Smithsonian Institution, Washington, DC, USA*

KEVIN MICHAEL KOCOT • *Department of Biological Sciences and Alabama Museum of Natural History, The University of Alabama, Tuscaloosa, AL, USA*

DELPHINE LALLIAS • *Institut National de la Recherche Agronomique (INRA), Unité Génétique en Aquaculture, Centre de Jouy-en-Josas, Jouy-en-Josas, France*

KATJA LEHMANN • *Centre for Ecology and Hydrology, Crowmarsh Gifford, Wallingford, UK*

MATTHIEU LERAY • *National Museum of Natural History, Smithsonian Institution, Washington, DC, USA*

SIGBJØRN LIEN • *Centre for Integrative Genetics (CIGENE), Department of Animal and Aquacultural Sciences, IHA, Norwegian University of Life Sciences, NMBU, Ås, Norway*

ULRIKA LIND • *Department of Marine Sciences, University of Gothenburg, Strömstad, Sweden*

ANDREW R. MAHON • *Department of Biology, Institute for Great Lakes Research, Central Michigan University, Mount Pleasant, MI, USA*

MIKKO NIKINMAA • *Department of Biology, University of Turku, Turku, Finland*

OLGA ORTEGA-MARTINEZ • *Department of Marine Sciences, University of Gothenburg, Strömstad, Sweden*

MARINA PANOVA • *Department of Marine Sciences, University of Gothenburg, Strömstad, Sweden*

RICARDO PEREYRA • *Department of Marine Sciences, University of Gothenburg, Strömstad, Sweden*

SEAN W.J. PROSSER • *Centre for Biodiversity Genomics, Biodiversity Institute of Ontario, University of Guelph, Guelph, ON, Canada*

NAIARA RODRÍGUEZ-EZPELETA • *AZTI, Marine Research Division, Sukarrieta, Bizkaia, Spain*

DIRK STEINKE • *Centre for Biodiversity Genomics, Biodiversity Institute of Ontario, University of Guelph, Guelph, ON, Canada*

KRISTIL KINDEM SUNDSAASEN • *Centre for Integrative Genetics (CIGENE), Department of Animal and Aquacultural Sciences, IHA, Norwegian University of Life Sciences, NMBU, Ås, Norway*

SYLVIE V.M. TESSON • *Department of Marine Sciences, University of Gothenburg, Gothenburg, Sweden*

FILIPA F. VALE • *Host-Pathogen Unit, Research Institute for Medicine, (iMed-ULisboa), Faculdade de Farmácia da Universidade de Lisboa, Universidade de Lisboa, Lisbon, Portugal; Instituto de Medicina Molecular, Faculdade de Medicina da Universidade de Lisboa, Universidade de Lisboa, Lisbon, Portugal*

ANDREA WAESCHENBACH • *Department of Life Sciences, Natural History Museum, London, UK*

STEPHEN B. WEISBERG • *Southern California Coastal Water Research Project Authority, Costa Mesa, CA, USA*

ROMAN WENNE • *Institute of Oceanology, Polish Academy of Sciences, Sopot, Poland*

PIERRE DE WIT • *Department of Marine Sciences, University of Gothenburg, Strömstad, Sweden*

ANNA-LISA WRANGE • *Department of Marine Sciences, University of Gothenburg, Strömstad, Sweden*

Chapter 1

Sampling of Riverine or Marine Bacterial Communities in Remote Locations: From Field to Publication

Katja Lehmann

Abstract

This protocol describes how to sample and preserve microbial water column samples from rivers that can be used for 16S or 18S metabarcoding studies or shotgun sequencing. It further describes how to extract the DNA for sequencing and how to prepare raw Illumina MiSeq amplicon data and analyze it in the R environment.

Key words Biodiversity, Riverine microbial communities, Community analysis, Illumina MiSeq

1 Introduction

High-throughput sequencing technologies have revolutionized biodiversity studies of prokaryotes and are increasingly used to study whole communities. In rivers, which are diverse environments with different sub-habitats that are closely linked to adjacent terrestrial biomes, the collection and analysis of eDNA offer unprecedented monitoring opportunities. Collection of viable riverine microbiological samples, however, is often confounded by the remoteness and inaccessibility of sampling sites. In addition to this, increasingly open access to research data creates a need for data interoperability and so a need for standardized procedures to ensure consistency between datasets. Mega-sequencing campaigns, such as the Earth Microbiome Project or Ocean Sampling Day (OSD) [1, 2], can help this goal by driving the development of cost-effective protocols and analysis methods.

Here, I describe the standardized procedures to collect and analyze DNA samples for River Sampling Day (RSD) (part of Ocean Sampling Day [2]), a simultaneous sequencing campaign collecting a time series of ocean and river microbial data from the June and December solstices each year in rivers worldwide on the same day. Low-cost, manual sampling tools are utilized to collect

Sarah J. Bourlat (ed.), *Marine Genomics: Methods and Protocols*, Methods in Molecular Biology, vol. 1452,
DOI 10.1007/978-1-4939-3774-5_1, © Springer Science+Business Media New York 2016

riverine water column samples, which can subsequently be extracted for 16S, 18S, metabarcoding, or shotgun sequencing. I then proceed to describe the preparation of raw Illumina MiSeq amplicon data for analysis, followed by a description of an analysis pipeline for the open-source statistics software package R. The sampling protocol is based on methods used in the Freshwater Biological Sampling Manual [3] and the methods used at the Western Channel Observatory in the UK [4].

2   Materials

2.1 Sample Collection

1. Sterivex 0.22 μm filter cartridge SVGPL10RC (male luer-lock outlet, Millipore, UK) or SVGP010 (male nipple outlet, Millipore, UK).
2. RNAlater (Thermo Fisher Scientific, Loughborough, UK, or Ambion Inc., Austin, Texas).
3. Luer-lock syringes, 3 mL (e.g., Medisave, Weymouth, UK).
4. High-pressure sampling bottle fitted with bicycle valve and tube outlet, 10% acid washed (e.g., Nalgene™ Heavy-Duty PPCO Vacuum Bottle, Thermo Fisher Scientific, Loughborough, UK). *See* Fig. 1 for illustration.
5. PTFE tubing.
6. Two hose clamps to secure PTFE tubes.
7. Bicycle pump.
8. Nitrile gloves.
9. 70% ethanol to clean gloves/equipment.
10. Sterilized sticky tac (e.g., Blu-Tac).

2.2 Sample Preparation

1. DNA extraction solution, e.g., a commercial kit
2. Sterile consumables and shakers/bead beaters/centrifuges required for DNA extraction method of choice.

2.3 Raw Data Preparation and Analysis

1. QIIME software (qiime.org).
2. R environment (www.r-project.org).

3   Methods

3.1 Sample Collection

Collect three replicate bacterial samples at each location. If sampling multiple locations, take the samples at each location within the same time frame. For specifics on safety, clean sampling, and record taking, *see* **Notes 1–3**.

3.1.1 Option A: Sampling Midstream

1. With a 10% acid-washed sampling bottle, wade into the river downstream from the point at which you will collect the sample.

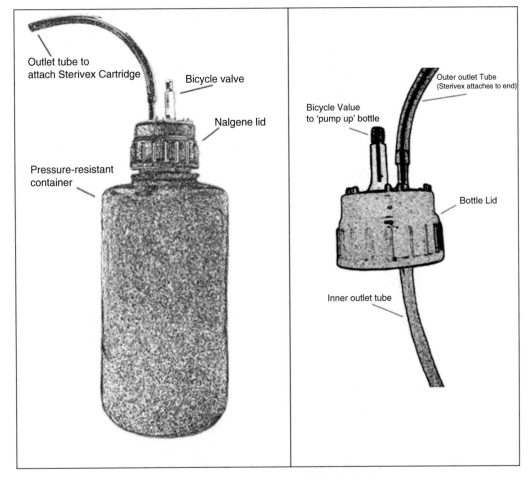

Fig. 1 Field sampling bottle with altered screw top to allow pressurized filtering

2. Wade upstream to the sample site. This ensures that you will not disturb sediments upstream from the sample point. Stand perpendicular to the flow and face upstream.

3. Remove the lid and hold it aside without allowing anything to touch the inner surface. With your other hand, grasp the bottle well below the neck.

4. Plunge it beneath the surface with the opening facing directly down; then immediately orient the bottle into the current.

5. Once the bottle is full, remove it from the water by forcing it forward (into the current) and upward.

3.1.2 Option B: Sampling from the Stream Bank

1. Secure yourself to a solid object on the shore.

2. Remove lid from a 10 % acid-washed sampling bottle.

3. Hold the bottle well below the neck. Reach out (arm length only) and plunge the bottle under the water, and immediately orient it into the current.

4. When the bottle is full, pull it up through the water while forcing it into the current.

3.1.3 Filtering

Now collect the microbial community by passing 1–5 L of the sampled water through a 0.22 μm filter using Sterivex cartridges. Filtration through the Sterivex filter should be done using the field sampling bottle:

1. Attach the Sterivex filter to the tube that comes out of the cap of your bottle (*see* Fig. 1). Secure the tube to the cap outlet and the Sterivex filter with two hose clamps.

2. Attach the bicycle pump to the valve on the bottle cap and pump up the bottle. If the water is very clear, you might need to refill the bottle and filter up to 5 L through the same filter. If you have to collect more water, place the bottle cap, and filter in sterile bags while you refill the bottle as described in Subheading 3.1. The filtration is done when the filter begins to clog up.

3. When the filtering is done, the Sterivex should be pumped free of standing water.

4. Seal the nipple side of the filter using sterilized sticky tac or similar; then use a 3 mL luer-lock syringe to fill the filter with RNAlater.

5. Seal the Sterivex filter using sterilized sticky tac or similar. Note that parafilm will crumble at temperatures below -45 °C and therefore should not be used.

3.1.4 Transport and Storage

1. Label the sample and place it in a sterile bag or tube. For transport from the sampling location to the lab, samples can be stored in the sealed bag in a cooling container. Samples in RNAlater can be kept at room temperature up to a week.

2. On arrival at the lab, provided the samples are stored in RNAlater, freeze samples at –20 °C (not –80 °C, or store in the refrigerator at 4 °C for up to a month if no freezer is available.

3.1.5 Metadata

A subset or all of the following metadata will greatly help to make sense of the microbial data, especially when multiple locations are being sampled. At minimum metadata should consist of sample volume, depth, temperature, lat/lon, time of day, and pH. Depending on the study, these should be supplemented by alkalinity, suspended sediment, soluble reactive phosphorus (SRP), total dissolved phosphorus (TDP), total phosphorus (TP), Si, F, Cl, Br, SO_4, total dissolved nitrogen (TDN), NH_4, NO_2, NO_3, dissolved organic matter (DOC), Na, K, Ca, Mg, B, Fe, Mn, Zn, Cu, and Al. The metadata measurements should be taken at or close to the date/time when the samples are collected.

3.2 Sample Preparation in the Lab

The DNA captured on the Sterivex filters needs to be extracted. For OSD/RSD, a commercial kit ensures consistency during extraction, but commercial kits are often not sold sterile, and some have been found to contaminate samples [5, 6]. This can confound sequencing results, especially when DNA concentration in the samples is expected to be low. Contamination of samples from a number of sources is a well-known danger at many stages of the extraction and sequencing process; it is therefore advisable to run a control alongside the samples during all steps, including the sequencing. Problems can also be caused by unexpected cross effects of preservative residues and kit reagents. It is advisable to do a test extraction first and verify DNA yield and quality on a gel. If necessary, an additional PEG precipitation prior to final cleaning steps on a kit spin filters might insure against DNA loss. Once the DNA is extracted, it can be amplified by PCR for 16S or any other amplicon analysis or transferred to the sequencing facility for shotgun sequencing as is. *See* Chapters 12 (Fonseca and Lallias), 13 (Bourlat et al.), and 14 (Leray et al.) for protocols detailing the preparation of amplicon libraries for Illumina sequencing. Here, we will focus on the analysis of 16S amplicon data derived from Illumina sequencing.

3.3 From Raw Sequencing Data to Operational Taxonomic Unit (OTU) Table

One of the most popular pipelines to process data derived from next-generation sequencing is QIIME [7], an open-source software wrapper that incorporates a great number of python scripts, including complete programs such as MOTHUR, in itself a comprehensive analysis pipeline [8], and USEARCH, a BLAST alternative [9]. For installation options, *see* **Note 4**. QIIME can process Illumina data, but also 454 and (with a bit of preprocessing) Ion Torrent data. We will focus on Illumina here, which has emerged as the predominant sequencing method in the last few years. To process any raw sequence data, QIIME requires a mapping file with metadata such as sample ID and primer- and barcode information (*see* Chapter 15 by Leray and Knowlton for further details on QIIME mapping file format). Depending on the format of the raw sequences, four scripts are required to process a set of Illumina-derived sequences in QIIME to obtain data that can be used for statistical analysis:

1. *join_paired_ends.py*, a script that joins paired end reads.
2. *validate_mapping_file.py*, a script which checks the soundness of the mapping file.

3. *split_libraries_fastq.py*, a script that divides the raw sequence library by barcode.

4. *pick_de_novo_otus.py*, a workflow that produces an OTU mapping file, a representative set of sequences, a sequence alignment file, a taxonomy assignment file, a filtered sequence alignment, a phylogenetic tree, and a biom-formatted OTU table.

Both the phylogenetic tree and the OTU table can then be exported into other programs for further analysis. In QIIME itself, further scripts allow for exploration of alpha diversity and beta diversity, notably:

5. *summarize_taxa_through_plots.py*, which creates taxonomy summary plots.

6. *alpha_rarefaction.py*, which calculates rarefaction curves.

7. *beta_diversity_through_plots.py*, which performs principle coordinates (PCoA) analysis on the samples.

For detailed instructions on performing diversity analyses with QIIME, *see* chapter 15 by Leray and Knowlton. QIIME also offers network analysis, which can be visualized in Cytoscape. QIIME has comprehensive help pages for each script (http://qiime.org/scripts/) and a number of tutorials (http://qiime.org/tutorials/index.html).

3.4 Basic Statistics in R

The open-source software package R [10] is a well-known statistics and scripting environment. It is available for Linux, Mac OS X, and Windows (www.**r**-project.org). Before starting the analysis, the following libraries need to be installed in R: biom [11], RColorBrewer [12], vegan [13], gplots [14], calibrate [15], ape [16], picante [17], Hmisc [18], BiodiversityR [19], psych [20], ggplot2 [21], grid [10], and biocLite.R [22].

3.4.1 Data Preparation

As a first step, the OTU table has to be imported into R either as text or as biom-formatted file with the following commands:

- Untransposed:
  ```
  otu.table=read.table("your_otu_table.txt ",
  sep="\t",header=T,row.names=1)
  ```
  transposed:
  ```
  otu.table=t(read.table("your_otu_table.txt", sep="\
  t",header=T,row.names=1))
  ```
- Or in biom format:
  ```
  1.  otu_biom="your_otu_table.biom"
  ```
  2.. Which needs to be transformed into a matrix:
  ```
  otu_biom=as(biom_data(otu_biom), "matrix")
  ```

Secondly, read in a mapping file:

```
otu.map=read.csv("your_map.csv",header=T)
```

Make sure to match the row order in your data matrix to that in your mapping file:

```
otu.map=otu.map[match(rownames(otu.table),otu.
map$OtuID),]
```

Save your original import as backup, in case you mess up your newly created dataframes at some point during the process:

```
otu.raw=otu.table
otu.map.raw=otu.map
```

Do a random rarefaction with the rrarefy function from the vegan package to reduce the number of sequences in each sample to that of the sample with the lowest number of sequences in the set (check your file or QIIME demultiplex log):

```
otu.table.rar<-rrarefy(otu.table, sample=x)
```

Now create factors—e.g., make the experimental treatment a factor (look at your mapping file to assess which factors you should create to make your analysis interesting or viable):

```
otu.map$Treatment=as.factor(otu.map$Treatment)
```

The data can now be analyzed statistically.

3.4.2 Exploring Alpha Diversity

In datasets, where abundance is represented in an unbiased way, it is easy to determine the most abundant OTU:

```
mostAbundantOtu<-which(colSums(otu.
table)==max(colSums(otu.table)))
```

It is then possible to calculate a rank-abundance curve for the data:

```
RankAbun.otus<- rankabundance(otu.table)
```

which is followed by plotting the results proportionally on a log scale. Set the plot panel (e.g., one row, two columns):

```
par(mfrow=c(1,2))
```

Assign x and y axes:

```
x<- RankAbun.otus [,1]
y<- RankAbun.otus [,2]/colSums(RankAbun.otus)[2]
```

Create labels manually:

```
l<- c("label 1", " label 2", "label 3")
```

Plot the data with labels:

```
plot(x, y, log="y", type="o", pch=16, xlab="Species
rank", ylab="Proportion", main="Rank Abundance, OTUs",
axes=FALSE)
textxy(x, y, labs=l, cex=0.8)
```

Now, traditional diversity indices can be calculated via the diversity function of the vegan package. Shannon-Wiener is set as default:

```
H<- diversity(otu.table)
```

Simpson and others can be calculated by specifying them especially:

```
S<- diversity(otu.table, index="simpson")
```

whereas related indices such as Pielou's J can be calculated with a simple function:

```
J<- H/log(specnumber(otu.table))
```

3.4.3 Exploring Beta Diversity

When working with a number of sites or treatments, the diversity indices can be presented next to each other in a boxplot for easy comparison.

First, create new objects for each treatment group or site:

```
H_resultsGroup1<-c(Result1, Result2, Result3, etc)

H_resultsGroup2<-c(Result1, Result2, Result3, etc)
```

The next step is to create a boxplot (with outliers represented as dots):

```
lmts<- range(H_resultsGroup1, H_resultsGroup2)
boxplot(H_resultsGroup1,H_resultsGroup2, ylim=lmts,
names=c("Group_1","Group_2"),          xlab="myExperiment",
main="Shannon diversity with SD")
```

It is also possible to test for significant differences between the calculated diversity indices with an ANOVA. Read in a matrix that lists samples/replicates in rows and diversity index results and treatment assignments per replicates in columns. To start the analysis, the linear model needs to be created first:

```
div.an<- lm(Shannon~factor(Treatment)+factor
(myFactor1)*factor(myFactor2), data=div.matrix)
```

The results can be printed in the console:

```
summary(div.an)
```

The ANOVA is then produced as follows:

```
anova(div.an)
```

A convenient way to explore differences between samples visually is by nonmetric multidimensional scaling (NMDS [23]). In an initial step, R has to produce a dissimilarity matrix (e.g., Bray-Curtis) as the basis:

```
otu.table.nmds=metaMDS(otu.table,distance="bray",tr
ymax=49)

sites=scores(otu.table.nmds, display="sites")
```

```
taxa=scores(otu.table.nmds, display="species")
```

If there are missing data points in the OTU table, it is good to remove them:

```
x1=range(sites[,1],taxa[,1],na.rm=T)y1=range(sites[,2],
taxa[,2],na.rm=T)
```

The NMDS results can be plotted in the following way:

```
plot(otu.table.nmds)
```

This has created a plot without labels and with crosses for species.

To create a plot with adjusted x and y axis ranges in which the dots are labeled by treatment, R can be instructed as follows:

```
plot(otu.table.nmds, type="n", xlim=x1, ylim=y1,
main="NMDS of bacterial samples, plotted by treatment")

points(sites,col=c("red","blue")[as.
numeric(otumap$Treatment)], pch=16, cex=1.0)
```

To create site labels, the following command can be used:

```
text(otu.table.nmds, display="sites", pos=4, cex=0.7,
offset=0.3)
```

R can also create species labels—if there are many species, this can make a plot far too busy:

```
text(otu.table.nmds, display="species", pos=4,
cex=0.7, offset=0.3)
```

The vegan package includes several multivariate statistical tests to test for differences between your treatments or locations.

Adonis (aka PERMANOVA [24]) is a multivariate equivalent to ANOVA. Any data needs to be checked for multivariate normality to make sure that the PERMANOVA is applicable:

```
adonis.otu=adonis(otu.table~otu.map$Treatment,method="
bray");adonis.otu
```

If a PERMANOVA is not permissible, there is another multivariate equivalent to ANOVA, called ANOSIM [25]. ANOSIM is a randomization-based method to analyze differences by comparing dissimilarity matrices of ranked data. It is less robust than PERMANOVA/Adonis, as it does not compare the distances directly. ANOSIM produces an R-statistic, which shows increasing differences in community composition on a scale of 0–1. The accompanying P-value shows if the R-value is significant or not. This is how the ANOSIM is called in R:

```
anosim.otu=anosim(vegdist(otu.table),grouping=otu.
map$Treatment,permutations=999)
```

This will produce a summary:

```
summary(anosim.otu)
```

And this will produce a boxplot of the result:

```
plot(anosim.otu)
```

Lastly, a simper analysis [25] can yield information about which OTUs contributed most to the observed dissimilarity between the treatments/locations. It is called as follows:

```
sim<- with(otu.map, simper(otu.table, Treatment))
```

The output can be assessed with the summary command:

```
summary(sim, ordered=TRUE, digits=3)
```

3.4.4 Further Analysis Options

This is only a small selection of analysis methods that can be performed in R and exploration is encouraged. Additionally, there are software packages such as MEGAN [26] or PICRUSt [27], which can offer additional workflows for data in biom format to explore metagenome data further.

4   Notes

1. If you collect from more than one location without being able to acid wash the equipment in between, please pump sterilized, deionized water through the equipment (bar filter) between locations. If that isn't possible, pump river water from the next location through your bottle before you start to filter (not recommended unless there is no better option).

2. Wherever practical, samples should be collected at midstream/offshore rather than nearshore. Samples collected from midstream/offshore reduce the possibilities of contamination (e.g., back eddies or seepage from nearshore soils). The most important issue to consider when deciding where the sample should be collected from is safety. If the flow is sufficiently slow and shallow for the collector to wade, e.g., into a stream without risk, then the sample can be collected at a depth where there is no risk that water might flow into the waders from above.

3. Record:

   • How much water you filtered

   • The time taken to filter the sample

   • Your observations about the color of the filter

   • If you collected from the stream bank or mid-river

4. QIIME can be installed natively on Linux (qiime.org) and Mac OS X (www.wernerlab.org/software/macqiime/) or can be run on Windows via VirtualBox (www.virtualbox.org). QIIME comes pre-installed and pre-configured on Bio-Linux, an open-source curated Linux distribution for bioinformaticians (environmentalomics.org/bio-linux/).

References

1. Gilbert JA, Jansson JK, Knight R (2014) The Earth Microbiome Project: successes and aspirations. BMC Biol 12(1):69

2. Kopf A et al (2015) The ocean sampling day consortium. GigaScience 4(1):1–5

3. Clark MJR (2003) British Columbia field sampling manual. Water, Air, and Climate Change Branch, Ministry of Water, Land, and Air Protection, Victoria, BC

4. Gilbert JA, Field D, Swift P, Thomas S, Cummings D, Temperton B, Weynberg K et al (2010) The taxonomic and functional diversity of microbes at a temperate coastal site: a 'multi-omic' study of seasonal and diel temporal variation. PLoS One 5(11), e15545

5. Evans GE, Murdoch DR, Anderson TP, Potter HC, George PM, Chambers ST (2003) Contamination of Qiagen DNA extraction kits with Legionella DNA. J Clin Microbiol 41(7):3452–3453

6. Salter SJ, Cox MJ, Turek EM, Calus ST, Cookson WO, Moffatt MF, Turner P, Parkhill J, Loman NJ, Walker AW (2014) Reagent and laboratory contamination can critically impact sequence-based microbiome analyses. BMC Biol 12(1):87

7. Caporaso JG, Kuczynski J, Stombaugh J, Bittinger K, Bushman FD, Costello EK, Fierer N, Gonzalez Pena A, Goodrich JK, Gordon JI, Huttley GA, Kelley ST, Knights D, Koenig JE, Ley RE, Lozupone CA, McDonald D, Muegge BD, Pirrung M, Reeder J, Sevinsky JR, Turnbaugh PJ, Walters WA, Widmann J, Yatsunenko T, Zaneveld J, Knight R (2010) QIIME allows analysis of high-throughput community sequencing data. Nat Methods 7(5):335–336

8. Schloss PD, Westcott SL, Ryabin T, Hall JR, Hartmann M, Hollister EB, Lesniewski RA et al (2009) Introducing mothur: open-source, platform-independent, community-supported software for describing and comparing microbial communities. Appl Environ Microbiol 75(23):7537–7541

9. Edgar RC (2010) Search and clustering orders of magnitude faster than BLAST. Bioinformatics 26(19):2460–2461

10. R Core Team (2015) R: a language and environment for statistical computing. R Foundation for Statistical Computing, Vienna, http://www.R-project.org/

11. McMurdie PJ, The Biom-Format Team (2014) biom: an interface package (beta) for the BIOM file format. http://biom-format.org/. R package version 0.3.12. http://CRAN.R-project.org/package=biom

12. Neuwirth E (2014) RColorBrewer: ColorBrewer palettes R package version 1.1-2. http://CRAN.R-project.org/package=RColorBrewer

13. Oksanen J, Blanchet FG, Kindt R, Legendre P, Minchin PR, O'Hara RB, Simpson GL, Solymos P, Stevens MHH, Wagner H (2015) vegan: community ecology package. R package version 2.3-0. http://CRAN.R-project.org/package=vegan

14. Warnes GR, Bolker B, Bonebakker L, Gentleman R, Huber W, Liaw A, Lumley T, Maechler M, Magnusson A, Moeller S, Schwartz M, Venables B (2015) "gplots: various R programming tools for plotting data. R package version 2.17.0. http://CRAN.R-project.org/package=gplots

15. Graffelman J (2013) calibrate: calibration of Scatterplot and biplot axes. R package version 1.7.2. http://CRAN.R-project.org/package=calibrate

16. Paradis E, Claude J, Strimmer K (2004) APE: analyses of phylogenetics and evolution in R language. Bioinformatics 20:289–290

17. Kembel SW, Cowan PD, Helmus MR, Cornwell WK, Morlon H, Ackerly DD, Blomberg SP, Webb CO (2010) Picante: R tools for integrating phylogenies and ecology. Bioinformatics 26:1463–1464

18. Harrell FE Jr., with Contributions from Charles Dupont and Many Others (2015) Hmisc: Harrell miscellaneous. R package version 3.16-0. http://CRAN.R-project.org/package=Hmisc

19. Kindt R, Coe R (2005) Tree diversity analysis. A manual and software for common statistical methods for ecological and biodiversity studies. World Agroforestry Centre (ICRAF), Nairobi. ISBN 92-9059-179-X

20. Revelle W (2015) psych: procedures for personality and psychological research. Version = 1.5.8. Northwestern University, Evanston, IL, http://CRAN.R-project.org/package = psych

21. Wickham H (2009) ggplot2: elegant graphics for data analysis. Springer, New York, NY

22. Huber W, Carey VJ, Gentleman R, Morgan M (2015) Orchestrating high-throughput genomic analysis with bioconductor. Nat Methods 12:115

23. Kruskal J (1964) Nonmetric multidimensional scaling: a numerical method. Psychometrika 29:115–129

24. Anderson M (2005) "PERMANOVA: a FORTRAN computer program for permutational multivariate analysis of variance, vol 24. Department of Statistics, University of Auckland, Auckland

25. Clarke KR (1993) Non-parametric multivariate analyses of changes in community structure. Aust J Ecol 18:117–143

26. Huson DH, Auch AF, Qi J et al (2007) MEGAN analysis of metagenomic data. Genome Res 17:377–386

27. Langille MGI et al (2013) Predictive functional profiling of microbial communities using 16S rRNA marker gene sequences. Nat Biotechnol 31(9):814–821

Chapter 2

DNA Extraction Protocols for Whole-Genome Sequencing in Marine Organisms

Marina Panova, Henrik Aronsson, R. Andrew Cameron, Peter Dahl, Anna Godhe, Ulrika Lind, Olga Ortega-Martinez, Ricardo Pereyra, Sylvie V.M. Tesson, Anna-Lisa Wrange, Anders Blomberg, and Kerstin Johannesson

Abstract

The marine environment harbors a large proportion of the total biodiversity on this planet, including the majority of the earths' different phyla and classes. Studying the genomes of marine organisms can bring interesting insights into genome evolution. Today, almost all marine organismal groups are understudied with respect to their genomes. One potential reason is that extraction of high-quality DNA in sufficient amounts is challenging for many marine species. This is due to high polysaccharide content, polyphenols and other secondary metabolites that will inhibit downstream DNA library preparations. Consequently, protocols developed for vertebrates and plants do not always perform well for invertebrates and algae. In addition, many marine species have large population sizes and, as a consequence, highly variable genomes. Thus, to facilitate the sequence read assembly process during genome sequencing, it is desirable to obtain enough DNA from a single individual, which is a challenge in many species of invertebrates and algae. Here, we present DNA extraction protocols for seven marine species (four invertebrates, two algae, and a marine yeast), optimized to provide sufficient DNA quality and yield for de novo genome sequencing projects.

Key words Genomic DNA extraction, Gastropod *Littorina*, Isopod *Idotea*, Barnacle *Balanus*, Brittle star *Amphiura*, Brown alga *Fucus*, Diatom *Skeletonema*, Marine yeast *Debaryomyces*

1 Introduction

With the development of next-generation sequencing (NGS) techniques, we can for the first time get comprehensive genomic information at a reasonable price for marine non-model organisms. However, the success of a genomic project greatly depends on the ability to obtain sufficient amounts of pure and high-molecular weight DNA from the target species. Purity is crucial for the library preparation step; longer insert size Illumina libraries (mate-pair libraries) and Pacific Biosciences (PacBio) sequencing require 5–20 μg of high-molecular weight DNA. As many marine species have large population sizes and, as a consequence, highly variable genomes [1], whole-genome sequencing projects are greatly facilitated by producing libraries using DNA from one single individual. Thus, optimization of DNA yield per extraction and per individual is a crucial initial task, especially given the small body size of many species. Furthermore, commercially available DNA extraction kits that perform well on vertebrate and plant material often fail to produce good-quality DNA for marine algae and invertebrates due to substances that co-purify with DNA and lead to low DNA yield and/or purity.

In this chapter, we present optimized DNA extraction protocols for seven marine species in the marine genome sequencing project of the Centre for Marine Evolutionary Biology (CeMEB), University of Gothenburg, Sweden [2]: the gastropod mollusk *Littorina saxatilis*, the isopod crustacean *Idotea balthica*, the barnacle crustacean *Balanus improvisus*, the brittle star echinoderm *Amphiura filiformis*, the brown algae *Fucus vesiculosus* (also tested on the closely related species *F. radicans*), the diatom *Skeletonema marinoi*, and the marine yeast *Debaryomyces hansenii*. All seven species are promising systems for studies of adaptation and speciation in the marine environment. However, progress has been impeded in the past by the lack of genomic information, and to remedy this, we undertook an ambitious project to sequence their genomes. (The genome of *D. hansenii* has already been sequenced [3], but our goal here was a comprehensive population genomics re-sequencing effort.) The first challenge was to develop robust and efficient genomic DNA extraction protocols for all these non-model marine species. For each species, the general strategy was to test several methods based on the literature and our previous experience, choose the method providing the highest yield of non-degraded DNA, and then further optimize the protocol to reach the NGS requirements for quantity and quality of DNA. For several of the species, further improvements increasing DNA yield and purity had to be made along the way in response to sequencing failures (see below).

1.1 *Littorina saxatilis* (Gastropod Mollusk)

Littorina saxatilis is a marine gastropod mollusk common on the rocky intertidal. Adult shell height is 1.2–25.8 mm; snail size varies between geographic populations and ecotypes [4]. The major challenge in DNA extraction from mollusk tissue is a high content of mucopolysaccharides that tend to co-purify with DNA [5]. In addition, some species including *L. saxatilis* are relatively small, and it is hard to obtain enough DNA from a single individual for a whole-genome sequencing project.

Using commercial kits such as the DNeasy Blood & Tissue Kit (Qiagen), DNeasy Plant Mini Kit (Qiagen), and E.Z.N.A. Mollusc DNA Kit (Omega Bio-tek) for *L. saxatilis* provides DNA suitable for routine PCR amplification of microsatellites, nuclear introns, and mitochondrial gene fragments, but the total yield (≤ 1 µg), concentration (≤ 10 ng/µL), and absorbance ratios are not compatible with NGS applications.

The protocol described here uses CTAB (cetyltrimethyl ammonium bromide) buffer, which binds proteins and polysaccharides at high salt concentration in combination with Proteinase K, which digests proteins. The DNA is extracted using chloroform: isoamyl alcohol, based on a method earlier suggested for mollusks [5], which has been modified to maximize the yield and improve the purity and integrity of the DNA and to include an RNase A treatment. Further, tissue homogenization in liquid nitrogen has been replaced by homogenization in the digestion buffer, since using liquid nitrogen with small tissues samples is difficult and may lead to loss and/or thawing of material.

We have successfully used this extraction method to prepare *Littorina* genomic DNA samples for comparative genomics hybridization [6], restriction site associated DNA (RAD) genome scans [7], and to obtain enough material for *L. saxatilis* de novo genome sequencing from one single specimen [2], where we combined sequencing of short- and long-insert Illumina libraries with PacBio sequencing.

One extraction typically gives ≥ 2 µg of genomic DNA at a concentration of 70–300 ng/µL. The DNA has a high-molecular weight (Fig. 1) and typical absorbance ratios are 1.95–1.99 at 260/280 nm and 2.0–2.22 at 260/230 nm. For de novo genome sequencing, we were able to obtain 70 µg of genomic DNA from a single individual by dividing tissues into 12 separate extractions.

1.2 *Idotea balthica* (Isopod Crustacean)

Idotea balthica is a marine isopod living on seaweeds in shallow waters. The average body length of adult animals is 20–30 mm. DNA extraction from arthropods is often difficult, especially from species with body pigmentation [8]. Different DNA extraction protocols have been tested mainly for insect species, e.g., [9]. In our work with *Idotea* species, DNA of a quality suitable for PCR amplification of nuclear and mitochondrial fragments is usually obtained using the Chelex method or the DNeasy Blood and Tissue Kit (Qiagen). However, both methods provide yields (<1 µg) and concentrations (<10 ng/µL) below NGS requirements. Here we suggest a protocol based on multiple phenol-chloroform extractions as this gives an approximately 50 times higher yield and high-molecular weight DNA. It includes two extractions with phenol:chloroform:isoamyl alcohol followed by two extractions with chloroform:isoamyl alcohol. In the development of this protocol, we also tried to use fewer extraction steps but this gave lower DNA purity (as estimated by spectrophotometric 280/260 ratios) without resulting in higher DNA yield.

DNA samples extracted with this protocol were successfully used to produce 2b-RAD [10] libraries. However, there were

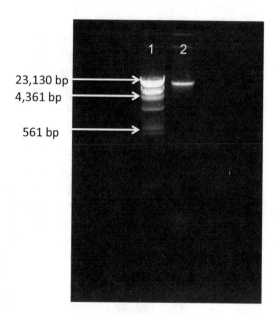

Fig. 1 Integrity of *Littorina saxatilis* DNA extracted by the CTAB method. Electrophoresis was performed in a 0.8 % agarose gel and 1× TAE buffer. DNA was stained with GelRed. *Lane 1*: Lambda DNA/HindIII Marker; *Lane 2*: 200 ng of *L. saxatilis* genomic DNA

problems with the Illumina TruSeq DNA library preparation that may be due to contaminants in the DNA preparations. To remedy this, after phenol-chloroform extraction, the DNA was additionally cleaned using Genomic DNA Clean & Concentrator-10 Kit (Zymo Research). This step removes the low-molecular weight smear (*see* Fig. 2) and contaminants. Using this two-step protocol and dividing the tissue from a large specimen into 24 extractions, we were able to obtain 41 µg of genomic DNA from a single individual that was used in our de novo genome sequencing project.

1.3 *Skeletonema marinoi (Diatom)*

Skeletonema marinoi is a microscopic chain-forming unicellular phytoplankton species. Cell valve diameter is 5–12 µm wide. Cell walls are made of silica and have a complex pore structure [11]. Silica is commonly utilized in commercial extraction kits to retain DNA. Thus, stringent conditions are needed to separate the DNA from the silica walls. The amount of genomic DNA required by any sequencing platform for whole-genome sequencing exceeds the amount available in a single cell (in the range of femtograms); thus, it is necessary to produce monoclonal cultures. We grow our strains in batch culture with F/2 medium supplemented with silica [12]. Culturing of microalgae, however, has several knock-on effects. First, there is a bias due to selection for culturable strains. Secondly, strains in laboratory cultures undergo physiological changes due to adaptation and selection of specific

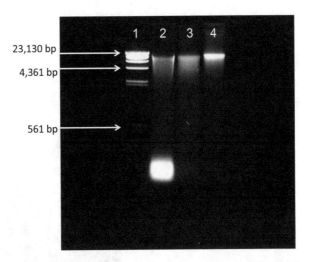

Fig. 2 Integrity of *Idotea balthica* DNA extracted by the CTAB:SDS method. Electrophoresis was performed on a 0.8 % agarose gel and 1× TAE buffer. DNA was stained with GelRed. *Lane 1*: Lambda DNA/HindIII Marker; *Lane 2*: 200 ng of *I. balthica* genomic DNA before the column purification; *Lane 3*: 200 ng of *I. balthica* genomic DNA purified with DNA Clean & Concentrator Kit; *Lane 4*: 200 ng of *I. balthica* genomic DNA purified with Genomic DNA Clean & Concentrator-10 Kit

cell lines and genetic changes due to mutations [13]. Thirdly, cultures also have the disadvantage of acquiring contaminants (e.g., bacteria or fungi), and foreign DNA is extracted together with DNA from the target species. To establish the de novo genome of *Skeletonema marinoi*, we treated the reference strain with antibiotics, as reported in [14, 15] before the DNA extraction. However, even after the antibiotic treatment, some bacterial contamination still remained.

For diatoms, CTAB extractions provide suitable genomic DNA for fingerprinting and fragment amplifications [16]. For de novo genome amplification, we modified the protocol to improve the quality and quantity and obtained an absorbance ratio of 1.8–2.0 at 260/280 nm, a unique high-molecular weight band of genomic DNA (Fig. 3), and a final amount of 10–30 μg of genomic DNA per billion antibiotic-treated cells. The best DNA was obtained when the culture was harvested by mild centrifugation in the exponential growth phase, the samples processed fast to avoid degradation, and the extracted DNA treated with RNase A.

This DNA extraction procedure has been used to prepare mate-pair and paired-end Illumina libraries and for PacBio sequencing. Additionally, the same DNA extraction protocol has been used for re-sequencing of non-axenic environmental isolates.

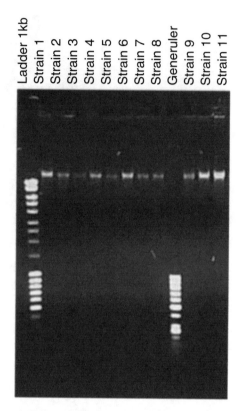

Fig. 3 Integrity of DNA extracted from 11 strains of *Skeletonema marinoi*. Electrophoresis was performed on a 0.7 % agarose gel and 1× TAE buffer; DNA was stained with Ethidium bromide

1.4 Amphiura filiformis (Brittle Star Echinoderm)

Amphiura filiformis is a small brittle star that lives on mud and sand bottoms. It has long arms and a small central disk (maximum diameter is 10 mm). Ophiuroids are highly calcified species with very little soft tissue. The viscera inside the disk are the exception, where internal organs of digestion and reproduction are located, along with a high amount of bacteria [17]. Initial DNA extraction on this species aimed to use a single adult male individual, reducing polymorphisms due to high variation among individuals. Using DNAzol (Invitrogen) for extraction of DNA from arms yielded just enough DNA for the project, but the resulting DNA preparation was colored brown, even after several ethanol washes, and the subsequent Illumina library preparation failed. Other protocols such as digestion with CTAB or SDS buffers and the NucleoSpin DNA extraction kit (Macherey-Nagel) did not provide suitable DNA for NGS applications.

Following the protocol routinely used for genomic DNA extraction from echinoderm sperm of many different species including that of the sea urchin *Strongylocentrotus purpuratus* [18], DNA was successfully extracted from *A. filiformis* sperm. This procedure was originally developed for fresh sperm recovered undiluted from spawning sea urchins. It can also be used for lyophilized sperm samples after grinding in dry ice, or frozen sperm.

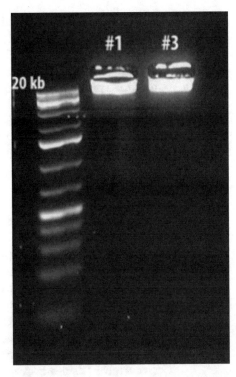

Fig. 4 Integrity of DNA extracted from *Amphiura filiformis* sperm. Electrophoresis was performed on a 0.8 % agarose gel and 1× TAE buffer. DNA was stained with GelRed. The *first lane* shows a 20 kb size DNA marker and the *second* and *third lanes* show two samples of *A. filiformis* genomic DNA

This protocol provided around 130 μg of genomic DNA at a concentration of 500–600 ng/μL and absorbance ratios 1.89 and 2.3 at 260/280 and 260/230 nm, respectively. The DNA had a high-molecular weight, as required by NGS service providers (Fig. 4).

1.5 Fucus vesiculosus (and F. radicans) Brown Macroalgae

Fucus seaweeds belong to the taxonomic order Fucales, which includes some of the most common littoral seaweeds. As with other organisms, one of the main challenges to obtain high-quality DNA from brown algae is to remove compounds constituting their cell walls and tissue. Alginates and fucose-containing sulfated polysaccharides are the main cell wall polymers in Fucales [19]. It has been shown that the amount of polysaccharides is directly correlated to the species' position on the shore, suggesting that high contents may confer an adaptive advantage to species frequently exposed to immersion [20]. The removal of these high amounts of polysaccharides is essential when attempting to extract high-quality DNA from these algae. Furthermore, additional polyphenolic compounds also complicate the extraction of pure and intact

DNA. The overproduction of polysaccharides is likely accompanied by the reinforcement of polyphenol-alginate complexes that consolidate further the cell wall architecture [19]. In high amounts, these phenolic compounds get co-washed during most DNA extraction procedures resulting in low-quality extractions and most commercial procedures only partially remove these compounds. Concomitantly, using large amounts of tissue also accumulates large amounts of "contaminant" chemical compounds that decrease the DNA yield per extraction.

Here, we present a combination of approaches that initially remove high contents of polyphenolic compounds using a solvent (acetone), followed by a CTAB-based extraction buffer solution containing chemical complexors of the "contaminant" metabolites (polyvinylpolypyrrolidone (PVPP) [21, 22], diethyldithiocarbamic acid (DIECA) [23], and a strong reductant of polysaccharides (β-mercaptoethanol). The method requires freshly harvested algal tissue or lyophilized tissue preserved in silica gel for no more than 2 months to avoid degradation of DNA. The DNA is extracted with the aid of the commercial extraction kit NucleoSpin Plant II (Macherey-Nagel) to effectively separate the contaminant proteins. However, it requires an extra cleanup step using DNA Clean & Concentrator (Zymo Research) after the DNA has been extracted to remove co-washed polysaccharides that become a viscous solution in the extract. Using this kit efficiently removes large amounts of undesired polysaccharides.

Given the accumulation of contaminating chemicals when large amounts of tissue are extracted at one time, the acquisition of high DNA yields and concentrations required for de novo genome sequencing is achieved by performing several extractions with low amounts of tissue in each. The typical amount of DNA obtained in one extraction is 2.5 μg, with high-molecular weight (Fig. 5) and absorbance ratios 1.9 and 1.8 at 260/280 and 260/230 nm, respectively.

1.6 Balanus improvisus (Barnacle Crustacean)

Balanus improvisus is a relatively small acorn barnacle [24] of only 5–12 mg of tissue in dry weight per individual [25]. It is thus challenging to get high amounts of good DNA from one single individual (*see* **Note 1**). Due to high genetic variation (roughly 4% sequence divergence between two alleles within one single individual, use of a single individual is highly recommended for whole-genome sequencing in order to optimize the final genome assembly process. Ideally we aim for 10–20 μg of DNA from one individual to enable the production of several small and large fragment libraries for sequencing.

In order to optimize the amount and quality of genomic DNA preparations from adult barnacles, we initially tested several methods: the E.Z.N.A. Mollusc DNA Kit (Omega Bio-tek), the CTAB method [5], the DNAzol kit (Life Technologies), and the E.Z.N.A. Blood DNA Mini Kit (Omega Bio-tek). The methods

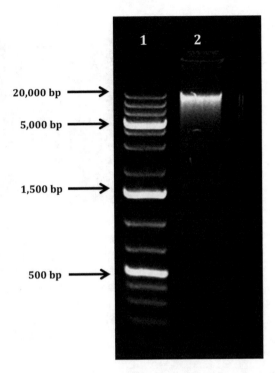

Fig. 5 Integrity of *Fucus vesiculosus* DNA. Electrophoresis was performed on a 0.8 % agarose gel and 1× TAE buffer. DNA was stained with GelRed. *Lane 1*: 1 kb ladder showing the 20 kb DNA size marker; *Lane 2*: 200 ng of *F. vesiculosus* genomic DNA

were independently tested at least twice, each time using 2–3 individuals. We found that the E.Z.N.A. Mollusc DNA Kit and the CTAB method resulted in either degraded DNA or a weak high-molecular weight DNA band together with an abundant low-molecular weight band that remained even after RNase treatment (Fig. 6a and *see* **Note 2**). DNAzol gave good DNA, but the DNA was very hard to dissolve in water or TE buffer, which is usually required by sequencing facilities/companies.

The E.Z.N.A. Blood DNA Mini Kit, however, gave good amounts of DNA with high integrity and purity (Fig. 6b). With this DNA kit, we obtained 8 ± 5 μg DNA per individual, but the individual variation was relatively large with a coefficient of variation (CV) of 58 % (Fig. 7a). We tested if this variation is the outcome of variable size (tissue weight) of the individual barnacles; however, even after normalizing for the variation in wet weight, we still see large individual differences in the amount of DNA obtained ($CV \approx 49$ %) (Fig. 7b). Thus, it is clear that tissue weight is not the only factor determining the amount of DNA per individual obtained. Preparing DNA from several barnacles and selecting the best preparation for sequencing is therefore recommended to ensure DNA of both high quantity and quality.

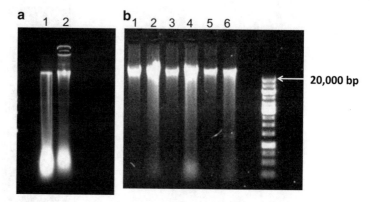

Fig. 6 Integrity of *Balanus improvisus* DNA extracted using two methods. (**a**) DNA extracted from two different adult *B. improvisus* individuals using the CTAB method. Only a small amount of the DNA appears as a high-molecular weight band and there is a large band of low-molecular weight material. B: DNA extracted from three different *B. improvisus* individuals, two elution steps each, using the E.Z.N.A. Blood DNA Mini Kit. *Lanes 1, 2*: Individual 1, first elution and second elution; *Lanes 3, 4*: Individual 2, first elution and second elution; *Lanes 5, 6*: Individual 3, first elution and second elution. *Last lane*: 20 Kb DNA size marker. Most of the DNA appears to be ≥20 Kb

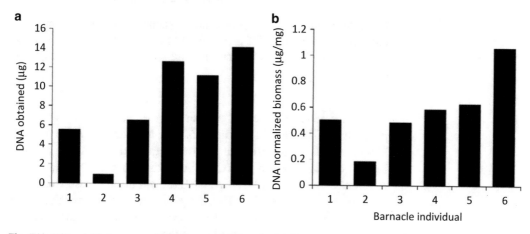

Fig. 7 Variable yields for genomic DNA preparations of adult *B. improvisus* individuals. The E.Z.N.A. Blood DNA Kit was used to prepare DNA from six different *B. improvisus* individuals. (**a**) The amount of DNA in μg obtained from each individual. (**b**) The amount of DNA obtained from each individual is normalized against the wet weight of the individual (wet weight per individual was in the range of 5–22 mg)

1.7 Debaryomyces hansenii (Marine Yeast)

Debaryomyces hansenii is a marine yeast that occurs globally with extreme tolerance to salt and dehydration stress. It is slightly halophilic and grows better in seawater compared to freshwater. Studies of *D. hansenii* will be important in our understanding of the evolution of osmoregulation in marine fungi. The genome sequence of *D. hansenii* has already been established and published for the type strain CBC767 [3]. In addition, genome contigs from an alternative strain, MTCC 234, were recently published [26]. However, in these genome publications, the method for DNA extraction has not been specified.

D. hansenii is quite distantly related to the common yeast model species *Saccharomyces cerevisiae*. Most of the of methodologies developed and applied to the model species work in *D. hansenii*; however, the marine yeast might require slight but important alterations to some of the commonly used yeast protocols. We initiated our population genomics project on *D. hansenii* by applying routine protocols extensively used for extracting DNA from *S. cerevisiae* (breakage of cells with glass beads and extraction with phenol:chloroform). However, we found that the amount of DNA, its quality, and purity were not sufficient when these standard protocols were applied to *D. hansenii*. Instead we found that more and better quality DNA was obtained from *D. hansenii* if some commercial kits were used. In order to test different protocols for efficiency and robustness on different strains, we extracted DNA from 17 different *D. hansenii* isolates (obtained from various geographical locations as well as sources) and two *S. cerevisiae* isolates (as controls). We found that the MasterPure Yeast DNA Purification Kit (Epicentre) yielded good DNA from 12 of the *D. hansenii* isolates (as well as from the two *S. cerevisiae* controls); however, the method provided rather low amounts for seven of the *D. hansenii* strains (Fig. 8). We then tested

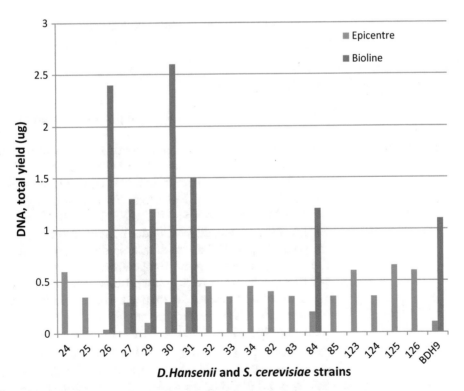

Fig. 8 DNA yield per strain in *Debaryomyces hansenii* and in *Saccharomyces cerevisiae* control. *Blue bars* show the amount of DNA in μg extracted using the MasterPure Yeast DNA Purification Kit (Epicentre) from 17 strain isolates of *D. hansenii* (numbers 24–124, and BDH9 [a transformation competent laboratory strain]) and from two strains of *S. cerevisiae* (numbers 125 and 126). Strains that yielded a rather low amount of DNA were also extracted using the ISOLATE II Genomic DNA Kit (Bioline) (*red bars*). For each extraction, 600 million cells were used

the ISOLATE II Genomic DNA Kit (Bioline), which is based on generating spheroplasts using the enzyme zymolyase in order to optimize the amount of DNA extracted. In our hands the Bioline kit yielded substantially higher amounts of DNA for all strains tested (Fig. 8) and would generally be recommended for extraction of DNA from a wide array of *D. hansenii* strains. The 260/280 nm ratio was sufficient using both kits (the recommended ratio is above 1.8), with the kit from Bioline providing somewhat higher purity (average 260/280 nm = 2.1 ± 0.06 [standard deviation]). The quality of the DNA obtained using both methods was high with low levels of degradation, and both yielded high-molecular weight DNA that resulted in good sequence reads.

2 Materials

Equipment and consumables required for all protocols:

1. 1.5 mL microcentrifuge tubes.
2. Centrifuge for 1.5 mL microcentrifuge tubes.
3. Vortex mixer.
4. Pipettes and filter tips of 100–1000, 2–200, and 0.1–1 µL.
5. Heat block or incubator.
6. Nanodrop.
7. Qubit (*see* **Note 3**).

Specific materials required for each protocol are given below.

2.1 Littorina saxatilis

1. CTAB buffer: 2% w/v cetyltrimethyl ammonium bromide (CTAB), 1.4 M NaCl, 20 mM EDTA, 100 mM Tris–HCl pH 8.0, 0.2% v/v β-mercaptoethanol. For 100 mL, weigh 2 g of CTAB and 8.2 g of NaCl; add 70 mL of double-distilled water, 10 mL of 1 M Tris–HCl pH 8.0, and 8 mL of 0.25 M EDTA. Let the salts dissolve under magnetic stirring and bring the volume up to 100 mL with double-distilled water. The solution can be stored at room temperature for 6 months (CTAB will precipitate in the refrigerator). Before the DNA extraction, add 2 µL of β-mercaptoethanol per 1 mL of CTAB buffer. This solution can be stored at room temperature for no more than a week (*see* **Note 4** for working with β-mercaptoethanol).
2. TE buffer: 10 mM Tris–HCl pH = 8.0, 1 mM EDTA. To prepare 50 mL, mix 0.5 mL of 1 M Tris pH 8.0 with 0.1 mL of 0.5 M EDTA pH 8.0 and adjust to 50 mL with distilled water. Use a sterile syringe and a 0.2 µm non-pyrogenic sterile filter to filter the solution. It is recommended to store the solution at 4 °C for short-term and at lower temperature for long-term storage.

For dissolving DNA, use 0.1× TE buffer (diluted 1:10 with double-distilled water). Alternatively, use nuclease-free water.

3. Proteinase K (20 mg/mL).

4. RNase A (100 mg/mL).

5. Chloroform:isoamyl alcohol 24:1 (CIA).

6. Isopropanol (2-propanol).

7. 70% ethanol.

8. Phase Lock Gel Heavy 2 mL columns (PGL columns; 5 Prime).

9. Safe-Lock tubes 1.5 mL (Eppendorf).

10. Fume hood.

11. Incubator at 60 °C with a shaking platform (e.g., Heidolph 1000).

12. Mixer Mill (e.g., Retsch MM301 with stainless steel balls).

13. Rotator (e.g., Stuart SB3).

14. Centrifuge for 1.5 mL tubes with cooling capacity (4 °C) and maximum speed ≥18,000 × g.

15. Tissue samples can be collected from live snails or snails fixed in 96–99% ethanol. For fixation, snails are left at −80 °C overnight, and then the shells are carefully crushed (facilitating the penetration of ethanol but avoiding damage to the tissues). The tissues are then placed in tubes filled with ethanol and stored at −20 °C. It is important to use a relatively large volume of ethanol (e.g., at least 20× the tissue volume) and to check the samples within one week after fixation. If the liquid has a yellow color (often the case when the digestive gland was damaged or when fixing large individuals), the ethanol should be changed. After that, the samples can be stored at −20 to −80 °C for a long period of time; we did not observe any sign of DNA degradation after 3 years of storage.

2.2   Idotea balthica

1. The SDS/CTAB buffer is a 1:1 mixture of CTAB and SDS (sodium dodecyl sulfate) buffers (*see* **Note 5**). For the recipe for CTAB buffer, *see* Subheading 2.1.

   SDS buffer: 0.7% w/v SDS, 10 mM NaCl, 10 mM Tris–HCl pH 8.0. For 300 mL buffer, add 2.1 g of SDS, 3 mL of 1 M Tris–HCl pH 8.0, and 6 mL of 0.5 M NaCl to 280 mL of double-distilled water. Let the SDS dissolve under magnetic stirring and bring the volume up to 300 mL with distilled water. The solution can be stored at room temperature for months. The day before the extraction, mix equal volumes of CTAB and SDS buffers and add 2 μL of β-mercaptoethanol per 1 mL of mixture (*see* **Note 4** for working with β-mercaptoethanol). Incubate the mixture at 60 °C overnight to dissolve the precipitate.

2. Proteinase K (20 mg/mL).

3. Protease (7.5 AU, Qiagen).

4. RNase A (100 mg/mL).

5. Phenol:chloroform:isoamyl alcohol 25:24:1 (PCIA).

6. Chloroform:isoamyl alcohol 24:1 (CIA).

7. Isopropanol (2-Propanol).

8. Glycogen (5 mg/mL).

9. 70% ethanol, 0.1× TE buffer (*see* Subheading 2.1) or nuclease-free water to dissolve the DNA.

10. Genomic DNA Clean & Concentrator-10 Kit (Zymo Research).

11. Phase Lock Gel Heavy 2 mL columns (PGL columns; 5 Prime).

12. Safe-Lock tubes 1.5 mL (Eppendorf).

13. Fume hood.

14. Incubator for 60 °C with a shaking platform (e.g., Heidolph 1000).

15. Mixer Mill (e.g., Retsch MM301 with stainless steel balls).

16. Rotator (e.g., Stuart SB3).

17. Centrifuge for 1.5 mL tubes with cooling capacity (4 °C) and maximum speed $\geq 18,000 \times g$.

18. Tissue samples can be collected from living animals or animals stored in 96–99% ethanol. For fixation, isopods are decapitated, placed in the tubes with ethanol, and stored at 4 to –20 °C. To prevent DNA degradation and improve purity of DNA, it is important to change the ethanol twice, first 1 day and then 1 week after fixation.

2.3 Skeletonema marinoi

1. CTAB buffer: 2% w/v CTAB, 1.41 M NaCl, 200 mM Tris–HCl pH 8.0, 50 mM EDTA. To prepare 50 mL of the buffer, mix 1 g of CTAB, 10 ml of 1 M Tris–HCl pH 8.0, 5 ml of 0.5 M EDTA, and 4.09 g of NaCl and add distilled water up to 50 ml. Dissolve the chemicals using a hot plate set at 65 °C and a magnetic stirrer. For sterilization, leave the solution overnight under UV radiation. Store the solution at room temperature. Precipitates may form at the bottom of the solution with aging; if so, stir the solution. If the precipitation is too dense, or the solution has become yellow, make a fresh stock.

2. 1 M Tris–HCl pH 8.0: add 121.1 g of Tris to 700 mL of distilled water. After dissolving, adjust to 900 mL with distilled water. Adjust the pH to 8.0 with concentrated HCl (ca. 50 mL) and bring the final volume of the solution to 1 L with distilled water.

3. 0.5 M EDTA pH 8.0: add 186.12 g of EDTA to 750 mL of distilled water. Gradually add 20 g of NaOH and adjust the pH to 8.0. EDTA is not soluble until the solution reaches pH 8.0. Bring the final volume to 1 L with distilled water.

4. Chloroform:isoamyl alcohol solution 24:1 (CIA).

5. β-mercaptoethanol.

6. RNase A (100 mg/mL).

7. Isopropanol.

8. Ice cold ethanol (75% final concentration diluted in double-distilled water).

9. 0.1× TE buffer (*see* Subheading 2.1) for DNA re-suspension.

10. 50 mL Falcon tubes.

11. 1.5 mL Safe-Lock tubes (Eppendorf).

12. Fume hood.

13. Centrifuge for 50 mL Falcon tubes.

14. 1.5 mL tube centrifuge with cooling capacity (4 °C).

15. Samples: after culturing, it is possible to harvest the phytoplankton cells on a membrane filter, or using multiple-centrifugation steps (recommended).

16. A plate reader (e.g., Varioskan TM Flash Multimode Reader, Thermo Scientific) to measure chlorophyll A fluorescence, used as a proxy for the abundance of cells in culture before extraction (*see* **Note 6**).

2.4 Amphiura filiformis

1. Sperm isolation buffer: 20 mM NaCl, 50 mM Tris pH 8.0, 20 mM EDTA. Dissolve the salts with magnetic stirring and bring the volume to 100 ml with distilled water. Filter sterilize and store at room temperature.

2. STE buffer: 40 mM NaCl, 10 mM Tris pH 8.0, 1 mM EDTA. Dissolve the salts with magnetic stirring and bring the volume to 100 ml with distilled water. Filter sterilize and store at room temperature.

3. 20% SDS (w/v in distilled water).

4. Phenol:chloroform:isoamyl alcohol 25:24:1 (PCIA).

5. Chloroform:isoamyl alcohol 24:1 (CIA).

6. RNase A 100 µg/mL.

7. Proteinase K (20 mg/mL).

8. 3 M sodium acetate.

9. 100, 95, and 75% ethanol.

10. 0.1× TE buffer or nuclease-free water to dissolve DNA.

11. Filtered sea water.

12. DNA Clean & Concentrator Kit (Zymo Research).

13. 5 mL Falcon tubes.

14. Fume hood.

15. Rotator (e.g., Stuart SB3).

16. Centrifuge for 5 mL Falcon tubes.

17. Shaking incubator.

2.5 Fucus vesiculosus and F. radicans

1. Extraction buffer: 2% CTAB, 3% polyvinylpyrrolidone (PVP-40 or 0.1% PVPP-"PVP-cross linked"), 1.4 M NaCl, 20 mM EDTA pH 8.0, 100 mM Tris–HCl pH 8.0, 1% β-mercaptoethanol. For 100 mL buffer, mix 2 g of CTAB, 10 mL of 1 M Tris–HCl pH 8.0, 4 mL of 0.5 M EDTA, 28 mL of 5 M NaCl (or 8.1 g of NaCl), and 3 g of PVP-40 (MW: 40,000). Add double-distilled water to a final volume of 100 mL. Heat with stirring to dissolve the CTAB (be careful not to boil over) and autoclave.

2. 3.5 mM diethyldithiocarbamic acid (DIECA).

3. 100% acetone.

4. RNase A (10 mg/mL).

5. NucleoSpin Plant II kit (Macherey-Nagel).

6. DNA Clean & Concentrator-25 Kit (Zymo Research).

7. Double-distilled or nuclease-free water to elute DNA.

8. Fume hood.

9. Mixer Mill (e.g., Retsch MM301 with stainless steel balls).

10. Rotator (e.g., Stuart SB3).

2.6 Balanus improvisus

1. E.Z.N.A. Blood DNA Mini Kit (Omega Bio-tek).

2. RNase A (100 mg/mL).

3. Isopropanol.

4. 100% ethanol.

5. Microcentrifuge tubes with corresponding pestles (VWR).

2.7 Debaryomyces hansenii

1. YPD medium: 2% w/v yeast extract, 1% w/v peptone, 2% w/v glucose.

2. 10 mM EDTA (ethylenediaminetetraacetic acid) pH 8.0.

3. MasterPure Yeast DNA Purification Kit (Epicentre).

4. ISOLATE II Genomic DNA Kit (Bioline).

3   Methods

3.1 Littorina saxatilis

1. Prepare 1.5 mL Safe-Lock tubes (*see* **Note 7**) with 500 µL of digestion buffer (CTAB-β-mercaptoethanol) and 20 µL of Proteinase K and place them in the heat block at 60 °C.

2. Dissect tissue samples of no more than $2 \times 2 \times 2$ mm in size (*see* **Note 8**) and place them directly upon dissection in the tubes with preheated digestion buffer.

3. Vortex the samples well and incubate at 60 °C on a shaking platform set at 150 rpm for 1 h (if an incubator with shaking platform is not available, *see* **Note 9**).

4. Homogenize the tissues in the Mixer Mill: add two steel balls per sample and shake for 5 min at 30 Hz/s (*see* **Note 10** for more information on tissue homogenization).

5. Incubate at 60 °C as in **step 3** for 30 min to let the bubbles and foam formed during homogenization disappear and then transfer the homogenate to a fresh tube using a pipette or by placing a magnet at the bottom of the tube to hold the metal balls in place while pouring out the homogenate.

6. Add 5 μL of RNase A (*see* **Note 11**), vortex, and incubate 1 h at 60 °C as in **step 3**.

7. Cool the samples for 5 min at room temperature. During this time, pre-spin the PGL columns (one for each extraction) for 1 min at $14,000 \times g$ at room temperature.

8. Add 500 μL of CIA (in the fume hood), close the lids tightly, and mix by inversion in the rotator for 10 min at 40 rpm.

9. Pour the mixture including the white precipitate into a PGL column and centrifuge for 5 min at $14,000 \times g$ at room temperature to separate the phases (if PGL columns are not available, phase separation can be done directly in the microcentrifuge tubes, *see* **Note 12**).

10. Carefully pour the upper phase into a new 1.5 mL microcentrifuge tube. If there is a thin gel layer on top of the upper phase, puncture it with a pipette tip to facilitate pouring.

11. Add 500 μL of room temperature isopropanol. Often one can see DNA threads precipitate. Mix slowly by inverting ten times and incubate for 5 min at room temperature.

12. Centrifuge for 30–40 min at maximum speed ($\geq 18,000 \times g$) and 4 °C to pellet the DNA. After centrifugation, there will be whitish DNA pellets visible at the bottom of the tubes.

13. Carefully decant or pipette out the liquid.

14. Add 1 mL of room temperature 70% ethanol and wash the pellets by inverting the tubes in the rotator for 5 min at 20 rpm.

15. Centrifuge for 5 min at $14,000 \times g$ at room temperature.

16. Carefully decant or pipette out the ethanol. It is not necessary to remove all the ethanol, just as much as can be removed without disturbing the DNA pellet. The pellets may float and it is important to make sure they are not lost during the washing steps. Repeat washing **steps 14** and **15** with 500 μL of 70% ethanol.

17. Remove all the ethanol: first decant as much liquid as possible and then spin briefly to collect the drops at the bottom and remove the rest using a 100 μL pipette.

18. Air-dry the pellets in the open tubes at room temperature. Avoid over-drying (*see* **Note 13**).

19. Add 50 μL of 0.1× TE buffer or nuclease-free water and let the pellets dissolve overnight at 4 °C.

20. Mix gently by inverting and tapping the tubes (vortexing of the DNA solution may lead to shearing of the DNA), spin briefly to collect the solution at the bottom of the tube, and proceed to quantification.

21. Samples can be stored at –20 to –80 °C for more than one year. (After 3 years, we did not observe any signs of DNA degradation, but multiple thawing-freezing cycles may lead to partial degradation.)

3.2 *Idotea balthica*

1. Prepare 1.5 mL Safe-Lock tubes (*see* **Note 7**) with 400 μL of the digestion buffer (CTAB:SDS:β-mercaptoethanol), 20 μL of Proteinase K, and 20 μL of Protease. Place them in the heating block at 60 °C.

2. Dissect tissue samples of approximately $2 \times 2 \times 2$ mm size, avoiding the gut and exoskeleton (*see* **Note 14**), and place them directly upon dissection in the tubes with preheated digestion buffer.

3. Vortex samples well and incubate at 60 °C on the shaking platform for 1 h at 150 rpm (if an incubator with a shaking platform is not available, *see* **Note 9**).

4. Homogenize the tissues in the Mixer Mill: add two steel balls per sample and shake for 5 min at 30 Hz/s (*see* **Note 9** for more information on tissue homogenization).

5. Incubate for 30 min at 60 °C as in **step 3** to let the bubbles and foam formed during homogenization disappear and then remove the metal balls used for homogenization with forceps or a magnet.

6. Add 5 μL of RNase A (*see* **Note 11**), vortex, and incubate for 1 h at 60 °C as in **step 3**.

7. Cool the samples for 5 min at room temperature. During this time, pre-spin the PGL columns (three per extraction) for 1 min at $14,000 \times g$ at room temperature.

8. Add 400 μL of PCIA, close the lids tightly and mix by inversion in the rotator for 15 min at 40 rpm.

9. Pour the mixture into PGL columns and centrifuge for 5 min at $14,000 \times g$ at room temperature to separate the phases (if PGL columns are not available, phase separation can be done in microcentrifuge tubes; *see* **Note 15**).

10. Add 400 μL of PCIA into the same PGL column, close the lids tightly and mix by inversion in the rotator for 10 min at 40 rpm.

11. Centrifuge for 5 min at $14,000 \times g$ at room temperature to separate the phases.

12. Pour the upper phase into a new PGL column, add 400 µL of CIA, and mix by inversion as in **step 10**.

13. Centrifuge as in **step 11.**

14. Transfer the upper phase into a new PGL column, add 400 µL of CIA, and mix by inversion as in **step 10**.

15. Centrifuge as in **step 11.**

16. Transfer the upper phase into a new microcentrifuge tube.

17. Add 2 µL of glycogen and 400 µL of room temperature iso-propanol. Mix by inverting slowly five times and incubate for 5 min at room temperature.

18. Centrifuge for 45 min at maximum speed ($\geq 18,000 \times g$) and 4 °C to pellet the DNA. At the end of centrifugation, there will be whitish DNA pellets visible at the bottom of the tubes.

19. Carefully decant or pipette out the liquid.

20. Add 1 mL of 70 % ethanol (room temperature) and wash the pellets by inverting the tubes in the rotator for 5 min at 20 rpm.

21. Centrifuge for 5 min at $14,000 \times g$ at room temperature.

22. Carefully decant or pipette out the ethanol. It is not necessary to remove all the ethanol, just as much as can be removed without disturbing the DNA pellet. The pellets may float and it is important to make sure they are not lost during the washing steps. Repeat washing **steps 19** and **20** with 500 µL of 70 % ethanol.

23. Remove all the ethanol: first decant as much liquid as possible and then spin briefly to collect the drops at the bottom and remove the rest using a 100 µL pipette.

24. Air-dry the pellets in the open tubes at room temperature. Avoid over-drying (*see* **Note 13**).

25. Add 50 µL of 0.1× TE buffer or nuclease-free water and let the pellets dissolve overnight at 4 °C.

26. Mix gently by inverting and tapping the tubes (vortexing of the DNA solution may lead to shearing of the DNA), centrifuge briefly to collect the solution at the bottom of the tubes, and measure the DNA concentration.

27. Use the Genomic DNA Clean & Concentrator-10 Kit according to the manufacturer's protocol to further clean the samples (*see* **Note 16** on amount and concentration of DNA in this step).

3.3 Skeletonema marinoi

Collection, storage, and lysis of cells:

1. Harvest the diatom cells through multiple-centrifugation steps: Initially centrifuge a larger volume of culture in 50 mL

falcon tubes for 10–20 min at $3900 \times g$. Subsequently, resuspend the pellet into a smaller volume and transfer it to 1.5 mL microcentrifuge tubes. A second centrifugation step for 6 min at $20,200 \times g$ at 4 °C will remove most of the supernatant. A third centrifugation step for 4 min at $20,200 \times g$ at 4 °C will remove the rest of the media. *See* **Note 17**.

2. To each 1.5 mL microcentrifuge tube, add a master mix composed of 500 μL of CTAB buffer, 4 μL of RNase A, and 12 μL of β-mercaptoethanol. Prepare the master mix containing CTAB and RNase A, mix, and add the β-mercaptoethanol under the fume hood. Add the total volume of 516 μL to each sample and securely close the cap of each tube before homogenization and transfer to the incubator.

3. Incubate the tubes for 1 h at 65 °C with a vortex agitation of a few seconds every 15 min. Check that the pellet is diluted at the start of the incubation.

4. Transfer the tubes on ice for approximately 1 min.

DNA extraction:

5. Add 500 μL of CIA under the fume hood and invert the tubes repeatedly until the two solutions are mixed.

6. Centrifuge for 10 min at $20,200 \times g$ at 4 °C. After centrifugation, put the tubes on ice, taking care not to disturb the three layers.

7. Transfer the upper phase to a fresh 1.5 mL microcentrifuge tube. Be careful not to pipette the white intermediate layer, or the greenish oily bottom layer.

8. Check visually that the upper phase is clear and homogeneous (without oily structures). If not, add 500 μL of CIA as in **step 5** and repeat **steps 6–7** with caution, as the three phases are shades of white.

DNA purification:

9. Add one volume (400–600 μL) of ice-cold isopropanol (pre-stored at –20 °C).

10. Invert the tubes several times and incubate the tubes at –20 °C for a minimum of 1 h, but preferably overnight. *Note*: when the concentration of genomic DNA is high, the solution can turn purple-pink and the DNA precipitates, forming milky trails.

11. Centrifuge for 30 min at $20,200 \times g$ at 4 °C. After centrifugation, put the tubes on ice, taking care not to disturb the DNA pellet.

12. Pour the liquid gently without disturbing the pellet. The pellet forms a white spot at the bottom of the tube. The size of the

pellet depends on the amount of DNA extracted and the color on its purity and humidity.

13. Add 400 µL of ice-cold 75 % ethanol (pre-stored at –20 °C).

14. Centrifuge for 15 min at 20,200×g at 4 °C. After centrifugation, put the tubes on ice, being careful not to disturb the DNA pellet.

15. Pour the liquid gently without disturbing the pellet.

16. Prepare a clean area with blotting paper under the hood. After pouring, turn each tube upside down to dry at room temperature.

Resuspension of DNA:

17. After 1–2 h, the dried pellet is dissolved in 25–50 µL of double-distilled H$_2$O, TE buffer, or nuclease-free water, *see* **Note 18**.

18. The tubes are gently agitated manually and stored at 4 °C overnight to dissolve the pellet. DNA can be stored at 4 °C for up to 1 week, at –20 °C for up to 1 month, or at –80 °C for a longer period.

3.4 *Amphiura filiformis*

Sperm collection:

1. Washed animals are spawned individually in around 20 mL of filtered sea water in 50 mL Falcon tubes by transferring them to the light after a night in the dark. Remove the animal when spawning is completed.

2. Filter the sperm through a 100 µm mesh to remove larger pieces of debris.

3. Transfer the solution into a 50 mL tube and centrifuge gently for 10 min at 1000×g.

4. Remove the supernatant, leaving a small amount of liquid; resuspend in the remaining liquid; and transfer to a 1.5 mL tube. Centrifuge again for 10 min at 1000×g.

5. Remove all supernatant; store the sample at –20 °C or proceed to DNA extraction.

DNA extraction:

6. Add 600 µL of sperm isolation buffer and 3 µL of fresh Proteinase K solution to the collected sperm in a 1.5 mL tube and vortex.

7. Add 15 µL of 20% SDS and shake vigorously by hand as sperm lyse (*see* **Note 19**). Pulse spin. If the suspension is too thick to flow easily, then add more buffer, Proteinase K, and SDS solution.

8. Incubate for 1 h at 65 °C, then at 37 °C overnight.

9. Add 3 µL of fresh Proteinase K and shake vigorously. (If you added more isolation mix at **step 7**, increase the amount of Proteinase K accordingly.) Incubate for 1 h at 65 °C.

10. Add an equal volume of PCIA and extract with gentle shaking in an incubator for 5–8 h at 37 °C.

11. Centrifuge for 5 min at maximum speed and transfer the clear aqueous phase to a fresh tube.

12. Add one volume of PCIA and leave overnight at room temperature on the rotator wheel.

13. Centrifuge for 5 min at 18,000×g. Transfer the clear aqueous phase to a new tube. Repeat this step again if the aqueous phase is not completely clear. Add one volume of CIA and incubate for 1 h at room temperature.

14. Centrifuge for 5 min at 18,000×g, transfer the clear aqueous phase to a new tube, add one volume of CIA, and incubate for 8 h at room temperature.

15. Centrifuge for 5 min at 18,000×g and transfer the clear aqueous phase to a new tube. Bring the volume up to 500 μL with STE buffer. Add 1 mL of 100% ethanol. (If you added more isolation mix at **step 7**, increase the volume proportionally.) Mix and precipitate for at least 30 min at room temperature (*see* **Note 20**).

16. Centrifuge for 15 min at 18,000×g and decant the supernatant.

17. Add 1 mL of 75% ethanol at room temperature and wash the pellets by inverting the tube by hand several times.

18. Centrifuge for 2 min at maximum speed and room temperature.

19. Decant the ethanol carefully. A small amount can be left in the tube. Be careful not to disturb the pellet or drop it when decanting.

20. Repeat washing **steps 17–19** with 95% ethanol.

21. Dry the pellet at 37 °C in the heating block with the tube open.

22. Resuspend in 100 μL 10% TE buffer with 20 μg/mL RNase A.

23. Incubate 3 h at 37 °C.

24. Add 100 μL of PCIA, shake quickly and vigorously, centrifuge for 5 min at 18,000×g, and transfer the aqueous phase to a fresh tube.

25. Add 100 μL of CIA, shake quickly and vigorously, centrifuge for 5 min at 18,000×g, and transfer the aqueous phase to a new tube.

26. Repeat **step 25**.

27. Precipitate the DNA by adding 1/10 volume of 3 M sodium acetate and two volumes of 100% ethanol.

28. Centrifuge for 15 min at 18,000×g and decant the supernatant.

29. Wash the pellets with 75% ethanol, then 95% ethanol, and dry the pellets as in **steps 17–21**.

30. Resuspend the DNA in 100 μL of 10% TE buffer.

DNA cleanup with the Zymo DNA Clean & Concentrator:

31. Preheat the nuclease-free water to 65 °C for the final elution (65 μL per extraction).

32. Add 100 μL of DNA Binding Buffer to each DNA sample. Mix 1 s in a vortex mixer.

33. Transfer the mixture to a Zymo-Spin column in a collection tube.

34. Centrifuge for 30 s at $14,000 \times g$. Discard the flow-through.

35. Add 200 μL of DNA Wash Buffer to the column. Centrifuge for 30 s at $13,000 \times g$ and discard the flow-through.

36. Repeat the washing step.

37. Place the Zymo-Spin column into a new 1.5 mL tube. Pipette 29 μL of nuclease-free water (preheated at 65 °C) onto the membrane. Incubate the column for 5 min at 65 °C. Centrifuge for 30 s at $13,000 \times g$ to elute the DNA. Repeat this step with the same volume and elute into the same tube.

3.5 *Fucus vesiculosus* and *F. radicans*

DNA extraction:

1. Place a small piece of algal tissue (10–15 mg) in a 1.5 mL microcentrifuge tube along with two small stainless steel ball bearings (5 mm) and close the lid. Place it into the Mixer Mill and pulverize the tissue for 1.5 min at 30 Hz/s.

2. To remove polyphenolic compounds, suspend the ground material in 1 mL of 100% acetone for 10 min in the rotator.

3. Centrifuge the samples for 1 min at $12,800 \times g$, pour out the acetone, and discard it.

4. Repeat **steps 2** and **3** and air-dry the samples for 5–10 min (avoid over-drying).

5. Add 500 μL of 2% CTAB extraction buffer to each tube. Use a pipette tip to scrape the tissue pellet off the tube wall.

6. Add 17.5 μL of 0.1 M DIECA, 5 μL of β-mercaptoethanol under a fume hood, and 10 μL of RNase A solution, vortex vigorously, and incubate the mixture for 1 h at 65 °C. Vortex the mixture every 10 min.

7. From this step onwards, the NucleoSpin Plant II Kit is used following the manufacturer's instructions. Preheat the nuclease-free water to 65 °C for the final elution (55 μL per extraction).

8. Place a NucleoSpin Filter (violet ring) into a new collection tube (2 mL) and load the crude lysate onto the column using wide-bore filter tips. Centrifuge for 2 min at $12,800 \times g$, collect the clear flow-through, and discard the Filter. If not all the

liquid has passed through the filter, repeat the centrifugation step. If a pellet is visible in the flow-through, transfer the clear supernatant to a new 1.5 mL tube using wide-bore pipette tips. Alternatively, place the NucleoSpin Filter into a new 1.5 mL tube and pass the pre-cleared supernatant through the filter once more to remove solid particles completely.

9. Add 450 μL of Buffer PC and mix thoroughly by gentle inversion a few times.

10. Place a NucleoSpin Plant II Column (green ring) into a new Collection tube (2 mL) and load a maximum of 700 μL of the sample. Centrifuge for 1 min at $12,800 \times g$ and discard the flow-through.

11. Add 400 μL of Buffer PW1 to the NucleoSpin Plant II Column. Centrifuge for 1 min at $12,800 \times g$ and discard the flow-through.

12. Add 700 μL of Buffer PW2 to the NucleoSpin Plant II Column. Centrifuge for 1 min at $12,800 \times g$ and discard the flow-through.

13. Add another 200 μL of Buffer PW2 to the NucleoSpin Plant II Column. Centrifuge for 2 min at $12,800 \times g$ and discard the flow-through.

14. Place the NucleoSpin Plant II Column into a new 1.5 mL tube. Pipette 50 μL of nuclease-free water (preheated to 65 °C) onto the membrane. Incubate the NucleoSpin Plant II Column for 5 min at 65 °C. Centrifuge for 1 min at $12,800 \times g$ to elute the DNA.

DNA cleanup:

15. From this point, we use the Zymo DNA Clean & Concentrator-25 Kit. Preheat the nuclease-free water to 65 °C for the final elution (65 μL per extraction).

16. Add 100 μL of DNA Binding Buffer to each DNA sample. Mix 1 s in a vortex mixer.

17. Transfer the mixture to a Zymo-Spin column in a collection tube.

18. Centrifuge for 30 s at $14,000 \times g$. Discard the flow-through.

19. Add 200 μL of DNA Wash Buffer to the column. Centrifuge for 30 s at $12,800 \times g$ and discard the flow-through.

20. Repeat the wash step.

21. Place the Zymo-Spin Column into a new 1.5 mL tube. Pipette 58 μL of nuclease-free water (preheated to 65 °C) onto the membrane. Incubate the NucleoSpin Plant II column for 5 min at 65 °C. Centrifuge for 30 s at $12,800 \times g$ to elute the DNA.

3.6 *Balanus improvisus*

1. Select large and short-term starved fresh individuals for DNA extraction (*see* **Note 21**). Clean the barnacle shell with a fine brush to minimize the risk of contamination from other species (e.g., bacteria, algae). Remove the top plates (tergum and scutum) using a pair of tweezers (Fig. 9a, b and *see* **Note 22**). Grab the animal and pull it out of the shell. Mostly, this results in the soma (body) and cirri appearing without the mantle (*see* **Note 23**).

2. Put the soma and cirri from one adult barnacle into 250 µL of ice-cold buffer EB from the E.Z.N.A. Blood DNA Mini Kit in a 1.5 mL microcentrifuge tube. Homogenize with the plastic pestle in roughly five strokes (*see* **Note 24**).

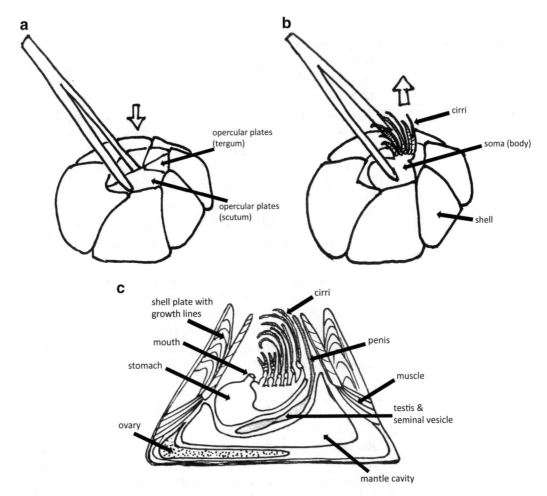

Fig. 9 Removing the body of an acorn barnacle from its shell. (**a**) Grab one of the top opercular plates by inserting tweezers gently through the aperture. Pull gently to remove the plate and to expose the animal. (**b**) Pull out the animal by grabbing the soma part below the cirri. (**c**) The overall anatomy of acorn barnacles. The mantle and potentially fertilized eggs (in the ovary) stay in the shell cavity when the body is pulled out and are discarded (they are not used for the DNA extraction)

3. Add 25 µL of protease solution OB, 250 µL of buffer BL and 2.5 µL of RNase A. Vortex for 15 s at full speed. Homogenize again with the plastic pestle (2–3 strokes).

4. Incubate the samples for 10 min at 65 °C. Vortex briefly 2–3 times during the incubation.

5. Centrifuge for 3 min at maximum speed.

6. Transfer the supernatant with a pipette into a new microcentrifuge tube.

7. Add 260 µL of 100% ethanol and vortex for 20 s at maximum speed.

8. For the remaining steps (chromatography, washing, and elution), follow the kit according to manufacturer's instructions.

3.7 Debaryomyces hansenii

1. Yeasts can be stored at –80 °C in a glycerol solution (20% v/v) almost indefinitely. Inoculate a loop-full of cells, directly taken from the frozen stock with a heated loop, onto YPD agar plates (*see* **Note 25**) and streak them out for single colony growth. Inoculate the plates for 48 h at 25–30 °C (*see* **Note 26**).

2. Inoculate a loop-full of yeast cells from a single colony on the agar plate into 10 mL of fresh YPD medium in a 50 mL Falcon tube. Incubate overnight at 25–30 °C with shaking. The optical density (600 nm) of the cultures is usually in the range of 2–6 optical units after roughly 17 h of incubation.

3. Harvest the cells by centrifugation for 10 min at $5000 \times g$. Wash the pellet with 1 ml of 10 mM EDTA, pH 8.0.

4. For both DNA kits, follow instructions from the manufacturer.

5. For the ISOLATE II Genomic DNA Kit, the enzyme zymolyase is used to produce spheroplasts. The seven strains tested with this protocol displayed somewhat different sensitivity to the zymolyase treatment, and for some of the strains, incubation had to be prolonged compared to the standard recommended time to complete spheroplast formation (*see* **Note 27**).

4 Notes

1. Barnacle species vary considerably in size. *B. improvisus* is a relatively small species and usually does not exceed 20 mm in diameter. The maximum wet weight obtained is about 30 mg. We have taken our individuals from laboratory cultures from the Swedish West Coast (from Tjärnö Marine Biological Station, Strömstad, Sweden, salinity ~30 psu).

2. For large fragment libraries that are used in particular for scaffolding and also for single-molecule long-read technologies such as PacBio, it is essential that the DNA has a high-molecular weight.

3. For quality control of the DNA sample, use a Nanodrop or any other spectrophotometric method to get an estimation of the 260/280 and 260/230 nm absorbance ratios of the sample, that indicate the amount of contamination with proteins and other organic compounds. Although spectrophotometric methods give an estimation of the concentration of DNA, it is highly recommended to measure the amount using Qubit (or similar DNA-specific methodology), which gives a more accurate determination of the concentration. In addition, it is important that the samples are run on a gel to estimate the amount in the low-molecular weight (degraded) and high-molecular weight DNA fractions. Ideally for sequencing, the DNA sample should be free of any degradation products and only contain material greater than 10–20 kb.

4. β-Mercaptoethanol has a characteristic unpleasant smell and is very toxic. It is extremely harmful if inhaled or swallowed and may be fatal if absorbed through the skin. While working with β-mercaptoethanol, wear protective gloves and perform all pipetting steps in a fume hood. When the tubes containing β-mercaptoethanol are taken out of the fume hood, their lids should be tightly closed. In the case of liquid spill on the surface of the tubes, wipe thoroughly with tissue, change gloves, and leave the tube in the fume hood until all smell disappears. Gloves, pipette tips, tissues, and plastic ware that have been in contact with β-mercaptoethanol should be disposed of as hazardous waste. Read the material safety data sheet before starting the work.

5. While most protocols use either CTAB or SDS buffer, a mixture of the two is sometimes used for DNA extractions in plants. In our tests, the SDS/CTAB mixture gave a better yield and purity of *Idotea* DNA than either of the buffers alone.

6. The plate reader can be used to rapidly assess the abundance of cells in culture before extraction in order to relate the amount of DNA extracted to the initial abundance of cells. Other alternative techniques are available. The extraction protocol works for small to large amount of *Skeletonema* cells and has been tested on a range from 0.31 to 1.8 billion cells counted before centrifugation using the plate reader. However, the purity of DNA (assessed by 230/260 absorbance ratio) decreases as the density of culture increases.

7. Safe-Lock tubes are recommended at this step. When the samples are mixed with chloroform:isoamyl alcohol, the pressure in the tubes may force the lid to open unexpectedly. If you use regular microcentrifuge tubes, after adding chloroform:isoamyl

alcohol, invert each tube a few times in the fume hood while holding the lid closed and then open the lid to release the pressure and close again tightly.

8. For one standard Illumina library, a single extraction from a piece of *Littorina* foot muscle of this size will be enough (DNA yield ≥ 2 µg). To obtain the maximum amount of DNA from a single individual, perform multiple extractions with the starting amount of tissue recommended in the protocol. Increasing the starting amount of tissue in a single extraction does not increase the yield proportionately and leads to lower DNA purity. Extractions from the digestive gland (hepatopancreas) give high yields but partially degraded DNA. Therefore we recommend carefully dissecting and discarding the hepatopancreas before collecting tissue samples for extraction. All other tissues and body parts (foot, head, mantle, all parts of the reproductive system) can be used for extraction of high-quality DNA. However, we recommend keeping different tissues separate in the extractions and assessing DNA integrity and purity for each extraction before pooling. Shell fragments should be avoided when collecting tissue samples for DNA extraction; they may result in a slightly pink coloration of the DNA solution due to co-purification of pigments (especially when the shell had a dark color).

9. If an incubator with a shaking platform is not available, incubate the sample in the heating block and vortex every 15–20 min.

10. Successful homogenization is crucial for high DNA yields. It is important to incubate the sample at 60 °C before the homogenization step. Normally no tissue pieces are visible after 5 min homogenization in the Mixer Mill. If tissue pieces are still visible, repeat the homogenization step for five more min (we never observed DNA shearing using this tissue homogenization method). If the Mixer Mill is not available, any other method of tissue homogenization can be used, including manual homogenization with pestles for Eppendorf tubes in the fume hood (although this is laborious for the processing of many samples).

11. To perform RNase A treatment directly in the digestion buffer, it is important to use a large amount of RNase A (5 µL of 100 mg/mL stock) and a long incubation time (1 h). On-column RNase A treatment after DNA extraction led to a loss of 50–90 % of the DNA.

12. If PGL columns are not available, phase separation can be done by centrifuging the tubes at **step 8.** After centrifugation, transfer them carefully to the fume hood (avoiding shaking) and collect the upper phase (approx. 500 µL) by pipetting. Be careful not to touch the white interphase. If the phases are mixed by mistake, repeat the centrifugation step.

13. At this step, it is important to allow the ethanol to evaporate without over-drying the pellet, because it will be difficult to dissolve. Depending on the size of the pellet and on how much ethanol was left in the tube, drying can take from 5 to 40 min. Check the pellets every 5–10 min. When dry, the DNA pellets look transparent; there should not be any ethanol drops left within the tube and no residual ethanol smell either.

14. In *I. balthica*, high-quality DNA can be extracted from the head and the abdominal muscle. Any pieces of the gut and its content should be avoided because it would yield highly degraded DNA. In addition, gut contents will lead to contaminant sequences. Before collecting tissue samples, cut the carapace along the dorsal side (being careful not to disturb the gut), remove the gut, and wash the animal in ethanol. Parts of the exoskeleton and the appendages should be avoided as well; pigments in the exoskeleton co-purify with the DNA and can inhibit downstream reactions such as amplification, ligation, etc.

15. If PGL columns are not available, all PCIA and CIA extraction steps can be performed in Safe-Lock or regular microcentrifuge tubes by centrifugation and pipetting of the upper phase into a new tube each time (being very careful not to disturb the phases). However, with four extraction steps, this will be time-consuming and using the PGLs column is recommended.

16. Column binding capacity in the Genomic DNA Clean & Concentrator-10 Kit is 10 μg. Measure DNA concentration and calculate the total amount of DNA in the samples before using the kit. Multiple extractions from the same individual can be pooled together before cleaning as long as the total amount of DNA is below 10 μg. If the amount of DNA is above 10 μg, split the sample into aliquots for cleaning. The kit can also help to concentrate DNA samples by using a small volume of elution buffer. Depending on DNA integrity, 50–90% of the DNA is recovered after cleaning with the kit (the recovery rate is lower when samples have a large fraction of short degraded fragments). Also, after extractions with phenol, the DNA samples may contain contaminants causing overestimation of the DNA concentration measured by the spectrophotometer. To avoid over-dilution of samples, it is better to use approximately ½ of the volume of elution buffer calculated from the total DNA amount applied to the cleaning column and dilute the samples afterwards if necessary. A second elution gives much lower DNA concentrations (10–20 ng/μL). If desired, it can be performed in a new tube.

17. During supernatant removal, the pellet will become loose, and therefore, it is important to split the last centrifugations into two steps. Always work under a clean hood. Pelleted cells can be stored at −80 °C. Keeping the cells at −80 °C prior to DNA

extraction facilitates the lysis of the cells. To avoid DNA degradation, we do not recommend repetitive thawing and freezing of the samples. Cells can also be concentrated on membrane filters (pore size 3 μm) and filters can be stored at −80 °C. However, we recommend the use of centrifugation on axenic cultures. We noticed that even gentle filtration breaks the cells with consequential DNA loss.

18. We recommend using nuclease-free water to resuspend the cleaned DNA pellet, because some genomic analyses require the absence of EDTA. The volume added depends on the size of the DNA pellet. For pellets of the size of a pen-tip or smaller, use 25 μL.

19. No automatic vortexing at this step.

20. You can stop the procedure here and keep the solution at 4 °C overnight and perform the next step on the next day.

21. Individuals used for DNA extraction were starved for at least 2 days. This is to avoid contamination with DNA of digested foods (*Artemia*, microalgae, etc.). We also tested using individuals preserved in ethanol at −20 °C. However, this procedure resulted in low DNA quality (degradation is seen more frequently). This is why we recommend using fresh samples.

22. When pulling out the first operculum plate, the whole animal is sometimes attached to it. If not, remove the other operculum plates to have easy access to the animal (Fig. 9a, b).

23. Sometimes parts of the mantle can be attached to the soma and cirri and be hard to remove. The mantle epithelium, ovary tissues, and sometimes fertilized eggs can be found inside the shell (Fig. 9c). To minimize genetic variation, we avoided including the eggs in the DNA preparation. Mantle and ovary tissues were also excluded to avoid the risk of gonad contamination.

24. Sonication can also be used to dissolve the tissues. However, care should be taken not to do this extensively since it will also result in DNA degradation. For this reason, we have abandoned sonication in favor of using the pestle, which is much more gentle to DNA.

25. The marine yeast *D. hansenii* can be grown on a wide variety of media. A frequently used medium is yeast nitrogen base (YNB; DIFCO), which is a synthetic defined medium used for cultivation of several different yeast species. This can be used for either solid (by adding agar) or liquid growth. Another commonly used rich medium is yeast peptone dextrose (YPD), which is less well defined but is used to obtain high biomass.

26. Model species of yeast, such as *S. cerevisiae* and *Schizosaccharomyces pombe*, are usually grown at 30 °C. This temperature also works for growth of *D. hansenii*, and since 30 °C rooms/incubators are found in most standard microbial laboratories, this temperature could be handy to work with. However, *D. hansenii*

grows better at slightly lower temperatures (25–27 °C), which should be preferred in physiological experiments. For the purpose of obtaining enough yeast cells for DNA extraction, either temperature works fine; here we have used 30 °C.

27. The efficiency of spheroplast formation is checked under the microscope as follows: roughly 5 µL of the cell suspension is applied to a microscopy slide and gently covered by a cover slip. A small drop of pure water is applied just at the edge of the cover slip, thereby gently diluting the cell suspension. This leads to a lowering of the concentration of the osmotic stabilizer (sorbitol), whereby proper spheroplasts become osmotically fragile and lyse (cells burst). If this is not observed, the incubation with zymolyase should be extended.

Acknowledgments

This work was funded by the Swedish Research Councils (VR and Formas) through the Linnaeus Centre for Marine Evolutionary Biology at University of Gothenburg. We thank Mikael Dahl, Sonja Leidenberger, and Pierre De Wit for sharing their experience on other DNA extraction protocols for *Idotea balthica* and Natalia Mikhailova for sharing her experience on DNA extraction methods for *Littorina saxatilis*.

References

1. Leffler EM, Bullaughey K, Matute DR, Meyer WK, Ségurel L, Venkat A, Andolfatto P, Przeworski M (2012) Revisiting an old riddle: what determines genetic diversity levels within species? PLoS Biol 10(9), e1001388. doi:10.1371/journal.pbio.1001388

2. IMAGO Genome Sequencing project within the Centre for Marine Evolutionary Biology, University of Gothenburg, Sweden. http://cemeb.science.gu.se/research/imago-marine-genome-projects. Accessed 10 Aug 2015

3. Dujon B, Sherman D, Fischer G, Durrens P, Casaregola S, Lafontaine I, De Montigny J, Marck C, Neuvéglise C, Talla E, Goffard N, Frangeul L, Aigle M, Anthouard V, Babour A, Barbe V, Barnay S, Blanchin S, Beckerich JM, Beyne E, Bleykasten C, Boisramé A, Boyer J, Cattolico L, Confanioleri F, De Daruvar A, Despons L, Fabre E, Fairhead C, Ferry-Dumazet H, Groppi A, Hantraye F, Hennequin C, Jauniaux N, Joyet P, Kachouri R, Kerrest A, Koszul R, Lemaire M, Lesur I, Ma L, Muller H, Nicaud JM, Nikolski M, Oztas S, Ozier-Kalogeropoulos O, Pellenz S, Potier S, Richard GF, Straub ML, Suleau A, Swennen D, Tekaia F, Wésolowski-Louvel M, Westhof E, Wirth B, Zeniou-Meyer M, Zivanovic I, Bolotin-Fukuhara M, Thierry A, Bouchier C, Caudron B, Scarpelli C, Gaillardin C, Weissenbach J, Wincker P, Souciet JL (2004) Genome evolution in yeasts. Nature 430(6995):35–44. doi:10.1038/nature02579

4. Reid DG (1996) Systematic and evolution of *Littorina*. The Ray Society, London

5. Winnepenninckx B, Backeljau T, De Wachter R (1993) Extraction of high-molecular-weight DNA from molluscs. Trends Genet 9(12):407. doi:10.1016/0168-9525(93)90102-N

6. Panova M, Johansson T, Canbäck B, Bentzer J, Alm Rosenblad M, Johannesson K, Tunlid A, André C (2014) Species and gene divergence in *Littorina* snails detected by array comparative genomic hybridization. BMC Genomics 15:687. doi:10.1186/1471-2164-15-687

7. Ravinet M, Westram A, Johannesson K, Butlin R, André C, Panova M (2015) Shared and non-shared genomic divergence in parallel ecotypes of *Littorina saxatilis* at a local scale. Mol Ecol. doi:10.1111/mec.13332

8. Nishiguchi MK, Doukakis P, Egan M, Kizirian D, Phillips A, Prendini L, Rosenbaum HC,

Torres E, Wyner Y, DeSalle R, Giribet G (2002) DNA isolation procedures. In: DeSalle R, Giribet G, Wheeler W (eds) Techniques in molecular systematics and evolution. Birkhaeuser Verlag, Berlin

9. Chen H, Rangasamy M, Tan SY, Wang H, Siegfried BD (2010) Evaluation of five methods for total DNA extraction from Western corn rootworm beetles. PLoS One 5(8), e11963. doi:10.1371/journal.pone.0011963

10. Wang S, Meyer E, McKay JK, Matz MV (2012) 2b-RAD: a simple and flexible method for genome-wide genotyping. Nat Methods 9(8):808–810. doi:10.1038/NMETH.2023

11. Hildebrand M (2008) Diatoms, biomineralization processes, and genomics. Chem Rev 108(11):4855–4874. doi:10.1021/cr078253z

12. Guillard RRL (1975) Culture of phytoplankton for feeding marine invertebrates. In: Smith W, Chanley M (eds) Culture of marine invertebrate animals. Plenum, New York, NY

13. Lakeman MB, von Dassow P, Cattolico RA (2009) The strain concept in phytoplankton ecology. Harmful Algae 8(5):746–758. doi:10.1016/j.hal.2008.11.011

14. Nagai S, Imai I, Manabe T (1998) A simple and quick technique for establishing axenic cultures of the centric diatom *Coscinodiscus wailesii* Gran. J Plankton Res 20(7):1417–1420. doi:10.1093/plankt/20.7.1417

15. Provasoli L, Shiraishi K, Lance J (1959) Nutritional idiosyncrasies of *Anemia* and *Tigriopus* in monoxenic culture. Ann N Y Acad Sci 77(2):250–261. doi:10.1111/j.1749-6632.1959.tb36905.x

16. Tesson S, Borra M, Kooistra WHCF, Procaccini G (2011) Microsatellite primers in the planktonic diatom *Pseudo-nitzschia multistriata* (Bacillariophyceae). Am J Bot 98(2):33–35. doi:10.3732/ajb.1000430

17. McKenzie JD, Kelly MS (1994) Comparative study of sub-cuticular bacteria in brittlestars (Echinodermata: Ophiuroidea). Mar Biol 120(1):65–80. doi:10.1007/BF00381943

18. Sea Urchin Genome Sequencing Consortium (2006) The genome of the sea urchin *Strongylocentrotus purpuratus*. Science 314(5801):941–952. doi:10.1126/science.1133609

19. Deniaud-Bouët E, Kervarec N, Gurvan M, Tonon T, Kloareg B, Herve C (2014) Chemical and enzymatic fractionation of cell walls from Fucales: insights into the structure of the extracellular matrix of brown algae. Ann Bot 114(6):1203–1216. doi:10.1093/aob/mcu096

20. Mabeau S, Kloareg B (1987) Isolation and analysis of the cell walls of brown algae: *Fucus spiralis*, *F. ceranoides*, *F. vesiculosus*, *F. serratus*, *Bifurcaria bifurcata* and *Laminaria digitata*. J Exp Bot 38(194):1573–1580. doi:10.1093/jxb/38.9.1573

21. McDevit DC, Saunders GW (2009) On the utility of DNA barcoding for species differentiation among brown macroalgae (Phaeophyceae) including a novel extraction protocol. Phycol Res 57(2):131–141. doi:10.1111/j.1440-1835.2009.00530.x

22. Toth GB, Pavia H (2001) Removal of dissolved brown algal phlorotannins using insoluble polyvinylpolypyrrolidone (PVPP). J Chem Ecol 27(9):1899–1910. doi:10.1023/A:1010421128190

23. Phillips N, Smith CM, Morden CW (2001) An effective DNA extraction protocol for brown algae. Phycol Res 49(2):97–102. doi:10.1046/j.1440-1835.2001.00229.x

24. Crisp DJ, Bourget E (1985) Growth in barnacles. Adv Mar Biol 22:199–244. doi:10.1016/S0065-2881(08)60052-8

25. Wrange AL, André C, Lundh T, Lind U, Blomberg A, Jonsson PJ, Havenhand JN (2014) Importance of plasticity and local adaptation for coping with changing salinity in coastal areas: a test case with barnacles in the Baltic Sea. BMC Evol Biol 14:156. doi:10.1186/1471-2148-14-156

26. Kumar S, Randhawa A, Ganesan K, Raghava GPS, Mondal AK (2012) Draft genome sequence of salt-tolerant yeast *Debaryomyces hansenii* var. *hansenii* MTCC 234. Eukaryot Cell 11(7):961–962. doi:10.1128/EC.00137-12

Chapter 3

High-Throughput Sequencing of Complete Mitochondrial Genomes

Andrew George Briscoe, Kevin Peter Hopkins, and Andrea Waeschenbach

Abstract

Next-generation sequencing has revolutionized mitogenomics, turning a cottage industry into a high throughput process. This chapter outlines methodologies used to sequence, assemble, and annotate mitogenomes of non-model organisms using Illumina sequencing technology, utilizing either long-range PCR amplicons or gDNA as starting template. Instructions are given on how to extract DNA, conduct long-range PCR amplifications, generate short Sanger barcode tag sequences, prepare equimolar sample pools, construct and assess quality library preparations, assemble Illumina reads using either seeded reference mapping or de novo assembly, and annotate mitogenomes in the absence of an automated pipeline. Notes and recommendations, derived from our own experience, are given throughout this chapter.

Key words Illumina, MiSeq, Long-range PCR, Shotgun sequencing, Mitogenomics, Multiplexing

1 Introduction

Animal mitochondrial (mt) genomes are circular molecules, typically ~15–17 kb long, which in most metazoans encode 37 genes (22 transfer RNAs, 2 ribosomal RNA genes, and 13 protein-coding genes); exceptions to this arrangement include the linear genomes of medusozoans (e.g., [1]), isopods (e.g., [2]), and certain sponges [3] and the lack of one of the protein-coding genes (atp8) in a number of animal phyla (*see* [4]). Their wide-ranging use as a source of molecular markers can be attributed largely to the varying levels of evolutionary and functional constraints acting on the different parts of the mitogenome, which results in mutational rate heterogeneity within and between genes [5]. Thus, depending on the level of sequence conservation, different parts of the mitogenome can be better used to study shallow divergences (e.g., phylogeography, population genetics, genus-level

Sarah J. Bourlat (ed.), *Marine Genomics: Methods and Protocols*, Methods in Molecular Biology, vol. 1452,
DOI 10.1007/978-1-4939-3774-5_3, © Springer Science+Business Media New York 2016

phylogeny) and deep evolutionary divergences (e.g., above genus-level phylogeny). However, there are well-known caveats associated with using mitochondrial data, especially when studying shallow divergences, which are linked to incomplete lineage sorting, introgression, selective sweeps, and background selection (*see* [6, 7]). In such cases, the gene genealogies of the mt data can conflict with those obtained using nuclear data (e.g., [8]). However, rather than providing conflicting phylogenetic signal, the concatenated use of mt and nuclear data can also provide complementary nodal support for the shallow and the deep nodes of a tree, respectively [9, 10]. Furthermore, the simplicity of transmission via maternal inheritance, combined with an absence (or low level) of recombination in most animal groups (but *see* [11]), the relative ease of PCR amplification due to the high copy number of mitogenomes, and the lack of paralogous copies (except for nuclear mitochondrial pseudogenes; *see* [12]) have made mtDNA a popular marker in evolutionary biology. Also, the small size and high conservation of gene content (*see* [13]) facilitate the usage of rare genomic changes such as gene order rearrangements. Rokas and Holland [14] estimated homoplasy of mt gene order to be low to moderate in animals, and although the extent of gene order rearrangement differs between and within phyla [13], it can be suitably variable to serve as synapomorphies for phylogenetic clades (e.g., [15, 16]) and for distinguishing between cryptic species [17]; but *see* also [3].

Whereas traditionally mitogenome sequencing involved time-consuming and sometimes troublesome long-range PCR, followed by cloning, Sanger sequencing and primer walking, next-generation sequencing (NGS) has revolutionized mitogenomics, turning a cottage industry into a high-throughput process (e.g., [18–22]). As the majority of our work has been conducted using the Illumina MiSeq platform, the methodology described below is geared toward this platform but it can easily be adjusted to others.

High-throughput sequencing of mitogenomes can be categorized as follows: (1) long-range PCR amplicon sequencing versus shotgun sequencing of genomic DNA (gDNA) and (2) indexed, multiplexed samples versus non-indexed, pooled samples (for a workflow overview, *see* Fig. 1). The decision whether to pursue long-range amplicon or gDNA shotgun sequencing is driven by a number of factors. In the case of shotgun sequencing, it is imperative to have gDNA extracts with a high proportion of double-stranded DNA (dsDNA) (for DNA extraction methods, *see* Subheading 3.1); long-range PCR (Subheading 3.2) uses single-stranded DNA (ssDNA) as template; thus, any gDNA extract with sufficiently long fragments will suffice. In cases where mt gene order is conserved among target organisms, suitable long-range PCR primers are available, and regions containing repeat motifs (which may interfere with PCR amplification) are not to be expected, NGS

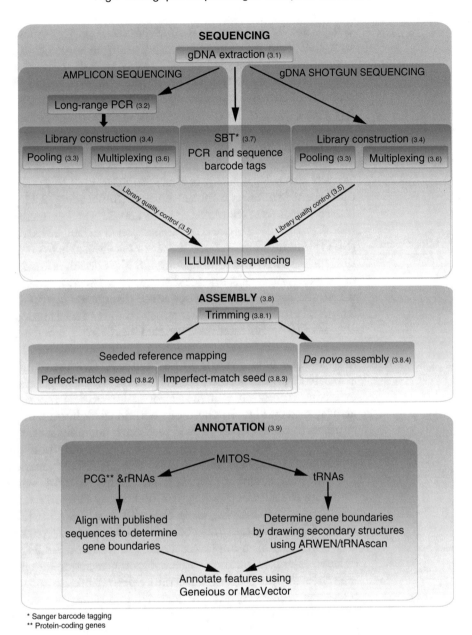

Fig. 1 Workflow outlining the procedure for next-generation sequencing of mitochondrial genomes using long-range PCR amplicons and genomic DNA shotgun sequencing. *Numbers* in *brackets* refer to chapter sections

sequencing of long-range PCR products is an effective strategy to minimize the proportion of nontarget reads, thus increasing the number of mitogenomes that can be sequenced on a given platform run. In most cases, multiple (typically 3), overlapping long-range PCRs are necessary to cover the complete mitogenome of a given target. In cases of unknown gene order, a lack of suitable long-range primers and/or the presence of repeat motifs which can complicate long-range PCR amplification, mitogenomes can be extracted from data generated using shotgun sequencing of total genomic double-stranded DNA. Because typically only ~0.5–1% of the reads obtained in this way are of mitochondrial origin, the large majority of the data remains redundant (although high copy number genes, such as the complete nuclear ribosomal RNA array and certain protein-coding genes, can easily be assembled from those data and can form useful complements to the mitogenome data).

The decision whether to multiplex PCR products or gDNA extracts into target-specific libraries (Subheading 3.6) or whether to pool them into an equimolar solution (Subheading 3.3) prior to library preparation (Subheadings 3.4 and 3.5) and extracting them bioinformatically using seed sequences, such as Sanger barcode tags (SBTs) (Subheadings 3.7 and 3.8.2) or data available from repositories, such as GenBank (Subheading 3.8.3), is driven primarily by the expected amount of sequence divergence between targets. In cases where the average expected sequence divergence is <5% over the length of a read, we would recommend a multiplexed approach; but also *see* [19] who assembled pooled reads from congeners. The advantage of the latter methodology is the much-reduced cost, as only a single library needs to be prepared. However, the caveats associated with this method are the necessity to either generate SBTs or having to rely on sequence information in data repositories to identify read contigs. Furthermore, additional bioinformatic effort is required to assemble the pooled reads into unambiguous, non-chimeric contigs, a process which is facilitated by only pooling PCR products and gDNA extracts from sufficiently distantly related taxa.

The read assembly process (Subheading 3.8), following read trimming (Subheading 3.8.1), can be broadly categorized into (1) seeded reference mapping using either SBTs, which provide a 100% match (Subheading 3.8.2), or published repository data, which may only provide an imperfect match (Subheading 3.8.3), and (2) de novo assembly (Subheading 3.8.4); no instructions are given for reference mapping using full-length, perfect-match mitogenome reference sequences, as our methodologies are geared toward sequencing non-model organisms for which full-length references sequences are not available. Subheading 3.9 outlines mitogenome annotation in the absence of an automated annotation pipeline.

2 Materials

2.1 DNA Extraction

1. Molecular grade ethanol (95–100%).

2. TE buffer (1×): 10 mM Tris–HCl, pH 7.5 and 1 mM ethylenediaminetetraacetic acid (EDTA), pH 8.0; adjust pH of final solution to 7.2, autoclave and filter-sterilize.

3. 1.5 ml microcentrifuge tubes (Axygen).

4. Tissue grinder pestles (Axygen) for 1.5 ml microcentrifuge tubes.

5. Isolate II Genomic DNA Kit (Bioline).

6. DNeasy Blood & Tissue Kit (Qiagen).

7. Rocking incubator (capable of 200 rpm motion).

8. Heating block or heated water bath.

9. Microcentrifuge (minimum of $16,000 \times g$ required).

2.2 Long-Range PCR

1. 0.2 ml PCR tubes.

2. TaKaRa LA Taq® DNA Polymerase (Mg^{2+} plus buffer) kit (Clontech).

3. Vortex mixer.

4. Microcentrifuge.

5. Thermal cycler.

6. Gel electrophoresis cast, tank, and power pack.

7. TBE buffer (1×): 89 mM Tris–HCl, pH 8.3; 89 mM boric acid; and 20 mM ethylenediaminetetraacetic acid (EDTA), pH 8.0; adjust pH of final solution to 8.3.

8. 0.8 % TBE agarose: 0.8 g agarose, 100 ml TBE (1×).

9. QIAquick PCR Purification Kit (Qiagen).

10. ZymoClean™ Gel DNA Recovery Kit (Zymo Research).

2.3 Equimolar Sample Pool Preparation

1. Qubit® fluorometer (Life Technologies).

2. Qubit® dsDNA broad-range or high-sensitivity assay kit (Life Technologies).

3. 2200 TapeStation (Agilent Technologies).

4. DNA and Genomic DNA Analysis ScreenTapes (Agilent Technologies).

5. Vacuum concentrator.

2.4 Library Preparation

1. Library preparation kits (TruSeq DNA PCR-Free, TruSeq Nano DNA, Nextera DNA, Nextera XT DNA; Illumina).

2. Agencourt AMPure XP PCR Purification Kit (Beckman Coulter).

3. Magnetic microcentrifuge tube rack for 1.5 ml microcentrifuge tubes.

4. Molecular grade ethanol (80 %).

5. Focused ultrasonicator (Covaris).

6. Thermal cycler.

2.5 Library Quality Control

1. FastStart Essential DNA Green Master Mix kit (Roche).

2. HPLC-purified qPCR primers (1.1: 5′-AATGATACGGCG ACCACCGAGAT-3′ and 2.1: 5′-CAAGCAGAAGACGGCA TACGA-3′).

3. PhiX Control v3 (Illumina).

4. Tween (0.1%): 50 ml sterile water and 50 μl Tween 20.

5. 1.5 ml microcentrifuge tubes.

6. 0.1 ml qPCR tubes.

7. Microcentrifuge.

8. Quantitative PCR instrument.

2.6 Sanger Barcode Tag (SBT) Generation

In addition to items 3–10 already listed in Subheading 2.2:

1. Illustra™ PuReTaq Ready-To-Go PCR beads (GE Healthcare).

3 Methods

3.1 DNA Extraction (Single Stranded vs. Double Stranded)

Two different approaches are presented here for DNA extractions depending on the subsequent downstream applications. The first maximizes recovery of dsDNA and is favored for shotgun sequencing (*see* **Note 1**), while the second provides a higher total yield of both ssDNA and dsDNA, thus providing more template for PCR enrichment. Samples referred to in this section have either been stored in 95–100% molecular grade ethanol or have been frozen at –80 °C (*see* **Note 2**):

1. Using a sterile scalpel blade, cut 25 mg of animal tissue into small pieces. If the sample is smaller than this, use the whole organism where possible (*see* **Note 3**).

2. If previously stored in ethanol, blot the tissue to remove excess liquid or allow the ethanol to evaporate. If it is necessary to rehydrate the tissue to improve DNA yield, soak in TE buffer (1×) for 12–24 h at room temperature.

3. Transfer the sample to a 1.5 ml microcentrifuge tube (*see* **Note 4**).

4. Homogenize the sample, if necessary, using a sterile tissue grinder pestle.

5a. If extracting DNA for shotgun sequencing, use the Isolate II Genomic DNA extraction kit following manufacturer's instructions including the following modifications:

   – Once the tissue has been homogenized, leave the pestle in the microcentrifuge while adding lysis buffer GL. This should remove any tissue remaining on the pestle.

   – Add 25 μl Proteinase K, vortex, and digest the samples at 56 °C for 3.5 h (*see* **Notes 5** and **6**).

5b. If extracting DNA for subsequent PCR enrichment, use the DNeasy Blood & Tissue Kit following manufacturer's instructions including the following modifications:

- Once the tissue has been homogenized, leave the pestle in the microcentrifuge tube while adding tissue lysis buffer ATL. This should remove any tissue remaining on the pestle.

- Add 20 µl of Proteinase K, vortex, and digest the tissue at 56 °C for 12–24 h) (*see* **Notes 5** and **6**).

- Following the addition of lysis buffer AL, heat the mix for 10 min at 70 °C using either a heating block or a heated water bath (*see* **Note 7**).

- Perform two elution steps, both in a volume of 100 µl of buffer AE (*see* **Note 8**)

3.2 Long-Range PCRs

Most of the long-range PCRs conducted by us used the TaKaRa LA Taq® DNA Polymerase (Mg^{2+} plus buffer) (*see* **Note 9**). As with most long-range PCR kits, the polymerase mix in the TaKaRa kit consists of *Taq* DNA polymerase and a proofreading enzyme. The proofreading enzyme ensures the removal of any misincorporated nucleotides by using $3' \rightarrow 5'$ exonuclease activity and therefore prevents premature termination of strand extension. However, synthesis using a proofreading enzyme is slow (~1–2 min for 1 kb), which is why it is combined with *Taq* polymerase, which can generate 1 kb in up to 10 s:

1. On ice, assemble the PCR master mix into a microcentrifuge tube in the following order (quantities are per 50 µl reaction volume): sterile water (to a final volume of 50 µl; exact volume depends on volume of primers and template DNA), 5 µl 10× LA PCR Buffer II (Mg^{2+} plus), 8 µl dNTP mixture (2.5 mM each), 2.0 µl of 10 mM of each primer (*see* **Note 10**), and 0.5 µl TaKaRa LA Taq (*see* **Notes 11** and **12**). Vortex briefly.

2. On ice, pipette aliquots of 50 µl, minus the volume of template DNA, into a 0.2 ml PCR tube, and add up to 100 ng of template DNA. Vortex very briefly at low to medium speed (*see* **Note 13**) and briefly spin down tubes in a microcentrifuge.

3. Transfer tubes to a preheated thermal cycler (*see* **Note 14**) and run the following PCR profile: initial denaturation at 94 °C for 2 min, followed by 40 cycles of 94 °C for 20 s, X for 30 s, and 68 °C for Y min; X denotes annealing temperature and Y denotes extension time. Finish with a final 10 min extension at 68 °C. *See* **Note 15** for further explanation of cycling profiles.

4. Visualize PCR products on a 0.8 % TBE agarose gel.

5. Purify PCR products using either the QIAquick PCR purification or Zymoclean™ Gel DNA Recovery Kit following manufacturer's instructions (*see* **Note 16**).

6. Sanger sequence both ends of the PCR products to verify their identity.

3.3 Equimolar Sample Pool Preparation

In cases where multiple samples, either as amplicons or gDNA, will be pooled in a single library preparation, it is important to produce an equimolar solution of template DNA in order to obtain even read coverage across and within samples (*see* **Note 17**). This requires accurate DNA concentration quantification using a fluorometer (*see* **Note 18**) and, in the case of amplicons, an assessment of fragment length prior to pooling of samples.

Amplicons

Combining different length amplicons at equal molarity requires longer amplicons to be added at a higher concentration; thus, the same number of fragments of each amplicon is being pooled:

1. Quantify amplicon concentrations using a Qubit® fluorometer.

2. If amplicon sizes are unknown, estimate them using a TapeStation.

3. Calculate the molarity of each sample as follows:

$$\text{Molarity}\,(\text{nM}) = \frac{\text{amplicon concentration}\,(\text{ng}\,/\,\mu l)}{660\,(\text{g}\,/\,\text{mol}) \times \text{amplicon length}\,(\text{bp})} \times 10^6,$$

where 660 is the weight of a single DNA base pair.

4. Add sufficient volume of each amplicon to produce an equimolar solution.

gDNA

1. Quantify gDNA extract concentrations using a Qubit® fluorometer.

2. Divide the total amount of DNA required for the library prep (*see* Subheading 3.4) by the number of samples being pooled (*see* **Note 17**).

3. Adjust the sample volumes to be added so that the amount of total gDNA for each sample is equal (*see* **Note 19**). The pool volume can be adjusted to suit the library preparation method by adding nuclease-free water or by drying down the sample using a vacuum concentrator.

3.4 Library Construction

Illumina offers two main types of DNA library preparation kits: those using mechanical fragmentation and those using enzymatic fragmentation. Kits using mechanical fragmentation require more DNA input but produce a more even coverage, so, where possible, those kits are preferential. Of those kits using mechanical fragmentation, TruSeq DNA PCR-Free and TruSeq Nano DNA require 2 µg and 200 ng of input DNA for the 550 bp insert protocol, respectively (see manufacturer's recommendations). Of those kits using enzymatic fragmentation, Nextera DNA and Nextera XT DNA require 50 and 1 ng of input DNA, respectively (see manufacturer's recommendations). If multiple library types are required, check these are compatible for use on a single Illumina sequencing run (*see* **Note 20**):

1. For gDNA samples, assess quantity and fragment length of DNA using a TapeStation (*see* **Note 21**).

2. Once a decision on library preparation kits has been made, dilute the pooled samples to the concentration and volume required for the chosen kit.

3. Construct the libraries following manufacturer's instructions (*see* **Note 22**). Note that **items 2–6** in Subheading 2.4 are necessary to follow the manufacturer's instructions.

4. Check library quality using real-time PCR (qPCR) using the FastStart Essential DNA Green Master Mix kit and HPLC-purified qPCR primers listed in Subheading 2.5 following manufacturer's instructions.

3.5 Library Quality Control

Following completion of library preparation, samples should be validated using qPCR and the size of the library fragments checked on a TapeStation (*see* **Note 23**):

1. For each sample, make two separate dilutions of 1:1000 and dilute one of the dilutions to 1:10,000. For the standards, make a 1:100 dilution of 2 nM PhiX in triplicate followed by five serial 1:10 dilutions (standards will range from 20 nm to 0.0002 nm). Make all dilutions using 0.1% Tween.

2. On ice, assemble FastStart Essential DNA qPCR master mix into a 1.5 ml microcentrifuge tube as follows (quantities are per 10 μl reaction volume): sterile water 2.8 μl, 5 μl Master Mix, 0.1 μl of 10 mM of each HPLC-purified qPCR primer. Vortex briefly.

3. On ice, pipette master mix aliquots of 8 μl into each 0.1 ml qPCR tube and add 2 μl of diluted template DNA. Vortex very briefly at low to medium speed (*see* **Note 13**) and briefly spin down tubes in a microcentrifuge.

4. Transfer tubes to the quantitative PCR instrument and run the following profile: initial denaturation at 95 °C for 10 min, followed by 45 cycles of 95 °C for 10 s, and 60 °C for 30 s.

3.6 Pooling of Target-Specific Libraries (Multiplexing)

Individual libraries can be labeled using indexed adaptor sequences, allowing the pooling of multiple libraries (*see* **Note 17**). Following the sequencing run, library-specific reads are de-multiplexed using the on-instrument software (Illumina). Currently, TruSeq and Nextera kits offer 24 and 6 single-indexed adaptor sequences, respectively. Higher levels of multiplexing can be done using dual indexing, where indexes are added to both ends of the library fragments. Currently TruSeq and Nextera preparation kits allow for dual indexing 96 and 384 samples, respectively. Thorough protocols and advice on pooling these indexes are included in the product manuals:

1. Calculate the concentration of the libraries to be pooled by multiplying qPCR values by 1000 or 10,000 depending on the dilution factor. Providing these values agrees and falls within the range of the qPCR standards; calculate the average concentration for each library.

2. To obtain size-corrected library concentrations, use the following formula:

$$\text{Corrected library concentration} = \frac{300}{\text{average library fragment length}} \times \text{average library concentration,}$$

where 300 is the average length of the PhiX Control v3 standard.

3. Based on these size-corrected values, dilute samples to the same concentration (commonly 2 or 4 nM) using Illumina EBT Buffer.

4. Add equal volumes of these diluted samples to the final sample pool for denaturing and dilution to MiSeq loading concentration.

3.7 Sanger Barcode Tag (SBT) Generation

Short, target-specific Sanger sequences can be used as starting seeds to assemble pooled NGS reads into target-specific contigs (Subheading 3.8.2). These are typically generated as follows:

1. Choose existing or develop new primers for short regions (~500–700 bp) situated in the mitogenome. In the case of overlapping long-range PCR amplicons (*see* Subheading 3.2), a single SBT can be generated within the overlapping region. If there is good overlap between amplicons, i.e., >800 bp, and the mitogenome sequences are sufficiently divergent, e.g., from congeners, two short identifying regions per mitogenome should suffice.

2. Carry out 25 μl PCR reactions (e.g., Illustra™ PuReTaq Ready-To-Go PCR beads) using 1.0 μl of 10 mM of each primer (*see* **Note 10**) and either 0.3 μl of the purified PCR products generated in Subheading 3.2 or up to 100 ng of gDNA as templates.

3. For PCR product visualization, purification, and sequencing, *see* Subheading 3.2.

3.8 Data Assembly

We describe two methods of NGS data assembly: seeded reference mapping and de novo assembly. The first involves aligning reads to a reference sequence, either a complete or partial mitochondrial genome (e.g., SBTs), using prespecified criteria (i.e., percentage of allowed mismatches, length of required overlap, etc.). The second method, de novo assembly, requires no reference sequence and instead relies on finding overlaps of reads through sequence alignment. This section outlines the assembly of reads which would have had their adaptor sequences already removed and which would have already been separated according to their Illumina indexes (de-multiplexed) using the on-instrument software (Illumina) (*see* **Note 24**).

3.8.1 Data Trimming

In almost all cases, NGS reads contain low-quality bases, which necessitate them to be trimmed prior to their assembly; if left untrimmed, these bases create mismatches during sequence alignment which can result in sequence ambiguity in the resultant contigs or reads being excluded from the assembly:

1. Transfer the single or paired read files to a new folder in Geneious (https://www.geneious.com [23]). This can be done either via the menu (File > Import > From File... and choosing FASTQ) or by dragging and dropping the files into the viewer (*see* **Note 25**).

2. With the required files highlighted, select Annotate & Predict > Trim Ends... and trim the reads from both the 5′ and 3′ ends by allowing no ambiguous bases and an error probability of 0.1 or less. This ensures masking of terminal regions with greater than 10% chance of being incorrect (*see* **Note 26**).

3. If required, the two read files (forward and reverse) can be paired using the Sequence > Set Paired Reads... function and choosing pairs of inward facing forward and reverse reads with an insert size of 550 bp (*see* **Note 27**).

3.8.2 Reference Mapping Using Perfect-Match Seed Sequences

Exact-match reference sequences, i.e., SBTs (*see* Subheading 3.7), can be used as seeds to start assembling data into taxon-specific contigs. Reads are mapped to these seeds and are used to extend contigs until the amplicons are complete. In the case of overlapping amplicons, reads derived from amplicons without seeds are used to extend seeded assemblies to produce contiguous sequences of overlapping amplicons. The reference mapping process in Geneious performs three steps which can be repeated iteratively: (1) derive a new reference sequence from previous mapping assembly, (2) use the newly derived reference sequence for in silico baiting, and (3) map baited reads to the newly derived reference sequence, thereby extending it. These steps are continued until the specified numbers of iterations have been completed or until no further reads can be mapped to the assembly based on the prespecified criteria (*see* **Note 28**):

1. Trim data as described in Subheading 3.8.1.

2. Load SBTs as FASTA format into the Geneious folder that contains the trimmed Illumina read files. This can be done

either via the menu (File > Import > From File… and choosing FASTA) or by dragging and dropping the files into the viewer.

3. With the required files highlighted (*see* **Note 29**), select Tools > Align/Assemble > Map to Reference… and using the "Custom Sensitivity" option, with settings of 2% maximum mismatches; 1% allowed gaps per read (maximum size of 3); 50 bp minimum overlap (95% overlap identity); word length 18 (index word length can be adjusted dependent on available memory); ignoring words repeated >12 times and a maximum ambiguity of 4, run 100 iterations ensuring the "Use existing trim regions" option is selected (*see* **Note 30**). If the full 100 iterations have been completed and the resulting contig is significantly smaller than expected, repeat the process using the newly extended sequence as seed reference in place of the SBT.

4. Check for circularity (completeness) by aligning ~1000 bp from both the start and end of the contig (*see* **Note 31**).

5. If the resulting contig is incomplete, reassemble the data, starting from **step 3** and using the newly extended sequence as seed reference in place of the SBT, adjusting the "Custom sensitivity" settings relevant to the situation. For example, when assembling low-complexity repeat regions, allowing for a larger percentage of mismatches can be beneficial, while enforcing a greater overlap and reduced acceptance of mismatches can be used if nontarget sequence is being incorporated in the assembled contig (*see* **Note 32**).

3.8.3 Reference Mapping Using Imperfect-Match Seed Sequences

In the absence of perfect-match seed sequences, i.e., SBTs (see Subheading 3.7), sequences from publically available databases can be used in their place. Reads can be mapped to small regions of conserved genes or complete mitochondrial genome sequences from closely related taxa. This method is not recommended for sequences derived from shotgun sequencing of non-multiplexed, pooled gDNA extracts as the required level of mismatch between the reference seed sequence and the reads may overlap with multiple samples and lead to the creation of chimeric sequences.

1. Trim data as described in Subheading 3.8.1.

2. Load reference sequence as FASTA format into the Geneious folder that contains the trimmed Illumina read files. This can be done either via the menu (File > Import > From File… and choosing FASTA) or by dragging and dropping the files into the viewer.

3. With the required files highlighted (see **Note 29**), select Tools > Align/Assemble > Map to Reference… and using the "Low Sensitivity" default settings, run a single iteration ensuring the "Use existing trim regions" option is selected (see **Note 30**). Depending on the degree of similarity between the

reads and the reference sequence, the assembly settings can be relaxed to incorporate increasingly dissimilar reads. The resulting contig can then be used as a new reference sequence under stricter parameters (see **Note 33**).

4. Using the newly extended sequence from the previous step, reassemble the data using the "Custom Settings" as described for SBT reference sequence seeds (Subheading 3.8.2) and run for 100 iterations.

5. Check for circularity by aligning ~1000 bp from both the start and end of the contig (*see* **Note 31**).

6. If the resulting contig is incomplete, reassemble the data (starting from **step 3**) using "Custom sensitivity" settings.

3.8.4 De Novo Assembly

If neither exact-match, i.e., SBTs (*see* Subheading 3.7), nor imperfect-match seed sequences are available or have been used unsuccessfully in a mapping assembly, de novo assembly methods can be used (*see* **Note 34**).

1. Trim data as described in Subheading 3.8.1.

2. With the required files highlighted (*see* **Note 29**), select Tools > Align/Assemble > De Novo Assemble… from the menu and using the "Custom Sensitivity" option change the settings to those given for conducting a reference assembly from SBT sequences (Subheading 3.8.2), ensuring the "Use existing trim regions" option is selected. The assembly process will end once no more reads can be mapped.

3. In order to distinguish mitochondrial from nuclear and/or other plasmid contigs, a custom BLAST search [24] can be run through Geneious (*see* **Note 35**). To do this, import the complete or partial mitochondrial genomes from closely related taxa into a new folder in Geneious. Select Tools > Add/Remove Databases > Set Up BLAST Services… and choose "Custom BLAST." Add the database by specifying the location of the file containing your reference sequences.

4. With the output of the de novo assembly highlighted, choose Tools > BLAST from the menu and select the newly set up custom database. As with the BLAST web server, different types of searches are permissible. In case of incomplete contig(s), positive BLAST search matches or "hits" can be used as references for mapping assemblies (as outlined in Subheading 3.8.2).

3.9 Mitogenome Annotation

In the absence of an automated bioinformatic pipeline, we suggest to follow the methodology for mitogenome annotation outlined below:

1. Upload the mitogenome sequences as FASTA format onto the MITOS web server ([25]; http://mitos.bioinf.uni-leipzig.de/

index.py), select the correct genetic code and run the software using default settings. If you are annotating multiple mitogenomes, select "Allow Multifasta" in the "Advanced" settings.

2. Load mitogenome sequence as FASTA file into Geneious and import BED file from the MITOS output.

3. In order to verify the gene boundaries of the protein-coding and ribosomal RNA genes, as given by MITOS, construct alignments (e.g., MAFFT; [26, 27]) with published mitogenomes from closely related taxa. In the case of protein-coding genes, check for alternative start and stop codons that minimize gene overlap and result in more conservative gene lengths (*see* **Note 36**). Consult the NCBI website for taxon-specific mitochondrial genetic codes, including start and stop codons (http://www.ncbi.nlm.nih.gov/Taxonomy/Utils/wprintgc. cgi#SG5). In the case of ribosomal RNA genes, check for alternative beginnings and ends that minimize gene overlap and that are in line with beginnings and ends of published data.

4. In order to verify the identity and gene boundaries of transfer RNAs (tRNAs), we recommend drawing their secondary structures. This can be done using (1) tRNAScan-SE ([28]; http:// selab.janelia.org/tRNAscan-SE/) using the "tRNAscan only" option in "Search Mode" and the "Mito/Chloroplast" option in "Source"; under "Extended Options," select the most appropriate genetic code from the "Genetic Code for tRNA Isotype Prediction" and/or (2) ARWEN [29] using default options; deselect "Search for mammalian mitochondrial tRNA genes" if not annotating mammalian data (*see* **Note 37**).

5. Adjust the annotation in Geneious accordingly.

4   Notes

1. In order to preserve the double-stranded helix of DNA, we strongly advise against heat-fixation of specimens.

2. These protocols can also be used for samples stored in RNAlater; however, RNAlater is not favored as a preservative for DNA by us as it does not preserve tissue integrity. Crucially, the chelating agents in RNAlater cause the dissolution of calcium carbonate. Thus, if RNAlater is to be used as preservative for calcium carbonate skeleton-forming organisms, it is imperative to prepare morphological vouchers. Many tissue types simply dissolve in RNAlater.

3. If extracting DNA from small organisms for direct shotgun sequencing, it may be preferable to pool multiple individuals in order to maximize the return of dsDNA. However, this must be balanced against the loss of intraspecific variation in

the final data (i.e., polymorphisms or SNPs can no longer be ascribed to an individual).

4. If not using Axygen 1.5 ml microcentrifuge tubes, ensure that a sterile plastic mortar can reach the bottom of the tube otherwise the tissue will not be fully homogenized in **step 4**.

5. Where possible use an incubator with a rocking platform set to 200 rpm. If a rocking platform is not available, vortex the samples for 5 s every 30 min or as often as possible if incubating overnight.

6. When dealing with organisms that have a calcium carbonate skeleton, following the digestion period, we advise to carry out a 1 min low-speed spin at $1000 \times g$ to sediment any remaining skeletal parts. Pipette the supernatant into a new 1.5 ml Eppendorf tube for further processing.

7. This step used to be part of the manufacturer's instructions but has now been removed. We recommend including this step, especially when dealing with small amounts of tissue.

8. For small specimens, in order to obtain a more concentrated DNA eluate, carry out two separate elutions of 100 µl, each. Use the first elution as working solution and the second elution as backup extract. The elution buffer can be heated to 70 °C to further increase recovery.

9. Of the large number of commercially available long-range PCR kits, we have experience using Elongase® Amplification System (Invitrogen), Expand 20kb^{Plus} PCR System (Roche), TaKaRa LA Taq® DNA Polymerase (Mg^{2+} plus buffer) (Clontech), and LongAmp® Taq PCR kit (New England BioLabs). In our experience, the TaKaRa LA Taq® DNA Polymerase (Mg^{2+} plus buffer) kit produces some of the most reliable results. However, the LongAmp® Taq PCR kit works out at roughly half the price of the TaKaRa kit and produced, in our opinion, comparable results. Furthermore, for difficult templates, we observed that conducing PCRs in 50 µl, as opposed to 25 µl volumes, produced stronger PCR products.

10. Double the amount of primer if they are degenerate.

11. When making a master mix, always make enough for $n+1$, where n is the number of reactions to be performed. Pipetting error almost invariably results in insufficient master mix for the last reaction if made for only n reactions.

12. The order in which components are added to the master mix is in order of least to most expensive. This reduces the risk of making costly pipetting errors.

13. In order to retain the integrity of long-template DNA fragments, vortex only very carefully or use a pipette tip to stir the mix. PCRs have also worked without any mixing.

14. Always preheat the PCR block to at least 85 °C. This minimizes mis-priming and nonspecific amplification.

15. The cycling profile given in **step 3**, Subheading 3.2, differs from that given in the TaKaRa LA Taq DNA Polymerase kit user manual as follows: we denatured at 94 °C instead of at 98 °C; we carried out the final extension at 68 °C rather than at 72 °C; we ran 40 instead of 30 cycles. These modifications are the results from previous optimizations using other kits. Because these conditions gave good results also with the TaKaRa kit, they were retained. Furthermore, we employed a three-step PCR profile, rather than the suggested two-step PCR profile in which annealing and extension are carried out in one step at 68 °C. The three-step profile allows for the use of primers with melting temperatures <73 °C (as a rule of thumb, annealing temperature should be ~5 °C below the lowest melting temperature of the primers). We have obtained fragments as large as 8.5 kb using annealing temperatures as low as 48 °C for primers with a melting temperature of 53 °C, although it is recommended to design long-range PCR primers with high-melting temperatures up to 73 °C. The extension time is determined by the size of the PCR product. We tended to give generous extension times, i.e., 1 min/kb + 1 min.

16. If the amplicons are longer than 10 kb, a greater proportion of DNA will be recovered using a non-column-based purification kit such as QIAEX II gel extraction kit (Qiagen).

17. In our experience, a minimum of six gDNA samples can be shotgun sequenced on a single Illumina flow cell using version 3 chemistry (paired end 2 × 300 bp; MiSeq Reagent Kit v3), with an expected ~100× coverage of the complete mitochondrial genome. However, for extracts with a high proportion of double-stranded mtDNA, the same coverage can be expected when multiplexing approximately 25 taxa.

18. It is important to note that the commonly used NanoDrop spectrophotometer (Thermo Scientific) does not give sufficiently accurate readings to quantifying DNA for NGS. The most commonly used method to quantify dsDNA is the Qubit® (Life Technologies) fluorometer, used in conjunction with either the Qubit® dsDNA broad-range assay kit (suitable for quantification of concentrations 100 pg μl^{-1} to 1000 ng μl^{-1}) or the Qubit® dsDNA high-sensitivity assay kit (suitable for quantification of concentrations 10 pg μl^{-1} to 100 ng μl^{-1}).

19. The simplest way of pooling gDNA is to vary the volume of each sample based on concentration. The total amount of gDNA added for each sample should be guided by the concentration of the strongest sample. Add at least 1 µl of this sample to avoid pipetting errors. Once finished, the pool can be quantified using

fluorometry and the intactness of the DNA assessed on a TapeStation. Ideally all samples being pooled will be of similar quality, so downstream treatment acts the same on all samples.

20. It is possible to combine any of the TruSeq DNA library preps on the same run as the indexes are in the same location and the same length. If combining Nextera and TruSeq libraries, it is necessary to do some additional demultiplexing.

21. A Bioanalyser (Agilent) can be used for all other validation steps but only the TapeStation instrument can accurately quantify large (>1.5 kb) DNA fragments.

22. If the protocol calls for mechanical fragmentation of DNA via ultrasonication, bear in mind the average fragment size of the input material. It is recommended to trial the fragmentation step and assess the lengths of fragments produced. Shorter amplicons and more heavily fragmented DNA will require shorter ultrasonication times (see instrument manufacturer's recommendations).

23. When quantifying libraries, it is recommended to conduct qPCRs, even for methods that suggest using fluorometry only, followed by subsequent analysis using a TapeStation. qPCR analysis gives a far better estimate of DNA fragments that are functional, i.e., those that contain adapters at both ends.

24. If the raw sequencing reads still contain the Illumina indexes, these can be removed by using the "Separate Reads by Barcode..." function in Geneious.

25. Geneious is preferred as a tool for quality assessment and data trimming as it allows visualization of the data and provides the ability to mask low-quality/ambiguous bases rather than simply removing them. This allows for subsequent reversal or editing of the trimmed data if necessary. If open-source software is required, Trimmomatic [30] can be used to trim the raw reads.

26. The error probability cutoff can be increased if the subsequent assembly proves difficult due to low-quality data or high error rates in the reads (e.g., long homopolymers or tandem repeats causing replication slippage during sequencing).

27. Working with paired-end reads can avoid misassembly of repetitive regions and misincorporation of nontarget DNA sequences (e.g., nuclear repeats).

28. If open-source software is required, the MITObim [31] pipeline for the MIRA assembler [32, 33] can be used to perform the same iterative mapping function.

29. This can include the FASTA SBT (to be used as seed reference) and either the paired read file, the two individual read files or a single read file.

30. By selecting "Custom sensitivity," it is possible to edit the advanced settings available under the "More options" tab. This provides a greater degree of flexibility and control over the assembly procedure.

31. This step assumes that the mitochondrial genome is circular and not linear as found in medusozoans, some isopods and sponges, and non-metazoans, such as fungi and plants (*see* [1, 3]).

32. Depending on how/if the amplicons were purified, small amounts of non-amplified gDNA will also be sequenced and will be present in the data.

33. It is advisable to translate any resulting contigs of protein-coding genes into amino acids to check for unexpected stop codons and frame-shift mutations, prior to using them as references for mapping assemblies, to ensure they are not nuclear mitochondrial pseudogenes.

34. If taxa are too closely related (i.e., there is low levels of sequence divergence between them), it is advisable to index each sample individually.

35. If open-source software is required, BLAST+ [34] can be used to locally search through the contigs produced by the de novo assembly.

36. These alignments are best viewed in a program that allows you to see the amino-acid translation alongside the nucleotide data. In the program Mesquite [35] codons can be shaded according to their inferred amino acids as follows: Load the alignment; in Show Matrix view, select characters to be translated; in List & Manage Characters view, if Genetic Code column is not visible, click on Columns > Current Genetic Code; to set the correct genetic code, click on Genetic Code > Genetic code > select code; to set codon position, click on Codon Position > Set codon position > Minimize stop codons; back in Show Matrix view, select Matrix > Colour Matrix Cells > Colour Nucleotide by Amino Acids. This amino-acid shaded view now allows the detection of alternative start and stop codons which may be more in line with beginnings and ends of published mitogenomes.

37. tRNAScan-SE provides more conservative estimates of tRNA secondary structures than ARWEN and should be used first. ARWEN can be used subsequently, to find tRNAs that were not found by tRNAScan-SE. ARWEN is likely to give several alternative drawings for the same tRNA, so care must be taken to chose the one that looks structurally most stable, has the correct anticodon, and which minimizes overlap with adjacent genes. Care must also be taken to differentiate between Serine 1 (codon AGN) and Serine 2 (codon UCN) and Leucine 1 (codon UUR) and Leucine 2 (codon UUU). In cases where neither MITOS nor tRNAScan-SE nor ARWEN were able to find missing

tRNAs (this is mostly the case when the typical four-arm clover-leaf tRNA structure is truncated and misses either the T- or D-stem), a manual search can be carried out for the conserved anticodon motif YUxxxR, where xxx denotes the anticodon, and by detecting adjacent stem and loop region by eye.

Acknowledgments

This work was partly funded by an NHM postdoctoral position to AB through the NHM Disease Initiative. The authors thank Tim Littlewood and Bonnie Webster for constructive comments on an earlier draft.

References

1. Kayal E, Bentlage B, Collins A, Kayal M, Pirro S, Lavrov D (2012) Evolution of linear mitochondrial genomes in medusozoan cnidarians. Genome Biol Evol 4:1–12

2. Doublet V, Raimond R, Grandjean F, Lafitte A, Souty-Grosset C, Marcade I (2012) Widespread atypical mitochondrial DNA structure in isopods (Crustacea, Peracarida) related to a constitutive heteroplasmy in terrestrial species. Genome 55:234–244

3. Lavrov DV, Pett W, Voigt O, Wörheide G, Forget L, Lang BF, Kayal E (2013) Mitochondrial DNA of *Clathrina clathrus* (Calcarea, Calcinea): six linear chromosomes, fragmented rRNAs, tRNA editing, and a novel genetic code. Mol Biol Evol 30:865–880

4. Podsiadlowski L, Mwinyi A, Lesný P, Bartolomaeus T (2014) Mitochondrial gene order in Metazoa – theme and variations. In: Wägele W, Bartolomaeus T (eds) Deep metazoan phylogeny: the backbone of the tree of life: new insights from analyses of molecules, morphology, and theory of data analysis. W. de Gruyter, Berlin, pp 459–474

5. Rubinoff D, Holland BS (2005) Between two extremes: mitochondrial DNA is neither the Panacea nor the Nemesis of phylogenetic and taxonomic inference. Syst Biol 54:952–961

6. Funk DJ, Omland KE (2003) Species-level paraphyly and polyphyly: frequency, causes, and consequences, with insights from animal mitochondrial DNA. Ann Rev Evol Syst 34:397–423

7. Ballard JWO, Whitlock MC (2004) The incomplete natural history of mitochondria. Mol Ecol 13:729–744

8. Shaw KL (2002) Conflict between nuclear and mitochondrial DNA phylogenies of a recent species radiation: what mtDNA reveals and conceals about modes of speciation in Hawaiian crickets. Proc Natl Acad Sci U S A 99:16122–16127

9. Pereira SL, Baker AJ, Wajntal A (2002) Combined nuclear and mitochondrial DNA sequences resolve generic relationships within the Cracidae (Galliformes, Aves). Syst Biol 51:946–958

10. Littlewood DTJ, Waeschenbach A, Nikolov PN (2008) In search of mitochondrial markers for resolving the phylogeny of cyclophyllidean tapeworms (Platyhelminthes, Cestoda) – a test study with Davaineidae. Acta Parasitol 53:133–144

11. White DJ, Wolff JK, Pierson M, Gemmell NJ (2008) Revealing the hidden complexities of mtDNA inheritance. Mol Ecol 17:4925–4942

12. Bensasson D, Zhang D, Hartl DL, Hewitt GM (2001) Mitochondrial pseudogenes: evolution's misplaced witnesses. Trends Ecol Evol 16:314–321

13. Gissi C, Iannelli F, Pesole G (2008) Evolution of the mitochondrial genome of Metazoa as exemplified by comparison of congeneric species. Heredity 101:301–320

14. Rokas A, Holland PW (2000) Rare genomic changes as a tool for phylogenetics. Trends Ecol Evol 15:454–459

15. Timmermans MJTN, Vogler AP (2012) Phylogenetically informative rearrangements in mitochondrial genomes of Coleoptera, and monophyly of aquatic elateriform beetles (Dryopoidea). Mol Phylogenet Evol 63:299–304

16. Webster BL, Littlewood DTJ (2012) Mitochondrial gene order change in *Schistosoma* (Platyhelminthes: Digenea: Schistosomatidae). Int J Parasitol 42:313–321

17. Waeschenbach A, Porter JS, Hughes RN (2012) Molecular variability in the *Celleporella hyalina* (Bryozoa; Cheilostomata) species complex: evidence for cryptic speciation from complete mitochondrial genomes. Mol Biol Rep 39:8601–8614

18. Rubinstein ND, Feldstein T, Shenkar N, Botero-Castro F, Griggio F, Mastrototaro F, Delsuc F, Douzery EJP, Gissi C, Huchon D (2013) Deep sequencing of mixed total DNA without barcodes allows efficient assembly of highly plastic ascidian mitochondrial genomes. Genome Biol Evol 5:1185–1199

19. Gillett CPDT, Crampton-Platt A, Timmermans MJTN, Jordal BH, Emerson BC, Vogler AP (2014) Bulk *de novo* mitogenome assembly from pooled total DNA elucidates the phylogeny of weevils (Coleoptera: Curculionoidea). Mol Biol Evol 31:2223–2237

20. Tang M, Tan M, Meng G, Yang S, Su X, Liu S, Song W, Li Y, Wu Q, Zhang A, Zhou X (2014) Multiplex sequencing of pooled mitochondrial genomes – a crucial step towards biodiversity analysis using mito-metagenomics. Nucleic Acids Res 42, e166

21. Tilak M-K, Justy F, Debiais-Thibaud M, Botero-Castro F, Delsuc F, Douzery EJP (2015) A cost-effective straightforward protocol for shotgun Illumina libraries designed to assemble complete mitogenomes from non-model species. Conserv Genet Resour 7:37–40

22. Timmermans MJTN, Viberg C, Martin G, Hopkins K, Vogler A (2016) Rapid assembly of taxonomically validated mitochondrial genomes from historical insect collections. Biol J Linn Soc 117:83–95

23. Kearse M, Moir R, Wilson A, Stones-Havas S, Cheung M, Sturrock S, Buxton S, Cooper A, Markowitz S, Duran C, Thierer T, Ashton B, Mentjies P, Drummond A (2012) Geneious Basic: an integrated and extendable desktop software platform for the organization and analysis of sequence data. Bioinformatics 28:1647–1649

24. Altschul SF, Gish W, Miller W, Myers EW, Lipman DJ (1990) Basic local alignment search tool. J Mol Biol 215:403–410

25. Bernt M, Donath A, Jühling F, Externbrink F, Florentz C, Fritzsch G, Pütz J, Middendorf M, Stadler PF (2013) MITOS: improved de novo metazoan mitochondrial genome annotation. Mol Phylogenet Evol 69:313–319

26. Katoh K, Misawa K, Kuma K, Miyata T (2002) MAFFT: a novel method for rapid multiple sequence alignment based on fast Fourier transform. Nucleic Acids Res 30:3059–3066

27. Katoh K, Standley DM (2013) MAFFT multiple sequence alignment software version 7: improvements in performance and usability. Mol Biol Evol 30:772–780

28. Lowe TM, Eddy SR (1997) tRNAscan-SE: a program for improved detection of transfer RNA genes in genomic sequence. Nucleic Acids Res 25:955–964

29. Laslett D, Canbäck B (2008) ARWEN: a program to detect tRNA genes in metazoan mitochondrial nucleotide sequences. Bioinformatics 24:172–175

30. Bolger AM, Lohse M, Usadel B (2014) Trimmomatic: a flexible trimmer for Illumina Sequence Data. Bioinformatics 30:2114–2120

31. Hahn C, Bachmann L, Chevreux B (2013) Reconstructing mitochondrial genomes directly from genomic next-generation sequencing reads—a baiting and iterative mapping approach. Nucleic Acids Res 41, e129

32. Chevreux B, Wetter T, Suhai S (1999) Genome sequence assembly using trace signals and additional sequence information. In: Computer science and biology. Proceedings of the German conference on bioinformatics (GCB)'99, pp 45–56

33. Chevreux B, Pfisterer T, Drescher B, Driesel AJ, Müller WE, Wetter T, Suhai S (2004) Using the miraEST assembler for reliable and automated mRNA transcript assembly and SNP detection in sequenced ESTs. Genome Res 14:1147–1159

34. Camacho C, Coulouris G, Avagyan V, Ma N, Papadopoulos J, Bealer K, Madden TL (2009) BLAST+: architecture and applications. BMC Bioinformatics 10:421

35. Maddison WP, Maddison DR (2015) Mesquite: a modular system for evolutionary analysis. Version 3.03. http://mesquiteproject.org

Chapter 4

Phylogenomics Using Transcriptome Data

Johanna Taylor Cannon and Kevin Michael Kocot

Abstract

This chapter presents a generalized protocol for conducting phylogenetic analyses using large-scale molecular datasets, specifically using transcriptome data from the Illumina sequencing platform. The general molecular lab bench protocol consists of RNA extraction, cDNA synthesis, and sequencing, in this case via Illumina. After sequences have been obtained, bioinformatics methods are used to assemble raw reads, identify coding regions, and categorize sequences from different species into groups of orthologous genes (OGs). The specific OGs to be used for phylogenetic inference are selected using a custom shell script. Finally, the selected orthologous groups are concatenated into a supermatrix. Generalized methods for phylogenomic inference using maximum likelihood and Bayesian inference software are presented.

Key words Phylogenomics, Transcriptomes, RNAseq, cDNA, Illumina, Phylogeny

1 Introduction

Over the last 10 years, phylogenomics has dramatically revised our understanding of metazoan relationships [1, 2]. In the broadest sense, phylogenomics refers to the inference of phylogenetic relationships based on large-scale molecular datasets. Although the original meaning of the term phylogenomics referred to the study of gene family evolution [3], popular usage now generally indicates the use of high-throughput sequencing of transcriptome or genome data for phylogenetic reconstruction. Most phylogenomic studies have used a shotgun sequencing approach, although a few have targeted specific genes [4], and there is a growing interest in 'anchored phylogenomics' that uses probes designed from diverse lineages within the target clade for targeted enrichment of loci [5–7]. Shotgun sequencing approaches tend to recover constitutively expressed 'housekeeping' genes no matter the source tissue that is sequenced, because these genes are vital to the function of the cell and are found across tissue types. Furthermore, these functionally important genes tend to be evolutionarily conserved, making them useful for inference of deep relationships.

Sarah J. Bourlat (ed.), *Marine Genomics: Methods and Protocols*, Methods in Molecular Biology, vol. 1452,
DOI 10.1007/978-1-4939-3774-5_4, © Springer Science+Business Media New York 2016

Early phylogenomic studies of animal relationships made use of expressed sequence tag (EST) data collected via Sanger-based methods [8–11]. Sanger-based EST methods required cloning randomly sheared cDNA fragments into bacterial vectors. The advent of massively parallel pyrosequencing methods such as 454 facilitated the collection of data from a broader subset of non-model organisms [12–14]. At present, Illumina sequencing offers lowest cost per base pair and has become the sequencing platform of choice for most phylogenomic studies [15–23]. The method presented later uses Illumina technology, although it can be modified to accommodate sequences generated using other methods.

After obtaining sequence data, phylogenomic dataset assembly consists of a series of bioinformatics steps. The essential steps are (1) de novo assembly of raw sequencing reads, (2) determination of orthologous groups of sequences, (3) selection of orthologous groups to be used in downstream analyses, (4) multiple sequence alignment, (5) concatenation, and (6) phylogenetic inference. To accomplish these steps, there are a myriad of phylogenomics programs available, many of which have similar functionalities, making choosing the most appropriate program for a given project a challenge. Several consistently updated pipelines such as Agalma [24], Osiris [25], and the unnamed pipeline of Yang and Smith [26] provide wrapper scripts for other existing software, offering a more seamless means to take raw reads through the stages of phylogenomic dataset assembly. These software options may be preferable for users with less bioinformatics experience, although these pipelines are open source and encourage user development and modification. Here we provide modified versions of scripts used in our previous publications (e.g., Kocot et al. [12] and Cannon et al. [15]), which can easily be adapted for other systems. The following steps represent a standard workflow that can be conducted on a local computer or remote cluster using the Linux operating system. Assembly, orthology determination, and phylogenetic inference will likely need to be performed on a high-performance computing cluster. This is one approach out of many possibilities, and we have pointed out alternatives where appropriate in the Subheading 4. New programs are released all the time, so it is important to check for updates and to read program manuals to make informed choices about the best approach for your particular system.

2   Materials

2.1   RNA Extraction

1. Solution for RNA stabilization and storage, or liquid nitrogen for tissue preservation.

2. Nuclease-free 1.5 ml Eppendorf tubes.

3. Trizol.

4. Homogenizer or liquid nitrogen and mortar and pestle.

5. Chloroform.

6. 100% isopropyl alcohol.

7. 75% ethanol.

8. RNase-free H_2O.

9. 4 °C centrifuge.

10. Quantification equipment—e.g., Nanodrop, Qubit, Agilent Bioanalyzer.

11. Gel electrophoresis apparatus.

12. RNA cleanup kit with DNase I.

13. Optional: commercial RNA extraction kit for small tissue samples.

2.2 cDNA Library Preparation

1. Clontech SMART cDNA Library Construction Kit.

2. Clontech Advantage2 PCR Kit.

3. 5′ Primer, 12 μM (5′-AAGCAGTGGTATCAACGCAGAGT-3′) (*see* **Note 1**).

4. RNase-free tubes and tips.

5. RNase inhibitor.

6. Thermal cycler.

7. PCR Purification kit.

8. 3M sodium acetate.

9. Quantification equipment—e.g., Nanodrop, Qubit, Agilent Bioanalyzer.

10. Gel electrophoresis apparatus.

11. Optional: vacuum centrifuge.

2.3 Sequencing

1. A sequencing facility with access to Illumina sequencing machines.

2.4 Bioinformatics: Dataset Assembly and Phylogenetic Inference

1. Linux computer or access to a remote server with the following software installed: Trinity [27], TransDecoder (http://transdecoder.sf.net), HaMStR [28], Mafft [29], Aliscore [30], and Alicut (https://www.zfmk.de/en/research/research-centres-and-groups/utilities), FastTreeMP [31], PhyloTreePruner [32], FASconCAT [33], RAxML [34], PhyloBayes [35].

2. Custom bash scripts available on GitHub at: https://github.com/kmkocot/springer_methods_chapter.

3   Methods

3.1   Extraction of Total RNA

Tissue to be used for RNA extraction should be fresh, preserved in RNA stabilization solution and stored in the freezer, or frozen at −80 °C. Numerous alternative protocols and kits exist for extraction of total RNA, and the best method for a given sample will depend on the size and composition of the tissue to be extracted. Useful discussion of RNA preparation methods can be found at the RNA-seqlopedia (rnaseq.uoregon.edu). In general, standard TRIzol-based methods work well for most macroinvertebrates, while for meiofauna or larvae, it may be necessary to use a commercial kit specifically designed for extracting RNA from cells or very small tissue samples. Cleanup of RNA extracted using TRIzol using a silica spin column-based kit that integrates removal of genomic DNA carryover using DNase I is recommended to reduce the carryover of phenol and genomic DNA that can negatively affect assembly. Final RNA should be resuspended in nuclease-free water and evaluated with available equipment, e.g., NanoDrop, Qubit, Bioanalyzer, and gel electrophoresis (*see* **Note 2**). RNA should be kept on ice while the quantity and quality are being checked, followed immediately by first-strand cDNA synthesis.

3.2   cDNA Synthesis

Again, several options are available for synthesis of complementary DNA from RNA. Illumina TruSeq library preparation kits incorporate Illumina library preparation steps including adding adaptors and indexing, eliminating the need for additional library preparation steps at the sequencing center. TruSeq kits currently require 0.1–4 μg input RNA; these kits may be preferred for large tissue samples. For microorganisms that yield smaller quantities of RNA, the SMART cDNA Library Construction Kit from Clontech can start with as little as 50 ng total RNA (*see* **Note 3**). Following is a suggested protocol using the SMART cDNA synthesis kit with slight modifications.

1. For very low amounts of starting RNA, samples may need to be concentrated in a vacuum centrifuge. Thoroughly clean the vacuum centrifuge before beginning, and as an added precaution, RNase inhibitor may be added to the sample before concentrating. Do not heat the sample during vacuum centrifugation.

2. Follow the manual of the SMART cDNA synthesis kit through first-strand synthesis.

3. For each first-strand cDNA product, perform an amplification test to determine the optimal number of PCR cycles. Volumes listed as follows are sufficient for the amplification test only; final amplification of cDNA will be completed in a subsequent amplification reaction. For each library combine the following in a 0.2 ml PCR tube on ice:

3.0 μl Diluted first-strand cDNA (from **step 2**)

21.0 μl PCR-grade H2O.

3.0 μl 10× Advantage 2 PCR Buffer.

0.75 μl dNTP mix.

1.4 μl 5′ PCR primer (12 μM).

0.6 μl 50× Advantage 2 Polymerase Mix.

Mix gently and then briefly spin down using a microcentrifuge. Place tube(s) in a thermal cycler that has been preheated to 95 °C and run the following program:

94 °C for 5 min (1 cycle).

94 for 40 s, 65 °C for 1 min, 72 °C for 5 min (15 cycles).

Hold at 6 °C.

4. After 15 cycles, remove and save 3 μl of the reaction mix, and subject the remaining mix to two additional cycles. Repeat this process until the reaction mix has been subjected to 25 cycles (*see* **Note 4**).

5. After cycling, analyze the reserved aliquots on an agarose gel. Estimate product concentration and size distribution in order to determine the optimal number of cycles. The cDNA should appear as a smear mostly between 500 bp and 3 kb, often with strong distinct bands representing abundant transcripts.

6. To ensure yield of >1 μg cDNA (required by most Illumina sequencing centers as of late 2015), run a final cDNA amplification as a series of multiple smaller reactions. Volumes are given as follows for 12 reactions per sample, although fewer reactions may be needed to reach 1 μg.

For each library combine the following in a 1.5 ml tube on ice:

36 μl Diluted first-strand cDNA (from step 2).

252 μl PCR-grade H2O.

36 μl 10× Advantage 2 PCR Buffer.

12 μl dNTP mix.

16.8 μl 5′ PCR primer (12 μM).

7.2 μl 50× Advantage 2 Polymerase Mix.

Aliquot 29.75 μl of this master mix into each of twelve 0.2 ml PCR tubes on an ice block.

Mix gently and then briefly spin down using a microcentrifuge. Place tubes in a thermal cycler that has been preheated to 95 °C and run the following program:

94 °C for 5 min (1 cycle).

94 for 40 s, 65 °C for 1 min, 72 °C for 5 min (n cycles).

Hold at 6 °C.

n = the optimal number of cycles for each library determined in step 3

7. Pool the 12 reaction products generated in **step 6**, and purify the amplified cDNA using a PCR purification kit following manufacturers protocols (*see* **Note 5**).

8. Analyze 3 μl purified cDNA on an agarose gel. Quantify cDNA concentration and purity using available equipment.

3.3 Sequencing

Prepared cDNA can be submitted as is to an Illumina sequencing facility. Depending on the sequencing depth required, multiple samples may be sequenced on a single lane of Illumina HiSeq (*see* **Note 6**). When following the protocol outlined earlier, it will be necessary for the sequencing center to perform Illumina library preparation steps, including adding adaptors and indexing samples.

3.4 Dataset Assembly

1. Download and make a secure backup of the raw sequencing data, which is typically provided in FASTQ format. For the commands listed as follows, we assume you are working in your home folder, have your data in a subfolder called "data," and the scripts in a separate subfolder called "scripts." Software listed in the materials section should be installed in your path. Please note that changes to this structure will require modifications of the commands.

2. Run Trinity to assemble reads into contigs, selecting appropriate memory and CPU options for your system (*see* **Note 7**).

```
Trinity.pl  --seqType  fq  --max_memory  50G
--CPU 8   --left

file_name_for_forward_reads_1.fastq.gz
--right

file_name_for_reverse_reads_2.fastq.gz
```

Trinity will produce a subdirectory with output files for each library, containing the completed assembly in fasta format. This file will be used for subsequent steps and should be moved to the home directory.

3. Translate assembled contigs using Transdecoder. The location of the Pfam-AB.hmm.bin file may vary depending on your system and installation of Transdecoder. Transdecoder will produce several output files, the translations with .pep file extensions (containing peptide sequences of predicted open reading frame regions in fasta format) should be carried forward to orthology determination.

```
TransDecoder    -t    Trinity_Output.fasta
--search_pfam  ~/bin/TransDecoder/pfam/Pfam-
AB.hmm.bin
```

4. Perform steps 2 and 3 on all raw RNAseq libraries to be included in your phylogenomic analysis, using unique file names.

5. Clean up intermediate files either by deleting or compressing and archiving, such as only the final translated Transdecoder .pep files are in the home directory.

6. Collect any additional translated amino acid sequences from sources other than raw Illumina data (e.g., predicted proteins from genome projects, publically available assemblies) that are to be used in the phylogenomic dataset, and place them in the home directory, using .pep file extensions. Nucleotide data from other sources must be translated as in step 6 prior to orthology determination.

7. Prepare translated sequences for orthology assignment. The script batch_prep_sequences.sh will remove line breaks from all translated fasta files using a script called nentferner.pl that is packaged with the HaMStR orthology determination software (*see* **Note 8**). This script will also remove special characters from fasta sequence headers that will cause errors in future steps, and move the unedited .pep files to a new directory titled "original_pep_files" that can be archived for future reference or discarded.

   ```
   ./scripts/batch_prep_sequences.sh
   ```

8. Categorize sequences into putatively orthologous groups (OG). Many software options are available for orthology determination (*see* **Note 9**). The following steps use HaMStR (Hidden Markov Model based Search for Orthologs using Reciprocity) version 13.2.3, with the "modelorganisms" core ortholog set and *Drosophila melanogaster* as the selected 'reference taxon' (*see* **Note 10**). It may be necessary to include the full path to the hamstr program and/or the hmmset, depending on your installation.

   ```
   hamstr -protein -strict -hmmset=modelorganisms_
   hmmer3 -refspec=DROME -sequence_file=Sequence_
   name.fa.nent -taxon=NAME
   ```

   Run HaMStR for each operational taxonomic unit (OTU) to be included in your dataset. Read the HaMStR manual for discussion of all flags. The -taxon flag gives each OTU a unique identifier to be supplied by the user for each OTU (here we have used the generic NAME, but you should select a unique four or five letter identifier for each species in your dataset). We advocate against the use of the -representative flag as it picks one sequence per taxon when two or more are present and can result in a final dataset including paralogs. We use a phylogenetic tree-based approach to select the best sequence from each taxon in these cases (see later).

9. Execute the bash script HaMStR_v13_concatenate.sh. HaMSrR_v13_concatenate.sh renames the files output by HaMStR into a format appropriate for orthology determination. Organisms included in the core ortholog set can be added or removed from each OG (see end of script). This script relies heavily on the Linux program rename, which works differently on different versions of Linux and may need to be modified (*see* **step 12**).

```
./scripts/HaMStR_v13_concatenate.sh
```

10. Execute the bash script phylogenomics_dataset_assembly.sh while in the folder containing the output of HaMStR_v13_concatenate.sh. The dataset assembly script takes the output of HaMStR and performs several steps to remove groups and sequences that are not suitable for phylogenomic analysis (*see* **Note 11**). The final product of this script is a set of trimmed amino acid alignments representing putatively orthologous groups suitable for phylogenomic analysis. The script requires GNU parallel be installed on your machine. There are several variables that must be modified for your purposes within the bash script. We suggest you examine the entire script carefully and modify it as needed. Input fasta file headers must be in the following format: >orthology_group_ID|OTU_abbreviation|annotation_or_sequence_ID_information (Example: >0001|LGIG|Contig1234). Fasta headers may not include spaces or nonalphanumeric characters except for underscores (pipes are OK as field delimiters only). If you have followed the earlier steps, your fasta headers should already be in this format.

```
./scripts/phylogenomics_dataset_assembly.sh
```

11. The output of the earlier script can be concatenated using FASconCAT. Before FASconCAT can be used, the fasta headers for each OTU in each OG alignment file must be made to match exactly. The simplest way to do this is to use the unique OTU identifier that was used in HaMStR. After executing the phylogenomics_dataset_assembly.sh script, the first field delimiter in your fasta headers should now be an @ symbol. If this is the case, type the following in the folder containing the individual orthogroup alignments, which will remove all characters following the first @ found on each line (*see* **Note 12**):

```
sed -i 's/\@.*//' *.fas
```

12. FASconCAT.pl will only work on files with the extension .fas, not .fa. You may need to rename .fa files to .fas. On Ubuntu Linux the command for this would be:

```
rename 's/.fa/.fas/g' *.fa
```

On Scientific Linux and some other distributions, the command would be:

```
rename .fa .fas *.fa
```

13. Create a concatenated total alignment matrix (*see* **Note 13**) using the program FASconCAT, which is an interactive program that offers many options for input and output files. To start FASconCAT, type the following in the folder containing the output sequences of the earlier script.

```
perl FASconCAT.pl
```

Select relaxed phylip output by typing "p" twice in the program menu. Once you have selected all the options that suit your downstream analysis, enter "s" in the program menu to start the concatenation (*see* **Note 14**).

14. Perform maximum likelihood phylogenetic inference with RAxML version 8. The following command executes a partitioned data analysis using the best-fitting model for each partition and the appropriate number of rapid bootstrap replicates. The partition data file should list "AUTO" as the model to use for each partition (*see* **Note 15**).

```
raxmlHPC-THREADS-AVX -T 16 -s Total_Alignment.
phylip -n RaxML.out -f a -N autoMRE -x 12345
-p 12345 -m PROTGAMMAAUTO -q partition_data.
txt
```

15. Perform Bayesian inference phylogenetic analysis using PhyloBayesMPI. The following commands execute four independent chains of **15,000** generations sampling one tree per generation under the site heterogeneous CAT + GTR model (*see* **Note 16**). More than 15,000 generations may be necessary for some datasets.

```
pb -x 1 15000 -cat -gtr -d Total_Alignment.
phy Chain1
pb -x 1 15000 -cat -gtr -d Total_Alignment.
phy Chain2
pb -x 1 15000 -cat -gtr -d Total_Alignment.
phy Chain3
pb -x 1 15000 -cat -gtr -d Total_Alignment.
phy Chain4
```

16. Assess convergence of the four chains using the bpcomp program packaged with PhyloBayes.

```
bpcomp -x 5000 Chain1 Chain2 Chain3 Chain4
```

This command discards one-third of all trees produced by the chains as burn-in, and compares the remaining lists of trees and outputs "maxdiff," a discrepancy index measuring how different the consensus trees produced by the four chains are.

The PhyloBayes manual recommends that the maxdiff value should be 0.1 or less, but 0.3 or less may be acceptable. bpcomp may be executed on currently running chains, so it is possible to check on progress of a run without stopping the analysis. bpcomp also produces a majority rule consensus tree.

4   Notes

1. The 5′ PCR primer is packaged with the Clontech SMART cDNA Library Construction kit at a concentration of 12 μM. We have found that the supply provided in the kit is often not sufficient to carry out the multiple amplification reactions recommended in our modified protocol, thus we recommend purchasing an additional supply and reconstituting it to 12 μM. Reconstituting to a more standard 10 μM will require modification to reaction volumes.

2. When working with very small samples (e.g., meiofaunal animals or marine invertebrate larval samples), visualization of RNA by gel electrophoresis will not be feasible. Synthesis of cDNA is usually successful even when measured quantities of RNA are extremely low or below the recommended starting amounts for the cDNA synthesis kit. If your samples are precious, proceed with cDNA synthesis and you will likely be rewarded. We have generated a successful cDNA library from an RNA sample that gave a negative reading on a Nanodrop.

3. We have had much success with the Clontech SMART cDNA Library Construction Kit with a variety of marine invertebrate samples. This kit can be used for as little as 50 ng total RNA up to 1 μg total RNA, so a single kit can be used if specimens in a range of sizes are to be processed. Keep in mind that indexing and Illumina library preparation steps will still need to be done at the sequencing center if submitting cDNA generated via the SMART kit. Clontech also manufactures kits that can start with as little as 100 pg RNA called "SMARTer Stranded RNA-Seq Kits—Strand-Specific Library Construction for Transcriptome Analysis on Illumina Platforms" that incorporate library preparation steps including indexing and adding adaptors, eliminating the need for downstream library preparation kits. We have no direct experience using this kit, but it may be a good option.

4. For most samples, 25 cycles will be sufficient. However, for some very tiny organisms, more cycles may be required. Fewer cycles will generally result in fewer nonspecific PCR products.

5. Most common PCR purification kits have a maximum yield of 10 μg per spin column, making it efficient to purify the replicate PCR products by pooling them and running the pooled products over a single silica spin column, loading multiple times. Double-check the maximum yield for your PCR

purification kit of choice before using this approach. The larger volumes of PCR master mix added to the purification kit buffers can affect pH, so we recommend that you use pH indicators included with your kit for all buffers to ensure efficient binding. If pH is too high, 3 M sodium acetate can be added to the buffer in order to lower pH to the optimal range.

6. We typically pool 6–8 transcriptomes in one lane of an Illumina HiSeq 2000 for phylogenomics. Use caution when combining samples across a single lane of Illumina HiSeq, as bleed-through has been demonstrated to occur. When multiple samples are sequenced in the same lane of an Illumina instrument, the data are sorted after sequencing by sequence 'barcodes' or 'indices' with a different code for each sample. Sometimes the barcode is misread. Usually, the misread barcode doesn't correspond to any of the samples being sequenced and that read is discarded. However, sometimes by random chance the barcode is misread as having the sequence of one of the other samples being processed so it gets put in the wrong 'bin.' If one of the samples has one or more really highly expressed genes (mitochondrial genes, nuclear ribosomal RNA, or other tissue-specific highly expressed genes), there might be so many reads from that transcript that end up incorrectly 'binned' that this gene ends up showing up in the assemblies of the other samples that were sequenced in parallel.

7. This command takes raw reads and assembles them directly. In many cases, it may be advisable to trim low quality reads and adaptor sequences prior to assembly. This can be accomplished using the Trimmomatic [36] program packaged with Trinity. Trinity can now also conduct digital normalization, which can significantly speed up assembly times. Normalization is not recommended if you have not used DNase treatment on your RNA prior to cDNA synthesis. Check the Trinity manual for details.

8. Many bioinformatics programs that manipulate sequence data in fasta format require that each sequence be listed on a single line (in other words, there are no line breaks within the sequence string). The perl script nentferner.pl is an extremely useful tool for removing line breaks in fasta files that is packaged with the HaMStR orthology determination program. This can also be accomplished with the fasta_formatter tool bundled with the FastX toolkit (http://hannonlab.cshl.edu/fastx_toolkit/index.html), and we highly recommend that you install one of these in your path.

9. There are several commonly used programs for orthology assignment. The program used here, HaMStR (Hidden Markov Model based Search for Orthologs using Reciprocity), generates profile hidden Markov models (pHMMs), each representing a set of orthologous genes for selected reference taxa from the InParanoid database [37] for which whole genomes are available. Sequences are searched against a reference taxon set, the

"model organisms" set in this example, which includes 1032 orthologous groups (OG) with sequences from *Homo sapiens*, *Ciona intestinalis*, *Drosophila melanogaster*, *Caenorhabditis elegans*, and *Saccharomyces cerevisiae*. Translated contigs are scanned for significant hits to each OG's pHMM. Matching sequences are then compared to the proteome of a selected primer taxon (*Drosophila melanogaster* in this example) using BLASTP (-strict option). If the *Drosophila melanogaster* amino acid sequence that contributed to the pHMM was the best BLASTP hit, then the sequence was assigned to that OG. If this reciprocity criterion is not met, the sequence is discarded. Other popular programs include OMA [38], FastOrtho [39] (a reimplementation of OrthoMCL [40]), and ab initio methods starting with all-by-all BLASTP searches followed by phylogenetic identification of orthologous sequences [13], implemented in programs such as ProteinOrtho [41] and Agalma [24].

10. HaMStR currently offers several precompiled core ortholog sets. The model organism set used here includes *Homo sapiens*, *Ciona intestinalis*, *Drosophila melanogaster*, *Caenorhabditis elegans*, and *Saccharomyces cerevisiae*, which works well in studies with broad taxon sampling across Metazoa. Also available are ortholog sets for Amniota, Arthropoda, basal metazoans, Chordata, Fungi, Insecta, Lophotrochozoa, and plants. It is also possible to use available genomic and transcriptomic data to build core ortholog sets from scratch for your taxonomic group of interest, although this process is arduous, and if none of the available core ortholog sets are appropriate for your study, it may be preferable to use an alternative orthology determination software program.

11. The input of this script is the putative orthologous groups generated by HaMStR. The script uses several other programs to produce individual trimmed alignments for each OG and to remove groups and sequences that are less suitable for phylogenomic analysis. The script is made up of a series of intermediate steps that are commented inside the script. A backup of all starting fasta files is created and placed into a new directory called "unedited_sequences." Next, newlines are removed from all files as described in **Note 7**. This process is repeated several times throughout the script. Sequences shorter than a set threshold are removed. This cutoff value is set in the program header using the variable MIN_SEQUENCE_LENGTH. OGs containing fewer taxa than a set threshold are removed and placed in a new directory called "rejected_few_taxa_1." This cutoff value is also set in the program header using the variable MIN_TAXA. Next, OGs are aligned using the program MAFFT [29]. Each OG is trimmed with the perl scripts Aliscore and Alicut [30] to remove columns with ambiguous alignment or little phylogenetic signal. Note that one recent study advocated against aggressive use of such alignment trimming software, particularly if it is trimming >20%

of aligned regions [42]. After trimming, spaces and gap only columns are removed, short alignments are discarded, and OGs containing too few taxa are removed and placed in a new directory called "rejected_few_taxa_2." Individual OG trees are generated using FastTreeMP [31] and the utility PhyloTreePruner [32] is used to screen for potential paralogs. PhyloTreePruner screens trees for instances where multiple sequences from the same OTU do not form monophyletic clades. Suspected paralogs are trimmed from the data matrix, leaving the maximally inclusive subtree in which sequences from each OTU form monophyletic clades or are part of the same polytomy. If an OG still possesses more than one sequence for an OTU (inparalogs), PhyloTreePruner is set to select the longest sequence for inclusion in the final concatenated alignment (-u option).

12. The sed -i flag will modify the file itself. To test the command prior to executing it, simply remove the -i option from the command and the output will appear in the terminal only.

13. The approach outlined here will generate a "total alignment" of all the OGs that pass through paralogy screening in PhyloTreePruner. In addition to conducting analyses of this total alignment, a number of approaches may be worth considering in an attempt to remove various sources of systematic error or "noise" from the data. Among others, MARE (matrix reduction) [43] maximizes information content of genes, taxa, and the overall alignment. BMGE (Block Mapping and Gathering with Entropy) [44] conducts trimming and recoding of alignments aimed at reducing artifacts due to compositional heterogeneity. TreSpEx [45] and BaCoCa [46] perform a variety of statistical calculations on individual taxa, OGs, or the total alignment to identify possible biases in phylogenomic datasets from sources such as long branch attraction, saturation, missing data, and rate heterogeneity. Combining these tools to generate multiple alignments can provide valuable insights into potential sources of bias in your data and strengthen your overall analysis.

14. By default, FASconCAT generates an .xls file containing single range information of each sequence fragment and a checklist of all concatenated sequences. The information in this file may easily be adapted to use in phylogenetic analyses to partition the concatenated matrix into gene regions for model specification, etc.

15. Model choice in phylogenomic analysis has been the subject of debate [47]. RAxML implements traditional site-homogenous models, or more recently developed LG4X and LG4M models [48] that integrate four substitution matrixes to improve modeling of site heterogeneity. The newest version of RAxML allows the user to choose to have the program select the best-fitting model for each partition in the concatenated matrix. We recommend either partitioning data by OG and selecting the best model of evolution for each group using RAxML or other

model selection software such as ProtTest [49], or partitioning sites using software such as PartitionFinder [50] over selecting a single substitution model across the concatenated matrix.

16. PhyloBayes implements the site-heterogeneous CAT model [51], which does not assume homogenous substitution patterns across an alignment. This assumption is likely to be violated in large, concatenated data matrices, so these models have been preferred over site homogenous models for phylogenomic datasets [47]. Bayesian inference under such complex models is extremely computationally expensive and will need to be carried out on a remote high performance computing cluster.

References

1. Giribet G (2015) New animal phylogeny: future challenges for animal phylogeny in the age of phylogenomics. Org Divers Evol 2015:1–8. doi:10.1007/s13127-015-0236-4

2. Telford MJ, Budd GE, Philippe H (2015) Phylogenomic insights into animal evolution. Curr Biol 25:R876–R887. doi:10.1016/j.cub.2015.07.060

3. Eisen JA, Fraser CM (2003) Phylogenomics: intersection of evolution and genomics. Science 300:1706–1707. doi:10.1126/science.1086292

4. Regier JC, Shultz JW, Zwick A et al (2010) Arthropod relationships revealed by phylogenomic analysis of nuclear protein-coding sequences. Nature 463:1079–1083. doi:10.1038/nature08742

5. Lemmon AR, Emme SA, Lemmon EM (2012) Anchored hybrid enrichment for massively high-throughput phylogenomics. Syst Biol 61:727–744. doi:10.1093/sysbio/sys049

6. Peloso PLV, Frost DR, Richards SJ et al (2015) The impact of anchored phylogenomics and taxon sampling on phylogenetic inference in narrow-mouthed frogs (Anura, Microhylidae). Cladistics 32:113–140. doi:10.1111/cla.12118

7. Prum RO, Berv JS, Dornburg A et al (2015) A comprehensive phylogeny of birds (Aves) using targeted next-generation DNA sequencing. Nature 526:569–573. doi:10.1038/nature15697

8. Philippe H, Lartillot N, Brinkmann H (2005) Multigene analyses of bilaterian animals corroborate the monophyly of Ecdysozoa, Lophotrochozoa, and Protostomia. Mol Biol Evol 22:1246–1253. doi:10.1093/molbev/msi111

9. Dunn CW, Hejnol A, Matus DQ et al (2008) Broad phylogenomic sampling improves resolution of the animal tree of life. Nature 452:745–749. doi:10.1038/nature06614

10. Delsuc F, Brinkmann H, Chourrout D, Philippe H (2006) Tunicates and not cephalochordates are the closest living relatives of vertebrates. Nature 439:965–968

11. Bourlat SJ, Juliusdottir T, Lowe CJ et al (2006) Deuterostome phylogeny reveals monophyletic chordates and the new phylum Xenoturbellida. Nature 444:85–88. doi:10.1038/nature05241

12. Kocot KM, Cannon JT, Todt C et al (2011) Phylogenomics reveals deep molluscan relationships. Nature 477:452–456

13. Smith SA, Wilson NG, Goetz FE et al (2011) Resolving the evolutionary relationships of molluscs with phylogenomic tools. Nature 480:364–367. doi:10.1038/nature10526

14. Telford MJ, Lowe CJ, Cameron CB et al (2014) Phylogenomic analysis of echinoderm class relationships supports Asterozoa. Proc Biol Sci 281(1786):pii: 20140479. doi:10.1098/rspb.2014.0479

15. Cannon JT, Kocot KM, Waits DS et al (2014) Phylogenomic resolution of the hemichordate and echinoderm clade. Curr Biol 24:2827–2832. doi:10.1016/j.cub.2014.10.016

16. Whelan NV, Kocot KM, Moroz LL, Halanych KM (2015) Error, signal, and the placement of Ctenophora sister to all other animals. Proc Natl Acad Sci 112:5773–5778. doi:10.1073/pnas.1503453112

17. Struck TH, Golombek A, Weigert A et al (2015) The evolution of annelids reveals two adaptive routes to the interstitial realm. Curr Biol 25:1993–1999. doi:10.1016/j.cub.2015.06.007

18. Weigert A, Helm C, Meyer M et al (2014) Illuminating the base of the annelid tree using transcriptomics. Mol Biol Evol 31:1391–1401. doi:10.1093/molbev/msu080

19. Laumer CE, Bekkouche N, Kerbl A et al (2015) Spiralian phylogeny informs the evolution of microscopic lineages. Curr Biol 25:2000–2006. doi:10.1016/j.cub.2015.06.068

20. Andrade SCS, Novo M, Kawauchi GY et al (2015) Articulating "Archiannelids": phylogenomics and annelid relationships, with emphasis on Meiofaunal taxa. Mol Biol Evol 32:2860–2875. doi:10.1093/molbev/msv157

21. Andrade SCS, Montenegro H, Strand M et al (2014) A transcriptomic approach to ribbon worm systematics (Nemertea): resolving the Pilidiophora problem. Mol Biol Evol 31:3206–3215. doi:10.1093/molbev/msu253

22. Laumer CE, Hejnol A, Giribet G (2015) Nuclear genomic signals of the "microturbellarian" roots of platyhelminth evolutionary innovation. eLife e05503. doi:10.7554/eLife.05503

23. Egger B, Lapraz F, Tomiczek B et al (2015) A transcriptomic-phylogenomic analysis of the evolutionary relationships of flatworms. Curr Biol 25:1347–1353. doi:10.1016/j.cub.2015.03.034

24. Dunn CW, Howison M, Zapata F (2013) Agalma: an automated phylogenomics workflow. BMC Bioinformatics 14:330. doi:10.1186/1471-2105-14-330

25. Oakley TH, Alexandrou MA, Ngo R et al (2014) Osiris: accessible and reproducible phylogenetic and phylogenomic analyses within the Galaxy workflow management system. BMC Bioinformatics 15:230. doi:10.1186/1471-2105-15-230

26. Yang Y, Smith SA (2014) Orthology inference in nonmodel organisms using transcriptomes and low-coverage genomes: improving accuracy and matrix occupancy for phylogenomics. Mol Biol Evol 31:3081–3092. doi:10.1093/molbev/msu245

27. Grabherr MG, Haas BJ, Yassour M et al (2011) Full-length transcriptome assembly from RNA-Seq data without a reference genome. Nat Biotechnol 29:644–652

28. Ebersberger I, Strauss S, von Haeseler A (2009) HaMStR: profile hidden markov model based search for orthologs in ESTs. BMC Evol Biol 9:157

29. Katoh K, Kuma K, Toh H, Miyata T (2005) MAFFT version 5: improvement in accuracy of multiple sequence alignment. Nucleic Acids Res 33:511–518

30. Misof B, Misof K (2009) A Monte Carlo approach successfully identifies randomness in multiple sequence alignments: a more objective means of data exclusion. Syst Biol 58:21–34

31. Price MN, Dehal PS, Arkin AP (2010) FastTree 2—approximately maximum-likelihood trees for large alignments. PLoS One 5, e9490

32. Kocot KM, Citarella MR, Moroz LL, Halanych KM (2013) PhyloTreePruner: a phylogenetic tree-based approach for selection of orthologous sequences for phylogenomics. Evol Bioinf Online 9:429–435. doi:10.4137/EBO.S12813

33. Kück P, Meusemann K (2010) FASconCAT: convenient handling of data matrices. Mol Phylogenet Evol 56:1115–1118. doi:10.1016/j.ympev.2010.04.024

34. Stamatakis A (2014) RAxML version 8: a tool for phylogenetic analysis and post-analysis of large phylogenies. Bioinformatics 30:1312–1313. doi:10.1093/bioinformatics/btu033

35. Lartillot N, Rodrigue N, Stubbs D, Richer J (2013) PhyloBayes MPI. Phylogenetic reconstruction with infinite mixtures of profiles in a parallel environment. Syst Biol 62:611–615. doi:10.1093/sysbio/syt022

36. Bolger AM, Lohse M, Usadel B (2014) Trimmomatic: a flexible trimmer for Illumina sequence data. Bioinformatics 30:2114–2120. doi:10.1093/bioinformatics/btu170

37. Östlund G, Schmitt T, Forslund K et al (2010) InParanoid 7: new algorithms and tools for eukaryotic orthology analysis. Nucleic Acids Res 38:D196–D203

38. Altenhoff AM, Schneider A, Gonnet GH, Dessimoz C (2011) OMA 2011: orthology inference among 1000 complete genomes. Nucleic Acids Res 39:D289–D294. doi:10.1093/nar/gkq1238

39. Wattam AR, Abraham D, Dalay O et al (2014) PATRIC, the bacterial bioinformatics database and analysis resource. Nucleic Acids Res 42:D581–D591. doi:10.1093/nar/gkt1099

40. Li L, Stoeckert CJ, Roos DS (2003) OrthoMCL: identification of ortholog groups for eukaryotic genomes. Genome Res 13:2178–2189. doi:10.1101/gr.1224503

41. Lechner M, Findeiß S, Steiner L et al (2011) Proteinortho: detection of (co-)orthologs in large-scale analysis. BMC Bioinformatics 12:124. doi:10.1186/1471-2105-12-124

42. Tan G, Muffato M, Ledergerber C et al (2015) Current methods for automated filtering of multiple sequence alignments frequently worsen single-gene phylogenetic inference. Syst Biol 64:778–791. doi:10.1093/sysbio/syv033

43. Meyer B, Meusemann K, Misof B (2010) MARE v0.1.2-rc

44. Criscuolo A, Gribaldo S (2010) BMGE (block mapping and gathering with entropy): a new software for selection of phylogenetic informative regions from multiple sequence alignments. BMC Evol Biol 10:210. doi:10.1186/1471-2148-10-210

45. Struck TH (2014) TreSpEx-detection of misleading signal in phylogenetic reconstructions based on tree information. Evol Bioinf Online 10:51–67. doi:10.4137/EBO.S14239

46. Kück P, Struck TH (2014) BaCoCa—a heuristic software tool for the parallel assessment of sequence biases in hundreds of gene and taxon partitions. Mol Phylogenet Evol 70:94–98. doi:10.1016/j.ympev.2013.09.011

47. Philippe H, Brinkmann H, Lavrov DV et al (2011) Resolving difficult phylogenetic questions: why more sequences are not enough. PLoS Biol 9, e1000602. doi:10.1371/journal.pbio.1000602

48. Le SQ, Dang CC, Gascuel O (2012) Modeling protein evolution with several amino acid replacement matrices depending on site rates. Mol Biol Evol 29:2921–2936. doi:10.1093/molbev/mss112

49. Darriba D, Taboada GL, Doallo R, Posada D (2011) ProtTest 3: fast selection of best-fit models of protein evolution. Bioinformatics 27:1164–1165. doi:10.1093/bioinformatics/btr088

50. Lanfear R, Calcott B, Ho SYW, Guindon S (2012) PartitionFinder: combined selection of partitioning schemes and substitution models for phylogenetic analyses. Mol Biol Evol 29:1695–1701. doi:10.1093/molbev/mss020

51. Lartillot N, Philippe H (2004) A Bayesian Mixture Model for across-site heterogeneities in the amino-acid replacement process. Mol Biol Evol 21:1095–1109. doi:10.1093/molbev/msh112

Chapter 5

SNP Discovery Using Next Generation Transcriptomic Sequencing

Pierre De Wit

Abstract

In this chapter, I will guide the user through methods to find new SNP markers from expressed sequence (RNA-Seq) data, focusing on the sample preparation and also on the bioinformatic analyses needed to sort through the immense flood of data from high-throughput sequencing machines. The general steps included are as follows: sample preparation, sequencing, quality control of data, assembly, mapping, SNP discovery, filtering, validation. The first few steps are traditional laboratory protocols, whereas steps following the sequencing are of bioinformatic nature. The bioinformatics described herein are by no means exhaustive, rather they serve as one example of a simple way of analyzing high-throughput sequence data to find SNP markers. Ideally, one would like to run through this protocol several times with a new dataset, while varying software parameters slightly, in order to determine the robustness of the results. The final validation step, although not described in much detail here, is also quite critical as that will be the final test of the accuracy of the assumptions made in silico.

There is a plethora of downstream applications of a SNP dataset, not covered in this chapter. For an example of a more thorough protocol also including differential gene expression and functional enrichment analyses, BLAST annotation and downstream applications of SNP markers, a good starting point could be the "Simple Fool's Guide to population genomics via RNA-Seq," which is available at http://sfg.stanford.edu.

Key words RNA-Seq, SNP, Transcriptome assembly, Bioinformatics, Alignment, Population genomics, NGS, Illumina

1 Introduction

1.1 Historical Background: From Sanger to RNA-Seq

Since the advent of DNA sequencing methods, and the discovery of genetic variation [1], there has been an interest in using this variation to understand evolutionary processes such as genetic drift, natural selection, and the formation of new species. Early on, gel electrophoretic markers such as AFLPs [2] and allozymes [3] provided some interesting insights into the genetic structures of populations. Later, the development of microsatellite markers further improved our understanding of neutral genetic variation in natural populations [4]. However, these markers are usually few

Sarah J. Bourlat (ed.), *Marine Genomics: Methods and Protocols*, Methods in Molecular Biology, vol. 1452,
DOI 10.1007/978-1-4939-3774-5_5, © Springer Science+Business Media New York 2016

and it cannot be known if they are representative of the genome as a whole. In addition, they are generally assumed to not be under any selection pressure [5]. Only recently, with the advent of high-throughput DNA sequencing methods, have we begun to gain insights into the genome-wide distribution of polymorphisms and the effects of natural selection on genome architecture.

1.2 Why Focus on the Transcriptome?

Even with the latest DNA sequencing technologies, putting together a genome sequence into full-length chromosomes from short read data is very difficult. The number of available genome sequences is ever increasing, but the list of well-assembled ("complete") genomes is to date still restricted to a few model taxa. Thus, it is many times desirable to focus on parts of the genome that contain the information of interest. There are many methods to do this, but they all fall within two categories: random and targeted methods. An example of a random method is RAD sequencing [6], in which the genomic DNA is fragmented using a restriction enzyme and regions flanking the restriction site are sequenced. These types of methods are useful for studying genome-wide distributions of genetic variation or for finding loci exhibiting interesting patterns. However, unless there is a well-annotated genome of the species of interest, it can be very difficult to gain an understanding of the function of the observed pattern. An example of a targeted method is RNA-Seq [7], whereby mature mRNAs are isolated and sequenced, usually with a poly-A binding method. While this method does not provide genome-wide observations, it focuses on the part of the genome that contains a large proportion of the functionally relevant information (how much is still an active debate, however). One might also argue that protein-coding sequences also have a larger chance of being affected by natural selection (both balancing and disruptive), while third codon positions and UTRs could be freer to evolve neutrally.

One very useful aspect of expressed sequence data is the relative ease of functional annotation due to the very conserved nature of protein evolution—by BLASTing to public databases one can in many cases gain an understanding of the function of an unknown sequence even in nonmodel systems where no genome sequence is available.

1.3 Issues with Transcriptomic SNPs

While characterizing the genetic variation present in and around protein coding regions allows for studies of natural selection and population genetics, there are some issues to keep in mind. First, the potential for background stabilizing selection can pose problems (even in UTRs and third codon positions linked to selected loci), as this process tends to disguise weak population structure [8]. Also, the assumptions of outlier analyses might be violated if most of the loci used in an analysis are under stabilizing selection [9]. Second, the very nature of mRNA can pose problems as there is great variation in transcript abundance, so in low-frequency transcripts it can be hard to separate sequencing errors from true SNPs [10]. In addition, patterns of allele-specific expression (ASE) can bias allele frequency estimates on pooled samples [11], or even cause incorrect genotyping if the difference in expression between alleles is too high [12]. It can also be difficult to separate out different isoforms of the same transcript from transcripts from paralog genes [13].

2 Materials

2.1 RNA Extraction Using Phenol/Chloroform

1. Solution for RNA stabilization and storage or liquid nitrogen for tissue preservation.
2. 1.5 ml Eppendorf tubes.
3. Trizol.
4. Chloroform.
5. Ball bearing beads.
6. 100 % isopropanol.
7. High salt buffer: 0.8 M Na citrate and 1.2 M Na chloride.
8. 75 % ethanol.
9. 4 °C centrifuge.
10. 55 °C heat block.
11. Tissue lyser or vortex mixer.

2.2 cDNA Library Preparation Using Illumina's TruSeq RNA Sample Prep Kit

1. Illumina TruSeq RNA sample preparation kit.
2. Magnetic beads for DNA purification (also called SPRI beads for solid-phase reversible immobilization).
3. Magnetic 96-well plate.
4. Reverse transcriptase.
5. Agilent Bioanalyzer or TapeStation.
6. QuBit high-sensitivity DNA assay.

2.3 Sequencing

1. A sequencing facility with access to Illumina sequencing machines.

2.4 Bioinformatics

1. Computer (Mac/Linux) with software installed: fastx toolkit, trinity, bwa, samtools (or access to a remote server with this software installed). Custom-made Python and bash scripts, GATK v 2.5 and Picard MarkDuplicates available on GitHub at: (https://github.com/DeWitP/SFG/tree/master/scripts/).

2.5 Validation

1. Primer 3 software.
2. PCR reagents: Oligonucleotides, dNTPs, BSA, $MgCl_2$, Water, Taq polymerase.
3. A sequencing facility for Sanger sequencing.

3 Methods

3.1 RNA Extraction

All Trizol steps should be done in a fume hood.

1. Thaw tissue (should be flash-frozen at time of sampling and stored at −80 °C, alternatively stored in RNA stabilization solution at −20 °C) on ice.

2. Cut tissue into small pieces with a clean razor blade, blot with tissue paper, and place in a 1.5 ml Eppendorf tube (*see* **Note 1**).

3. Add ball bearing beads, then 1 ml Trizol (in fume hood). Shake in a Tissue lyser (or Vortex on high speed) for 2 min until tissue has been homogenized.

4. Incubate at room temperature for 5 min.

5. Spin for 10 min at 12,000×*g*, 4 °C. Transfer liquid to clean tube.

6. Add 200 μl chloroform and shake vigorously for 15 s by hand.

7. Incubate for 2–3 min at room temperature.

8. Spin for 15 min at 12,000×*g*, 4 °C, then transfer the top phase (RNA) to a clean tube. DNA and proteins are in the bottom phase and can be stored at −20 °C until validation of markers is required.

9. If contamination occurs (part of the inter- or bottom phase are transferred), add 100 μl chloroform, shake for 15 s by hand, then repeat **step 8**.

10. Add 250 μl 100% isopropanol and 250 μl high salt buffer, shake.

11. Precipitate at room temp for 5–10 min.

12. Spin for 10 min at 12,000×*g*, 4 °C, then discard supernatant.

13. Wash pellet in 1 ml 75% ethanol. Spin for 5 min at 7500×*g*, 4 °C.

14. Discard supernatant, air dry for 5–10 min (30 s on 55 °C heat block).

15. Resuspend in nuclease-free water (12 μl) and incubate for 10 min at 55–60 °C. 1 μl can be used for QuBit concentration measurement and to examine RNA integrity (*see* **Note 2**).

16. Flash freeze in liquid nitrogen and store at −80 °C overnight, or continue directly with Subheading 3.2.

3.2 cDNA Library Prep

1. Standardize the amount of starting material, usually about 1 μg of total RNA produces good results.

2. Follow exactly the manual of the TruSeq kit (*see* **Note 3**).

3. Determine the fragment size distributions in the samples with an Agilent Bioanalyzer or TapeStation.

4. Measure the DNA concentration using a QuBit high-sensitivity DNA assay (the TapeStation measurements are usually not accurate enough).

5. The molarity can then be calculated as follows:

Molarity = Concentration   (ng/ml)/(0.66 × mean   fragment length (bp)).

6. Pool the samples equimolarly by calculating the required volume of each sample required so that the number of moles in each sample is identical. Illumina sequencing machines typically require a pool DNA molarity of 2–10 nM. The final pool volume should ideally be at least 20 μl (*see* **Note 4**).

3.3 Sequencing

1. Choose a sequencing center (*see* **Note 5**).

2. Send samples on ice, providing the center with information on DNA concentration and fragment size distribution.

3.4 Data Download and QC

1. Make a safety backup of the data, and upload the data to the location where you will be doing the analyses. This can either be on your local computer if it has enough capacity or preferably on a remote computer cluster.

2. Once the data is located in the right place, we want to control the quality (*see* **Note 6**). In this chapter, we assume that you are working in your home folder and have your data located in a subfolder called "data" and the Python scripts in a subfolder called "scripts." If you change this, please adjust the following instructions accordingly.

3. Move into the "data" folder:
```
cd ~/data
ls
```

4. Execute the bash script TrimClip.sh (*see* **Note 7**) by typing:
```
sh ../scripts/TrimClip.sh
```
while in the folder containing your data. Make note of how many reads are being trimmed and clipped through the screen output.

5. Calculate the fraction of duplicate and singleton reads, using the bash script CollapseDuplicateCount.sh (*see* **Note 8**), by typing:
```
sh ../scripts/CollapseDuplicateCount.sh
```
while in the folder containing your data. Results will be located in text files named with your original file name with *.duplicate-count.txt* appended.

6. Summarize quality score and nucleotide distribution data, then plot, by typing:
```
sh ../scripts/QualityStats.sh
```
in order to summarize your data files. Then execute the plotting software by typing:
```
sh ../scripts/Boxplots.sh
```

the software creates individual .png files for each sample, then combines them into one file called "Boxplots.pdf" (see Note 9).

3.5 Assembly (See Note 10)

1. Concatenate the sample files into one, using the cat command:
```
cat *.trimmed.clipped.fastq > assembly_
ready.fastq
```

2. Run Trinity to create a de novo assembly (*see* **Note 11**):
```
Trinity.pl --seqType fq --JM 1G \
--single assembly_ready.fastq --output as-
sembly
```

3. Summarize the statistics of the assembly, using the count_fasta. pl script, by typing:
```
../scripts/count_fasta.pl ./assembly/
Trinity.fasta \ > assembly/trinityStats.txt
```

4. Examine the statistics of the assembly (*see* **Notes 12** and **13**) by typing:
```
nano assemblyTest/trinityStats.txt
```

3.6 Mapping (See Note 14)

1. Open the BWAaln.sh script in nano, by typing:
```
nano ../scripts/BWAaln.sh
```
The default parameters are currently set as:

–n .01 –k 5 –l 30 –t 2

You can change them to something else if you like (*see* **Note 15**).

2. Execute the BWAaln.sh script (*see* **Note 16**) by typing:
```
sh ../scripts/BWAaln.sh
```

3. Convert your .sam files to .bam (*see* **Note 17**), sort and remove duplicate reads, by executing the script convert_to_bam_and_dedup.sh (*see* **Note 18**). Type:
```
sh ../scripts/convert_to_bam_and_dedup.sh
```

3.7 SNP Detection and Filtering (See Notes 19 and 20)

1. Create a tab-delimited text file called rg.txt, which is located along with your data files. This file provides critical information for GATK to keep the individuals apart in the merged file (*see* **Note 21**). It should be formatted like this (new line for each sample):
```
@RG     ID:READ_GROUP     SM:SAMPLE_
NAME     PL:Illumina
```

2. Merge your deduplicated .bam files:
```
samtools merge -h rg.txt merged.bam *dedup.
bam
```

3. Index your merged .bam file so that GATK will be able to search through it:

```
samtools index merged.bam
```

4. Realign around InDels using GATK, by typing (*see* **Note 22**):

```
sh ../scripts/realigner.sh
```

5. Detect variant sites, using the script SNP-detection.sh, by typing (*see* **Note 23**):

```
sh ../scripts/SNP_detection.sh
```

6. Recalibrate the SNPs, using the GATK VQSR algorithm, by typing (*see* **Note 24**):

```
sh ../scripts/VQSR.sh (see Note 25)
```

7. Extract genotypes of all individuals at all variable sites from the .vcf file into a format useable by Microsoft Excel, using a genotype quality threshold, by typing (*see* **Note 26**):

```
python ../scripts/getgenosfromvcf.py VQSR_
PASS_SNPS.vcf \ Genotypes.txt rows 20
```

8. Use the bash command 'grep' to create a new file with only SNPs with high-quality genotypes for all samples:

```
grep -v "\." Genotypes.txt > genotypes_
shared_by_all.txt
```

3.8 In Silico Validation

1. Test for deviations from Hardy–Weinberg equilibrium, especially for cases where all individuals are heterozygotes (*see* **Note 27**).

2. Another way is to use phase information to examine contigs for linkage disequilibrium—long linked stretches with fixed nucleotide differences could be signs of paralogous genes (but could also be a sign of a selective sweep).

3.9 Validation: Designing Primers, Sanger Sequencing (See Note 28)

1. Design primers by copy-pasting your protein-coding DNA sequence into the online portal Primer3 (http://bioinfo.ut. ee/primer3-0.4.0/) (*see* **Note 29**).

2. Make sure that the primer binding site does not contain any nucleotide variation.

3. Once you have sequences, you can easily order primers online.

4. Conduct a PCR using the annealing temperature specified by Primer3 (*see* **Note 30**) (Table 1).

5. Send off the PCR product to a sequencing facility for Sanger sequencing.

6. Confirm the genotypes using the Sanger chromatograms.

Table 1
Example of enzyme amounts to use for a 20 μl PCR reaction

Reagent	×1	×4
ddH_2O	9.8	39.2
10× buffer (comes with Taq)	2	8
BSA	2	8
$MgCl_2$	1.6	6.4
F primer	1	4
R primer	1	4
dNTPs	0.4	1.6
Taq polymerase	0.2	0.8
Template DNA	2	8
Total	20	80

4   Notes

1. Make sure that the lab space used is very clean. It is good to wash benches with RNAse-away or a similar RNAse remover beforehand.

2. Integrity of the RNA can be determined using denaturing MOPS agarose gels or a Bioanalyzer.

3. The Illumina TruSeq kits come with positive controls, which can be used to investigate where things have gone wrong during library preparation. These known sequences, if used, will have to be removed bioinformatically postsequencing.

4. Depending on the desired sequencing depth per sample, samples can in most cases be combined in one sequencing reaction. In this case, it is essential to use the barcoded adapters provided with the kit, and to not mix two samples with the same barcode.

5. Illumina sequencing is with few exceptions conducted by a sequencing center. When choosing which sequencing center to use, there are three important considerations: (a) Communication—do the technical staff answer to emails within a reasonable time? (b) Queue—how long will it take before your data will be available? (c) Price—is the sequencing possible considering the available budget?

6. There are many different potential quality control protocols, but the most important is to examine the distribution of base call qualities along the short Illumina reads, and to remove any artifacts from the sample preparation procedure. Artifacts can consist of either remains of adapter sequences or as PCR duplicates.

The objectives of this section are to (a) remove all bases with a Phred quality score of less than 20, (b) remove any adapter sequences present in the data, (c) graph the distributions of quality scores and nucleotides, and (d) calculate the fractions of duplicate and singleton reads in the data.

7. The bash script TrimClip.sh first invokes the quality trimmer, which scans through all reads, and when it encounters a base with a quality score of less than 20, trims off the rest of the read and then subsequently removes reads shorter than 20 bases. A temporary file is created, which is then used as an input file for the adapter clipper. The clipper removes any read ends that match the defined adapter sequences and then removes reads that after clipping are shorter than 20 bases.

8. The bash script CollapseDuplicateCount.sh first uses fastx_collapser to combine and count all identical reads. A temporary FASTA-formatted file called YOURFILE_collapsed.txt is created, which is then used as an input file for a python script (fastqduplicatecounter.py) that calculates the fractions of duplicate reads and singletons. This file is removed at the end of the program since it was just an intermediate step.

9. The easiest way to view the plots is by copying this file to your local drive and opening it there. The plots should look something like Fig. 1a, b. If the mean quality scores are low throughout or if the nucleotides are nonrandomly distributed, something could have gone wrong during sample preparation or sequencing.

10. RNA-Seq reads represent short pieces of all the mRNA present in the tissue at the time of sampling. In order to be useful, the reads need to be combined—assembled—into larger fragments, each representing an mRNA transcript. These combined sequences are called "contigs," which is short for "contiguous sequences." A de novo assembly joins reads that overlap into contigs without any template (i.e., no reference genome/transcriptome).

11. Building a de novo assembly is a very memory-intensive process. There are many programs for this, some of which are listed later. We are using Trinity [14] in this section, an assembler that is thought to work very well for transcriptomes, as opposed to others that are optimized for genome assembly. Trinity uses *De Bruijn graphs* to join reads together (*see* Fig. 2a). De Bruijn graphs summarize sequence variation in a very cost-effective way, speeding up the assembly process. Nevertheless, it is a very memory-intensive step, and having access to a computer cluster might be necessary if the number of reads is high.

12. When comparing the lengths and numbers of contigs acquired from de novo assemblies to the predicted number of transcripts from genome projects, the de novo contigs typically are shorter and more numerous. This is because the assembler cannot join contigs together unless there is enough overlap and coverage in the reads, so that several different contigs will match one

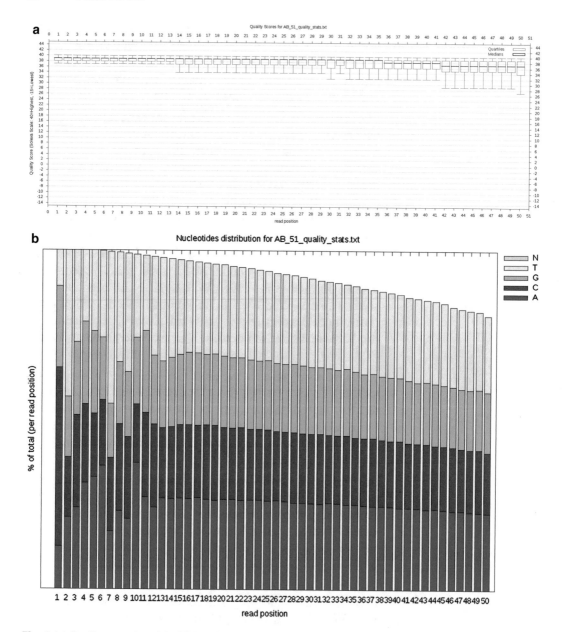

Fig. 1 (**a**) Quality score boxplot of 50-bp Illumina reads (after quality trimming, $Q < 20$), summarized by read position. Lower scores at the beginning of the reads are due to an artifact of the software used to calculate base quality scores. (**b**) Nucleotide distribution chart of 50-bp Illumina reads, summarized by read position. A nonrandom distribution in the first 12 bases is common and is thought to be an artifact of the random hexamer priming during sample preparation

mRNA transcript. Biologically, alternative splicing of transcripts also inflates the number of contigs when compared to predictive data from genome projects. This is important to keep in mind, especially when analyzing gene expression data based on mapping to a de novo assembly. To minimize this issue, we want to use as many reads as possible in the assembly

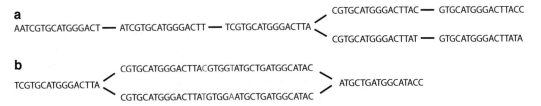

Fig. 2 (**a**) An example De Bruijn graph with k-mer size 16 and 5 nodes. (**b**) A bubble caused by two SNPs or sequencing errors. Shorter k-mers will decrease bubble size, but could increase fragmentation if coverage is not high enough

to maximize the coverage level. We therefore pool the reads from all our samples, which means that no information about the individual samples can be extracted from the assembly. In order to get sample-specific information, we need to map our reads from each sample individually to the assembly once it has been created (next section).

13. There are several parameters one can vary when assembling a transcriptome or genome. Perhaps the most important one is the k-mer (word) length of the De Bruijn graphs. Longer k-mers can help resolve repeat regions in genome assemblies and can be useful to resolve homeolog genes in polyploid species, whereas shorter one can increase performance in polymorphic sequences (*see* Fig. 2b). As Trinity focuses on transcriptome assembly, the k-mer length is preset to 25. In other assemblers, it can vary considerably.

14. Mapping refers to the process of aligning short reads to a reference sequence, whether the reference is a complete genome, transcriptome, or a de novo genome/transcriptome assembly. The program that we will utilize is called BWA [15], which uses a Burrow's Wheeler Transform method, with the goal of creating an alignment file also known as a Sequence/Alignment Map (SAM) file for each of your samples. This SAM file will contain one line for each of the reads in your sample denoting the reference sequence (genes, contigs, or gene regions) to which it maps, the position in the reference sequence, and a Phred-scaled quality score of the mapping, among other details [16].

15. There are several parameters that can be defined for the alignment process, including: the number of differences allowed between reference and query (–n), the length (–l) and number of differences allowed in the seed (–k), the number allowed and penalty for gap openings (–o, –O), and the number and penalty for gap extensions (–e, –E). Changing these parameters will change the number and quality of reads that map to reference and the time it takes to complete mapping a sample. For a complete list of the parameters and their default values, go to http://bio-bwa.sourceforge.net/bwa.shtml.

16. We will map the reads from each of your trimmed and clipped FASTQ files to the de novo reference assembly that you created in the previous section. Specifically, we will (a) create an index for the reference assembly (just once), which will help the aligner (and other downstream software) to quickly scan the reference; (b) for each sample, map reads to the reference assembly; and (c) convert the resulting file into the SAM file format and append "read group" names to the SAM file for each sample. Steps b and c are "piped," or put together feeding the output of one program in as the input for the next program. The read groups, which can have the same names as your sample names, will be appended to each file and will become critical for the downstream SNP detection step. The read group name in each SAM file will connect the reads back to individual samples after files have been merged for SNP detection. All of the earlier steps for all samples can be "batch" processed at once by editing the bash script BWAaln.sh. We then want to remove all duplicate reads, for which we need to use the MarkDuplicates program from the software package "Picard." Picard uses the binary equivalent of SAM files, BAM, as input, so first we need to convert the files using SAMtools. These steps are performed by the convert_to_BAM_and_dedup.sh bash script.

17. From now on, we will work with the binary equivalent of the SAM file format: BAM. BAM files take up less place on a hard drive and can be processed faster. Most SNP detection software are made to process BAM files. The drawback is that they cannot be examined directly in a text editor. Our first task is to remove any duplicate reads from the alignments, for which we also need to sort our aligned reads by alignment position. Identical, duplicate reads can be a result of biology and represent highly expressed transcripts. However, they are also quite likely to be an artifact of the PCR step in the sample preparation procedure. Artifactual duplicates can skew genotype estimates so they must be identified for SNP estimation.

18. The convert_to_bam_and_dedup.sh script has two elements: (a) It converts the .sam file to a binary bam file and sorts the reads within it. (b) It marks and removes duplicate reads using the MarkDuplicates program from the Picard package.

19. For all the data processing steps within this section, I have chosen to follow the recommendations of the Broad Institute, created for the Genome Analysis Toolkit (GATK): http://www.broadinstitute.org/gatk/guide/topic?name=best-practices [17]. I highly recommend keeping an eye on the instructions of this site for more information and updated protocols. They also have an excellent forum for posting technical questions. The only step in their protocol that we do not use is the Base Quality Score recalibration, as this step requires a list of known variant sites as input. If you do have access to this

type of data, it is highly recommended to follow the instructions on the GATK site.

20. The objectives of this section are to (1) merge your alignment files and realign poorly mapped regions, (2) detect variant sites and filter out true sites from false positives, (3) extract genotype information for all individuals at all variant sites.

21. There are three major steps to this section of the protocol. First, we need to process our alignment files slightly. We start by merging all the deduplicated .bam files from Subheading 4 into one file called merged.bam, which will be our base for SNP discovery. At this step, it is crucial that the "read group" headings for your samples (which we specified in the previous section) are correct, as they will be used to keep track of the samples within the merged .bam file. We then index our merged .bam file and search through the file for areas containing indels, where the initial mapping might be of poor quality. By using information from all samples in the merged file in a realignment step, we improve our chances of correctly aligning these regions. The merged realigned .bam file is what we will use in the next step, variant (SNP) detection and genotyping. An initial search for only very high-quality variant sites outputs a .vcf file, which is a list of all variant sites and the genotypes of all individuals for those sites. For information about the vcf file format, *see* http://www.1000genomes.org/node/101. We will consider the high-quality variants "true" sites for further processing. An additional search for variant sites, now with a lower quality threshold, is then conducted and by using our "true" variant sites from the first search we can build a Gaussian mixture model to separate true variants from false positives using a log-odds ratio (VQSLOD) of a variant being true vs. being false: (http://www.broadinstitute.org/gatk/gatkdocs/org_broadinstitute_sting_gatk_walkers_variantrecalibration_VariantRecalibrator.html). Following this, we can extract the genotype information for each individual from the .vcf file, while specifying a genotype quality threshold, and use this information to calculate allele and genotype frequencies. For simplicity we will use $Q=20$ ($p=0.99$) as a threshold.

22. There are two parts to the realigner.sh script: (a) call on RealignerTargetCreator to search for poorly mapped regions near indels and save those intervals in an output.intervals file. (b) Call on IndelRealigner to realign the intervals specified in step 1, and save the realigned file as merged_realigned.bam.

23. The SNP_detection.sh script has three elements: It calls on the GATK HaplotypeCaller to only call variant sites with a Phred scale quality of more than 20 (probability of being a true variant site >0.99). This will be used as a set of "true" variant sites to train the Gaussian mixture model used by the Variant Quality Score Recalibrator (VQSR) in the next step. The VQSR depends on a set of true variant sites, so if you are working with an organism for

which a validated set of variants exist, it is recommended to use that data here. However, as we are working with nonmodel organisms, we cannot assume that this data will always be available so let's assume that we have no prior knowledge in this case. You will want the quality threshold to be as high as possible at this point, but with out limited dataset, we will have to settle for $Q=20$ as a threshold. The script then calls on the HaplotypeCaller to call SNPs with a threshold that is largely determined by the sequencing depth. As we have low coverage due to our truncated fastq files, we will use a low-quality threshold here ($Q=3$). In reality, you would want to maximize this to reduce the chance of false positives. Finally, the script uses the VariantAnnotator to add annotations to the .vcf file output. The high-quality variant sites are stored in a file called: raw_snps_indels_Q20.vcf, while the variants that should be used for the final call set are in a file called: raw_snps_indels_Q3_annotated.vcf.

24. The VQSR.sh script has five elements: (a) It uses the high-quality SNP dataset to train a model that can be used for filtering the true SNPs from false positives in our call dataset. (b) It uses the high-quality InDel dataset to train a model that can be used for filtering the true InDels from false positives in our call dataset. (c) It applies the SNP model to the call data and flags all SNPs failing the filter. (d) It applies the InDel model and flags all InDels failing the filter. (e) It saves only the variant sites that have passed the VQSR into a new file called VQSR_PASS_SNPS.vcf.

25. If you get an error message when running the VQSR.sh script, try changing the settings for -percentBad, -minNumBad, and --maxGaussians in the first two commands of VQSR.sh using nano, then resaving and rerunning the script.

26. The final argument of the getgenosfromvcf.py script specifies a genotype Phred quality score cutoff of 20 (99 % probability of being true). This parameter can be changed according to your needs. The "rows" argument specifies that SNPs will be output in rows, with two columns per individual, one for each allele (specifying "cols" would return the same output, but with SNPs as columns, two columns per SNP).

27. There are many different software and methods to do this, so I will not go into much detail here.

28. The true test of a putative SNP is whether it can be validated using different methods. There are a variety of methods available for this, but we will focus on a traditional way, which is to design primers and to amplify and sequence fragments using PCR and Sanger sequencing.

29. Design primers: RNA-Seq data does unfortunately not contain any information about intron–exon boundaries, so the safest place to design primers is within the coding regions. It is also

possible to do this outside of coding frames, but in this case it can be nice to have access to a genome of a closely related species, in order to minimize the risk of designing primers that span over an intron.

30. Choosing samples for Sanger sequencing validation: Use DNA preferably from individuals indicated as homozygotes for the reference and alternative alleles at the SNP site of interest. It is possible to use heterozygotes as well, with an expectation of a double peak in the Sanger chromatogram, but PCR artifacts can potentially obscure this pattern.

References

1. Barton NH, Keightley PD (2002) Understanding quantitative genetic variation. Nat Rev Genet 3(1):11–21

2. Vos P, Hogers R, Bleeker M, Reijans M, Vandelee T, Hornes M, Frijters A, Pot J, Peleman J, Kuiper M, Zabeau M (1995) AFLP – a new technique for DNA-fingerprinting. Nucleic Acids Res 23(21):4407–4414

3. Richardson BJ, Baverstock PR, Adams M (1986) Allozyme electrophoresis: a handbook for animal systematics and population studies. Academic, San Diego, CA

4. Slatkin M (1995) A measure of population subdivision based on microsatellite allele frequencies. Genetics 139(1):457–462

5. Selkoe KA, Toonen RJ (2006) Microsatellites for ecologists: a practical guide to using and evaluating microsatellite markers. Ecol Lett 9(5):615–629

6. Baird NA, Etter PD, Atwood TS, Currey MC, Shiver AL, Lewis ZA, Selker EU, Cresko WA, Johnson EA (2008) Rapid SNP discovery and genetic mapping using sequenced RAD markers. PLoS One 3(10)

7. Wang Z, Gerstein M, Snyder M (2009) RNA-Seq: a revolutionary tool for transcriptomics. Nat Rev Genet 10:57–63

8. Beaumont MA, Nichols RA (1996) Evaluating loci for use in the genetic analysis of population structure. Proc R Soc B Biol Sci 263(1377):1619–1626

9. Charlesworth B, Nordborg M, Charlesworth D (1997) The effects of local selection, balanced polymorphism and background selection on equilibrium patterns of genetic diversity in subdivided populations. Genet Res 70(2):155–174

10. Martin JA, Wang Z (2011) Next-generation transcriptome assembly. Nat Rev Genet 12(10):671–682

11. Konczal M, Koteja P, Stuglik MT, Radwan J, Babik W (2013) Accuracy of allele frequency estimation using pooled RNA-Seq. Mol Ecol Resour 14:381–392

12. Skelly DA, Johansson M, Madeoy J, Wakefield J, Akey JM (2011) A powerful and flexible statistical framework for testing hypotheses of allele-specific gene expression from RNA-seq data. Genome Res 21:1728–1737

13. De Wit P, Pespeni MH, Palumbi SR (2015) SNP genotyping and population genomics from expressed sequences - current advances and future possibilities. Mol Ecol 24(10):2310–2323

14. Grabherr MG, Haas BJ, Yassour M, Levin JZ, Thompson DA, Amit I, Adiconis X, Fan L, Raychowdhury R, Zeng Q, Chen Z, Mauceli E, Hacohen N, Gnirke A, Rhind N, di Palma F, Birren BW, Nusbaum C, Lindblad-Toh K, Friedman N, Regev A (2011) Full-length transcriptome assembly from RNA-Seq data without a reference genome. Nat Biotechnol 29(7):644–U130

15. Li H, Durbin R (2009) Fast and accurate short read alignment with Burrows-Wheeler transform. Bioinformatics 25(14):1754

16. Li H, Handsaker B, Wysoker A, Fennell T, Ruan J, Homer N, Marth G, Abecasis G, Durbin R (2009) The sequence alignment/map format and SAMtools. Bioinformatics 25(16):2078

17. DePristo MA, Banks E, Poplin R, Garimella KV, Maguire JR, Hartl C, Philippakis AA, del Angel G, Rivas MA, Hanna M, McKenna A, Fennell TJ, Kernytsky AM, Sivachenko AY, Cibulskis K, Gabriel SB, Altshuler D, Daly MJ (2011) A framework for variation discovery and genotyping using next-generation DNA sequencing data. Nat Genet 43:491–498

Chapter 6

SNP Arrays for Species Identification in Salmonids

Roman Wenne, Agata Drywa, Matthew Kent, Kristil Kindem Sundsaasen, and Sigbjørn Lien

Abstract

The use of SNP genotyping microarrays, developed in one species to analyze a closely related species for which genomic sequence information is scarce, enables the rapid development of a genomic resource (SNP information) without the need to develop new species-specific markers. Using large numbers of microarray SNPs offers the best chance to detect informative markers in nontarget species, markers that can very often be assayed using a lower throughput platform as is described in this paper.

Key words SNP array, Salmon, Genotyping, Brown trout, Rainbow trout

1 Introduction

The development of high-throughput sequencing and genotyping technologies has enabled the detection and analysis of a large number of genetic markers (single nucleotide polymorphisms, SNPs) in species that have to date had limited genetic resources. SNP microarrays especially allow for Genome Wide Association Studies (GWAS), population structure analysis, and exploration of the effects of natural and artificial selection at the level of the genome [1]. A DNA microarray was developed and used for identification of some fish species at various stages of the life cycle including larvae and eggs [2] and analysis of the structure of the population from different geographical regions in order to improve compliance with and enforcement of fishing regulations [3].

The first Atlantic salmon (*Salmo salar*) SNP microarray (V1) available was used for (a) pedigree assignment [4, 5], (b) genetic differentiation of farmed and wild populations of Atlantic salmon in Norway [6], and (c) to construct a high resolution genetic map of Atlantic salmon and reveal the striking differences in recombination rates between male and female fish [7]. A year later, these same data were used to compare linkage maps of Atlantic salmon originating from Europe and North America [8]. Five families of

Sarah J. Bourlat (ed.), *Marine Genomics: Methods and Protocols*, Methods in Molecular Biology, vol. 1452, DOI 10.1007/978-1-4939-3774-5_6, © Springer Science+Business Media New York 2016

Canadian Atlantic salmon were studied in order to identify QTL (quantitative trait loci) associated with body weight [9].

In 2010, a second version (V2) of the array was developed containing a selection of 5.5K SNPs from the V1 array and a small number of untested novel markers. This was used to analyze 35-year-old dried scales stored at room temperature [10], to compare sedentary and migrating North American Atlantic salmon [11], in a study of neutral and adaptive loci among 54 North American populations of Atlantic salmon [12], to assess the efficacy of pooling samples from individuals of the north-European Atlantic salmon [13], and to analyze the cumulative introgression of hatchery salmon into wild populations of the Atlantic salmon [14]. The V2 array has also been used to explore important questions related to aquaculture including investigating the effect of genetic variation on the quality of salmon filets [15]. Other research using the array has included (a) exploring the genetic basis for differences in age of wild salmon populations migrating from the sea to a river for spawning [16], (b) investigating changes in genetic structure of salmon isolated in time and space in the River Namsen [17], and (c) searching for signatures of selection pressure related to the presence of parasites in wild Atlantic salmon populations, which was performed using microarray 6K [18]. Both of these arrays (V1 and V2) were developed using Illumina's Infinium technology [19, 20].

The V1 and V2 Atlantic salmon SNP arrays were designed and developed by researchers at the Center for Integrative Genetics, located at the Norwegian University of Life Sciences, NMBU [5]. For the V1 array, developed in 2006, roughly half the SNPs were detected within existing databases of ESTs (Expressed Sequences Tags), with the other half being detected through sequencing eight Atlantic salmon individuals from commercial hatchery populations in Norway using 454 technology. The V1 SNP array contained tests for 15,225 SNP markers and was used to genotype pedigreed samples ($n = 3297$) from a commercial breeding program in Norway (Aqua Gen AS, Norway), together with 1431 wild samples collected from 1977 to 2008 from 38 populations (31 populations from Europe, 7 from North America). All SNPs were classified according to the following categories (Fig. 1):

1. "SNP," presenting typical diploid behavior with AA, AB, and BB genotypes.

2. "MSV3" or multisite variant-3 where the locus is likely present as two copies within the partially tetraploid genome, but where the polymorphism is present at just one site giving, for example, an (AA)-AA, (AA)-AB, (AA)-BB allele behavior.

3. "MSV5" or multisite variant-5 where the locus is likely present as two copies within the partially tetraploid genome, and where the polymorphism is present at both sites giving, for

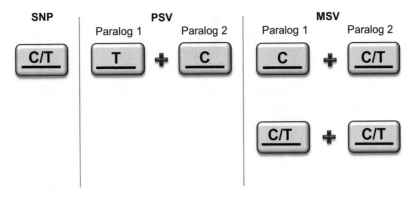

Fig. 1 Differences between SNP, PSV, and MSV

example, an AA-AA, AA-AB, AA-BB, AB-BB, and BB-BB allele behavior.

4. "PSV" or paralogous site variants, similar to MSV but each copy is fixed for opposite alleles giving (AA)-(BB) genotypes which consistently behave as heterozygous.

5. "failed" assays, where the chemistry fails to produce useful results.

6. "mono" or monomorphic, where the SNP was most likely a false positive and is in fact nonpolymorphic.

The relatively recent divergence of the salmonids means that some SNPs in extant species will predate speciation and can be used in multiple species, while other markers will be polymorphic on one species as a result of speciation. We have proposed that Atlantic salmon SNPs can be used to differentiate brown and rainbow trout in a similar manner to Smith et al. [21] who used the sequences derived from Atlantic salmon and rainbow trout SNP markers for the detection of Pacific salmon.

2 Materials

2.1 DNA Extraction

To extract Genomic DNA, the DNeasy Blood & Tissue Kit (Qiagen) was used according to the manufacturer's instructions. All chemicals were provided by the manufacturer:

1. Buffer ATL.

2. Buffer AL.

3. Buffer AW1.

4. Buffer AW2.

5. Buffer AE: 10 mM Tris–HCl, 0.5 mM EDTA, pH 9.0.

6. Proteinase K.

7. Ethanol 96%

2.2 DNA Quality

1. Agarose gel loading buffer (10×): 0.21% bromophenol blue, 0.21% xylene cyanol FF, 0.2 M EDTA, pH 8.0 and 50% glycerol or, Sigma loading buffer (6×): 0.05% bromophenol blue, 40% sucrose, 0.1M EDTA (pH 8.0) and 0.5% SDS.

2. TAE gel running buffer (1×): 40 mM Tris, 20 mM acetic acid, 1 mM EDTA. Dilute 20 ml TAE (50×) stock solution into 980 ml deionized water to make a 1× solution.

3. Agarose (1%): Dilute 1 g agarose in 100 ml TAE (1×). Heat in a microwave oven for about 1 min to dissolve the agarose.

4. Redsafe™ nucleic acid staining solution (20,000×) (iNtRON Biotechnology).

5. GeneRuler™ DNA Ladder Mix (Fermentas).

6. Agarose Gel Electrophoresis system.

2.3 DNA Quantification

1. Nano Drop ™ (Thermo Scientific).

2. Spectrophotometer.

3. Plate reader.

4. Quant-iT™ Pico Green® ds DNA reagent (Invitrogen).

5. TE buffer (20×): 200 mM Tris–HCL, 20 mM EDTA, pH 7.5.

6. Lambda DNA standard: 100 µg/ml in TE.

7. Tubes.

8. Plates.

2.4 Illumina Infinium Genotyping

1. Infinium HD Assay reagents are supplied by Illumina [22].

3 Methods

3.1 Collection of Fish Samples and Isolation of DNA

1. Collect fin clips from salmonid fish such as Atlantic salmon (*Salmo salar*), brown trout (*Salmo trutta*), or rainbow trout (*Oncorhynchus mykiss*).

2. Preserve the samples in 96% ethanol.

3. Store the samples at –80 °C.

4. Extract genomic DNA using Qiagen Dneasy Blood & Tissue Kit or any equivalent kit.

5. Resuspend isolated DNA in distilled water.

6. Store the isolates at 4 °C until further analysis.

3.2 DNA Quality: Agarose Gel Electrophoresis

Check the quality of the DNA using a 1% agarose gel electrophoresis in TAE buffer (*see* **Note 1**).

1. Prepare a 1% agarose gel solution with TAE buffer and mix thoroughly. Heat in a flask in the microwave oven until the

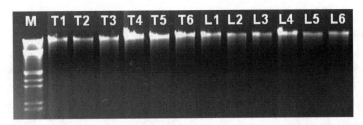

Fig. 2 Example of agarose gel electrophoresis of DNA samples extracted from fin clips. Lines T1–T6—sea trout samples; L1–L6—salmon samples, M—ladder (GeneRuler™ DNA Ladder Mix (Fermentas). *See* **Note 1**

solution is completely clear and no floating particles are visible (about 2–3 min).

2. Add 1 μl Redsafe per 100 ml agarose solution. Swirl the flask gently to mix the solution and avoid forming bubbles.

3. Pour the agarose solution into the gel tray containing comb teeth.

4. Allow the agarose gel to cool until solidified. Mix the DNA and loading buffer in 5:1 proportion (5 μl DNA and 1 μl dye).

5. Once the gel is solidified, place the agarose gel into the gel tray and fill with 1× TAE until gel is covered.

6. Carefully load the molecular weight ladder into the first well of the gel.

7. Carefully load the samples into the additional wells on the gel.

8. Run the gel at 100 V for 40 min.

9. Visualize the bands in UV light at frequency $\lambda = 365$ nm.

10. Document the gels using a photo or video gel documentation system (Fig. 2).

3.3 **DNA**
Quantification

3.3.1 Spectrophotometer

Use a Nano Drop™ or a similar instrument to measure DNA concentrations. DNA absorbs at 260 nm, proteins absorbs at 280 nm. The A260/A280 ratio gives an indication of protein contamination and pure DNA has an expected A260/A280 ratio of 1.8. Use nuclease-free water as blank sample.

3.3.2 Fluorometer

The major disadvantage of using an absorbance-based method like the NanoDrop is the large contribution of nucleotides and single-stranded nucleic acids to the signal and the inability to distinguish between DNA and RNA. Contaminants commonly found in nucleic acid preparations will also affect the measurements. Quant-iT™ PicoGreen® dsDNA reagent is a sensitive fluorescent nucleic acid stain for quantitating double-stranded DNA (dsDNA) in solution. Since the protocol is very sensitive, it is highly recommended to use pipetting robots and run both standards and samples in triplicate. We also recommend performing the analysis in 96-well format (not single tubes) and measuring using a plate reader. A DNA standard curve should be prepared with every 96-plate.

Table 1
Protocol for preparing a standard curve

Dilution step	Position in 96-well plate	Volume (µl) of TE	Volume (µl) of DNA	Final DNA concentration in Quant-iT™ PicoGreen® assay (ng/µl)
1	A1, A2, A3	286.7	13.3[a]	400
2	B1, B2, B3	150	150[b]	200
3	C1, C2, C3	150	150[b]	100
4	D1, D2, D3	150	150[b]	50
5	E1, E2, E3	150	150[b]	25
6	F1, F2, F3	150	150[b]	12.5
7	G1, G2, G3	150	150[b]	6.25
8	H1, H2, H3	150	0[b]	Blank

[a]λ DNA (100 ng/µl)

[b]DNA from previous dilution step

Prepare the standards:

1. Prepare a standard curve with concentrations from 6 to 400 ng/µl from the lambda DNA standard (100 µg/ml) provided in the Quant-iT™ PicoGreen® Kits.

2. Make three parallels of each dilution (300 µl each) in 1.5 ml Eppendorf tubes according to Table 1.

3. Mix thoroughly between each dilution step.

4. Transfer the diluted DNA to a 96-well "standards" plate according to Table 1. This plate can be used as a source of standard curve DNA for approximately 45 measurements and can be frozen between uses.

Dilutions and measurements:

1. Allow the Quant-iT™ PicoGreen® reagent to warm up to room temperature before opening the vial.

2. Prepare an aqueous working solution of the Quant-iT™ PicoGreen® reagent by making a 200-fold dilution of the concentrated DMSO solution in 1× TE buffer: Add 79.4 µl Quant-iT™ PicoGreen® reagent and 21.823 ml 1× TE buffer in a 50 ml Falcon tube and mix thoroughly.

3. Transfer 280 µl Quant-iT™ PicoGreen® working solution to wells A1-H3 in a 96-well plate and 210 µl Quant-iT™ PicoGreen® working solution to well A4-H12.

Protect the plate from light and use within a few hours.

4. Use a pipetting robot for best reproducibility in the following pipetting steps. If a robot is not available, use multichannel pipettes.

5. Add 178 μl of nuclease-free water to quadrants 1–3 in a 384-deepwell plate.

6. Add 2 μl of DNA from a 96-well plate to quadrants 1–3 in the 384-deepwell plate to make DNA dilutions in triplicate.

7. Mix the contents of each well in the 384-well plate containing DNA and water ten times with 100 μl volume. Spin the plate to avoid bubbles.

8. Transfer 52 μl of Quant-iT™ PicoGreen® working solution to quadrants 1–4 in a black 384-OptiPlate (or similar).

9. Transfer 2 μl of diluted DNA to quadrants 1–3 in the 384-Optiplate containing Quant-iT™ PicoGreen® working solution, mix ten times with 20 μl volume.

10. Transfer 2 μl of standards (from the standards plate described earlier) in triplicate to columns 1–3 in quadrant 4, mix ten times with 20 μl volume.

11. Seal the 384-Optiplate with film and spin down.

12. Incubate for 10 min protected from light.

13. Read the plate with a fluorescence microplate reader using 480 nm excitation wave length and 520 fluorescence emission wavelength.

14. Calculate DNA concentrations in an Excel document using values from the standard curve as a reference.

15. Normalize DNA samples with nuclease-free water to a final concentration of 50 ng/μl.

3.4 Genotyping

The Illumina infinium genotyping protocol can be obtained from [22].

Briefly, fragments of genomic DNA containing SNP alleles are hybridized to complementary synthetic probes immobilized to a microarray. A single base extension reaction incorporates fluorophore-labeled nucleotides and, after image capture and analysis, reveals the nature of the SNP alleles (Fig. 3).

Although most of the reagents are proprietary and their specific identities and functions are reserved by Illumina, some additional details about the specific steps in this process are included as follows:

1. High quality genomic DNA is first quantified using fluorometric methods (e.g., picogreen), and 200ng is Whole Genome Amplified (WGA) in an overnight reaction.

2. The following day, the WGA product is fragmented enzymatically before being precipitated using isopropanol and a colorized coprecipitant carrier. DNA pellets are thoroughly dried and resuspended in a hybridization solution containing formamide before being pipetted onto the array surface.

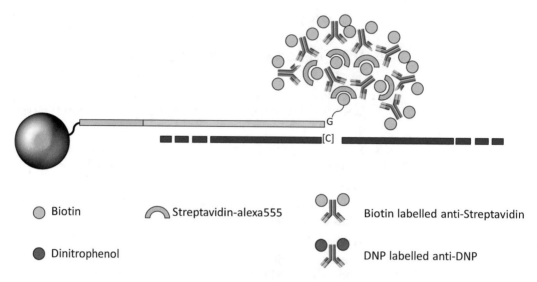

Fig. 3 Capture probes (approx. 50 nucleotides) are manufactured and linked to micro-spheres which are immobilized to the array surface (not shown). Fragmented gDNA hybridizes to the probe and the polymerase incorporates a single base at the 3′ end of the probe. Cytosine and guanine nucleotides are chemically modified with a biotin group, which, in the protocols' color development and signal amplification step, is bound by a fluorescently tagged streptavidin molecule. This in turn is bound by an antistreptavidin antibody labeled with additional biotins which, in an immunological sandwich-type assay, are bound by additional streptavidins. In the case of adenine and thymine, the fluorophore (2,4-dinitrophenol) is directly bound to the nucleotide eliminating the need for an intermediary molecule such as strepavadin. Instead, DNP-labeled antibodies bind directly to the nucleotide. Irrespective of the nucleotide, the signal is amplified through repeated cycles of antibody hybridization to ensure a strong detection signal above background

3. The array (typically in a 24-sample format) is kept in a humidified chamber and incubated overnight to allow all genomic DNA to hybridize to its specific capture probe sequence.

4. The following day, the arrays are washed to remove unbound probe and subjected to a series of liquid treatments, which include the single base extension of the probe (extension is dependent on the allele present in the genomic strand), and an antibody-based sandwich assay designed to amplify the color signal. The final liquid treatment includes coating the array with a viscous solution designed to protect the surface from physical and chemical assault, and drying it. Once dry the array can be scanned using an iScan instrument to produce the files required by Genome Studio.

3.5 Assessment of Genotyping Data Quality

As described earlier, all markers on the SNP array have been subjectively classified into one of six categories (SNP, MSV-3, etc.), based on their cluster performance within a large sample set (*see* **Note 2**). In this study, only markers classed as "SNP" and "MONO" on the basis of Atlantic salmon locus classification are used. Aside from subjective classification, some empirical measurements can be used to assess the quality of individual genotypes.

A GenCall score (GC) is assigned to each SNP assay and is a measure of confidence in the result. The GC score is between 0 and 1, with values below 0.15 indicating a failed assay, and values between 0.15 and 0.7 reflecting low to high assay performance, respectively. Values above 0.7 correspond to well-separated genotypes which are useful for the analysis [23, 24]. In addition to GC, the number of missing genotypes, MAF (Minor Allele Frequency), and the Hardy–Weinberg equilibrium (HWE; Hardy–Weinberg Equilibrium) can all be used to filter SNP loci and ensure that only the highest quality data is included in downstream analyses.

For a level of significance $p > 0.05$ [25], loci with GC values lower than 0.15 should be removed from further analysis. To avoid problems of missing data, resulting from the inability to determine the genotype for a given SNP, it is recommended to set the low quality DNA or ambiguous signal intensity threshold for missing data at the level of 5%. However, a lower level can be accepted in the case of a small number of individuals analyzed.

SNPs with a MAF below a certain threshold can be rejected. Depending on the purpose of the research, loci with MAF values below 0.01 can be omitted. Deviations from HWE can be determined by a chi-squared test using a random algorithm MCMC (Markov chain Monte Carlo) with significance level $p < 0.05$ [26]. To detect outlier loci, the hierarchical model of the island can be applied [27], using for instance 50,000 simulations for 100 subpopulations and 50 groups in the ARLEQUIN software v. 3.5.1.2 [28].

3.6 Population Genetics Statistical Analyses

Loci polymorphic for the salmonid species are to be selected from the results of the custom-designed Illumina iSelect SNP genotyping microarray for Atlantic salmon (see **Note 3**).

For this purpose, a molecular analysis of variance (AMOVA) locus-by-locus approach with 10,000 permutations can be used. Differentiation between species can be analyzed using a global-weighted average F between loci and between pairs of species [29, 30] at $p < 0.05$ using 1000 permutations. The ARLEQUIN software v. 3.5.1.2 [28] can be used to perform the tests.

The identification of putative species and assignment to these taxa can be performed with the Evanno method [31] using the software STRUCTURE v. 2.3.3 [32]. Individuals are attributed to the predefined population K (clusters) ($K = 1$–6) using ten independent waveforms for each K after 10,000 steps MCMC repeated 200,000 times, wherein each K was characterized as a set of allele frequencies at each locus. For the analysis, a mixed model can be chosen without giving any prior information on the origin of the fish. Individuals are attributed probabilistically to one or more clades if their genotypes have admixed genotypes of other taxon populations. To select the most optimal K value for the species compared, the incidence of probability logarithm can be used between successive values: K–Pr (X/K). The actual value of K will be estimated according to the method described by Evanno et al. [31] using HARVESTER [33].

Correspondence within and between species can be determined using a two-dimensional factorial correspondence analysis in the GENETIX software v. 4.05.2 [34, 35]. This method, based on the relationship between two variable allele frequencies of the SNP can be adapted to specific groups of individuals without indicating their origin.

The ability of a set of outlier markers to assign individuals to the most likely species can be evaluated using the software ONCOR [36]. Individual assignment tests to each group (population) can be carried out with the leave-one-out method. The samples are divided into two groups—the baseline and the mixture. The genotypes of individuals from the mixed sample are assigned to the base population without any a priori information about their origin. The method used to estimate the origin of individuals belonging to the mixed group has been described by Rannala and Mountain [37]. During assessment of the correctness of the individual fish identifications in the leave-one-out method, the genotype of each individual in each population is subsequently removed (one at a time) to estimate its origin, using the remaining baseline group.

3.7 Example Data

Samples of *S. salar*, *S. trutta*, and *O. mykiss* smolts from the Department of Salmonid Fish Breeding at the Inland Fisheries Institute in Rutki, Poland collected in May 2009 were used for analysis [38]. Among the "SNP" and "MSV" categories, 6112 markers showed an overall MAF > 0.01 (Fig. 4). These and another 64 markers, in total 6171 markers (6K), which had an overall MAF lower than 0.01 but had a MAF > 0.05 in at least one of the populations were subjected to further analysis. In the following analysis, this number was reduced to 5568 (version 1, V1) and 5349 (version 2, V2) markers (5.5K).

Twenty-four samples of brown (sea) trout *S. trutta* from weakly differentiated populations in Vistula and Slupia rivers, Poland were genotyped with the Atlantic salmon custom-designed Illumina iSelect SNP array containing 15,225 markers. One hundred and eight polymorphic loci were chosen for further analysis of brown trout specimens as a result of an AMOVA analysis. After applying all the quality control steps, 39 loci with F_{ST} for pairwise comparison greater than 0 were found [39]. These 39 loci were included in the assays of 442 samples of sea trout from the southern Baltic designed for 62 candidate SNPs [40]. A diagnostic panel of 23 SNPs was constructed successfully for the analysis of Southern Baltic populations of sea trout. Analysis of the example results suggests that the use of the Atlantic salmon SNP array designed mainly for one species enables the analysis of data from other closely related species (e.g., sea trout and rainbow trout), without the need to develop new species-specific markers (Fig. 5). This is particularly important for study species whose genome is still largely unknown.

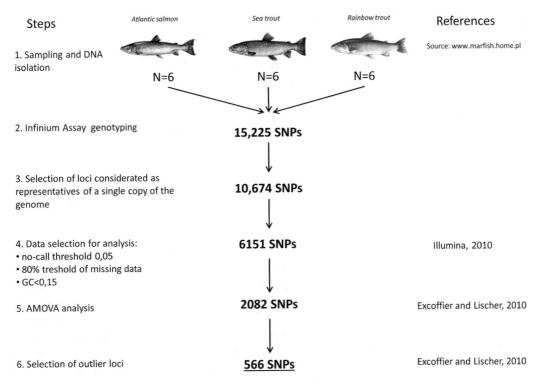

Fig. 4 Selection of SNPs for identification of three salmonid species (Figure reproduced from [38] with permission of Elsevier, modified)

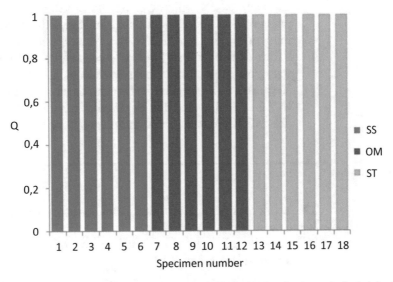

Fig. 5 Chart estimated value of Q (estimated rate of each individual belonging to each cluster) for the number of the analyzed groups *K*= 3 [38]. Each subject is represented in the graph as a vertical bar. SS—*S. salar* (1-6 individuals, blue); OM—*O. mykiss* (7–12 individuals, *red*); ST—*S. trutta* (13–18 individuals, *green*)

4 Notes

1. A key element in the success of Illumina genotyping is *DNA quality*. Extracted DNA should always be run on a 0.9–1% agarose gel and compared to a control sample or molecular weight ladder to confirm that the material has a predominance of high molecular weight material. A degraded sample will perform poorly in the whole genome amplification step and result in a low signal to noise in the analysis. DNA quantity is less crucial, and although the protocol demands 200 ng of DNA, we have found that performance is unaffected by amounts ranging from 100 to 300 ng, but this assumes that the DNA is of good quality.

2. For custom arrays, especially in organisms that are not typical diploids, *manual examination* (and perhaps adjustment) of SNP cluster patterns is the best way to differentiate high-confidence genotypes from low. This can be very laborious and various metrics (such as call rate, pedigree errors) within GenomeStudio can be used to sort SNPs and draw your attention to those markers that have potentially the most problems. However, a thorough investigation of all markers (or at the very least those that stand out in your analysis, e.g., F_{st} outliers) is worth the effort.

3. The same SNP will not necessarily perform identically when genotyped on a different technology platform. A natural outcome from high-density genotyping is the selection of a few candidate SNPs which can be more cheaply genotyped in a larger number of samples using an alternative technology like Sequenom, Fluidgm, KASP, etc. Our experience has been that if four of five SNPs "transfer" successfully and return usable genotypes, this should be regarded as a success. Of course there are a number of tricks that can be employed if a particular SNP is crucial to transfer, but the basic fact is that all technologies are different and expectations must be realistic.

Acknowledgements

This work was partially funded from statutory topic IV.1. in the Institute of Oceanology PAS and project No. 397/N-cGRASP/2009/0 of the Ministry of Science and Higher Education in Poland to R.W.

References

1. Bourret V, Kent MP, Primmer CR, Vasemägi A, Karlsson S, Hindar K, McGinnity P, Varspoor E, Bernatchez L, Lien S (2013) SNP-array reveals genome-wide patterns of geographical and potential adaptive divergence across the natural range of Atlantic salmon (*Salmo salar*). Mol Ecol 22(3):532–551. doi:10.1111/mec.12003

2. Kochzius M, Nölte M, Weber H, Silkenbeumer N, Hjörleifsdottir S, Hreggvidsson GO, Marteinsson V, Kappel K, Planes S, Tinti F, Magoulas A, Garcia VE, Turan C, Hervet C, Campo FD, Antoniou A, Landi M, Blohm D (2008) DNA microarrays for identifying fishes. Mar Biotechnol 10(2):207–217. doi:10.1007/s10126-007-9068-3

3. Martinsohn JT, Ogden R (2009) FishPopTrace Consortium. FishPopTrace—developing SNP-based population genetic assignment methods to investigate illegal fishing. Forensic Sci Int-Gen 2(1):294–296. doi:10.1016/j.fsigss.2009.08.108

4. Dominik S, Henshall JM, Kube PD, King H, Lien S, Kent MP, Elliott NG (2010) Evaluation of an Atlantic salmon SNP chip as a genomic tool for the application in a Tasmanian Atlantic salmon (*Salmo salar*) breeding population. Aquaculture 308(Suppl 1):56–61. doi:10.1016/j.aquaculture.2010.05.038

5. Gidskehaug L, Kent M, Hayes BJ, Lien S (2011) Genotype calling and mapping of multisite variants using an Atlantic salmon iSelect SNP array. Bioinformatics 27(3):303–310. doi:10.1093/bioinformatics/btq673

6. Karlsson S, Moen T, Lien S, Glover KA, Hindar K (2011) Generic genetic differences between farmed and wild Atlantic salmon identified from a 7K SNP-chip. Mol Ecol Res 11(Suppl 1):247–253. doi:10.1111/j.1755-0998.2010.02959.x

7. Lien S, Gidskehaug L, Moen T, Hayes BJ, Berg PR, Davidson WS, Omholt SW, Kent MP (2011) A dense SNP-based linkage map for Atlantic salmon (*Salmo salar*) reveals extended chromosome homologies and striking differences in sex-specific recombination patterns. BMC Genomics 12:615–625. doi:10.1186/1471-2164-12-615

8. Brenna-Hansen S, Jieying I, Kent PM, Boulding EG, Dominik S, Davidson WS, Lien S (2012) Chromosomal differences between European and North American Atlantic salmon discovered by linkage mapping and supported by fluorescence in situ hybridization analysis. BMC Genomics 13:432–444. doi:10.1186/1471-2164-13-432

9. Gutierrez AP, Lubieniecki KP, Davidson EA, Lien S, Kent MP, Fukui S, Withler RE, Davidson WS (2012) Genetic mapping of quantitative trait loci (QTL) for body-weight in Atlantic salmon (*Salmo salar*) using a 6.5 K SNP array. Aquaculture 358–359:61–70. doi:10.1016/j.aquaculture.2012.06.017

10. Johnston SE, Lindqvist M, Niemelä E, Orell P, Erkinaro J, Kent MP, Lien S, Vähä J-P, Vasemägi A, Primmer CR (2013) Fish scales and SNP chips: SNP genotyping and allele frequency estimation in individual and pooled DNA from historical samples of Atlantic salmon (*Salmo salar*). BMC Genomics 14:439–451. doi:10.1186/1471-2164-14-439

11. Perrier C, Bourret V, Kent MP, Bernatchez L (2013) Parallel and nonparallel genome-wide divergence among replicate population pairs of freshwater and anadromous Atlantic salmon. Mol Ecol 22(22):5577–5593. doi:10.1111/mec.12500

12. Bourret V, Dionne M, Kent MP, Lien S, Bernatchez L (2013) Landscape genomics in Atlantic salmon (Salmo salar): searching for gene-environment interactions driving local adaptation. Evolution 67(12):3469–3487. doi:10.1111/evo.12139

13. Ozerov M, Vasemägi A, Wennevik V, Niemelä E, Prusov S, Kent MP, Vähä J-P (2013) Cost-effective genome-wide estimation of allele frequencies from pooled DNA in Atlantic salmon (*Salmo salar* L.). BMC Genomics 14:12–23. doi:10.1186/1471-2164-14-12

14. Glover KA, Pertoldi C, Besnier F, Wennevik V, Kent MP, Skaala Ø (2013) Atlantic salmon populations invaded by farmed escapees: quantifying genetic introgression with a Bayesian approach and SNPs. BMC Genet 14:74–92. doi:10.1186/1471-2156-14-74

15. Sodeland M, Gaarder M, Moen T, Thomassen M, Kjøglum S, Kent M, Lien S (2013) Genome-wide association testing reveals quantitative trait loci for fillet texture and fat content in Atlantic salmon. Aquaculture 408–409:169–174. doi:10.1016/j.aquaculture.2013.05.029

16. Johnston SE, Orell P, Pritchard VL, Kent MP, Lien S, Niemelä E, Erkinaro J, Primmer CR (2014) Genome-wide SNP analysis reveals a genetic basis for sea–age variation in a wild population of Atlantic salmon (*Salmo salar*).

Mol Ecol 23(14):3452–3468. doi:10.1111/mec.12832

17. Sandlund OT, Karlsson S, Thorstad EB, Berg OK, Kent MP, Norum ICJ, Hindar K (2014) Spatial and temporal genetic structure of a river-resident Atlantic salmon (*Salmo salar*) after millennia of isolation. Ecol Evol 4(9):1538–1554. doi:10.1002/ece3.1040

18. Zueva KJ, Lumme J, Veselov AE, Kent MP, Lien S, Primmer CR (2014) Footprints of directional selection in wild Atlantic salmon populations: evidence for parasite-driven evolution? PLoS One 9(3), e91672. doi:10.1371/journal.pone.0091672

19. Shen R, Fan JB, Campbell D, Chang WH, Chen J, Doucet D, Yeakley J, Bibikova M, Garcia EW, McBride C, Steemers F, Garcia F, Kermani BG, Gunderson K, Oliphant A (2005) High-throughput SNP genotyping on universal bead arrays. Mutat Res 573(1-2):70–82. doi:10.1016/j.mrfmmm.2004.07.022

20. Steemers FJ, Gunderson KL (2007) Whole genome genotyping technologies on the BeadArray™ platform. Biotechnol J 2(1):41–49. doi:10.1002/biot.200600213

21. Smith MJ, Pascal CE, Grauvogel Z, Habicht C, Seeb JE, Seeb LW (2011) Multiplex preamplification PCR and microsatellite validation enables accurate single nucleotide polymorphism genotyping of historical fish scales. Mol Ecol Resour 11(Suppl 1):268–277. doi:10.1111/j.1755-0998.2010.02965.x

22. http://support.illumina.com/content/dam/illumina-support/documents/myillumina/05340b1f-c179-495d-b790-fa91ecbb6ff2/inf_hd_super_assay_ug_11322427_revc.pdf

23. Fan JB, Oliphant A, Shen R, Kermani BG, Garcia F, Gunderson KL, Hansen MM, Steemers F, Butler SL, Deloukas P, Galver L, Hunt S, Mcbride C, Bibikova M, Rubano T, Chen J, Wickham E, Doucet D, Chang W, Campbell D, Zhang B, Kruglyak S, Bentley D, Haas J, Rigault P, Zhou L, Stuelpnagel J, Chee MS (2003) Highly parallel SNP genotyping. Cold Spring Harb Symp Quant Biol 68:69–78. doi:10.1101/sqb.2003.68.69

24. Oliphant A, Barker DL, Stuelpnagel JR, Chee MS (2002) BeadArray technology: enabling an accurate, cost-effective approach to high-throughput genotyping. Biotechniques 32:56–61

25. Illumina (2010) Infinium genotyping data analysis. Technical Note: Illumina DNA analysis. Publication Number 970-2007-005, January 2010

26. Guo SW, Thompson NEA (1992) Performing the exact test of Hardy–Weinberg proportion for multiple alleles. Biometrics 48:361–372

27. Slatkin M, Voelm L (1991) FST in a hierarchical island model. Genetics 127(3):627–629

28. Excoffier L, Lischer HEL (2010) Arlequin suite ver 3.5: a new series of programs to perform population genetics analyses under Linux and Windows. Mol Ecol Resour 10(3):564–567. doi:10.1111/j.1755-0998.2010.02847.x

29. Weir BS, Cockerham CC (1984) Estimating F-statistics for the analysis of population structure. Evolution 38(6):1358–1370

30. Weir BS (1996) Genetic data analysis II: methods for discrete population genetic data. Sinauer Press, Sunderland, MA, 376 pp

31. Evanno G, Regnaut S, Goudet J (2005) Detecting the number of clusters of individuals using the software STRUCTURE: a simulation study. Mol Ecol 14(8):2611–2620. doi:10.1111/j.1365-294X.2005.02553.x

32. Pritchard JK, Stephens M, Donnelly P (2000) Inference of population structure using multilocus genotype data. Genetics 155(2):945–959

33. Earl DA, vonHoldt BM (2012) STRUCTURE HARVESTER: a website and program for visualizing STRUCTURE output and implementing the Evanno method. Conserv Genet Resour 4(2):359–361. doi:10.1007/s12686-011-9548-7

34. Belkhir K, Borsa P, Chikhi L, Raufaste N, Bonhomme F (2000) GENETIX 4.05, logiciel sous Windows TM pour la génétique des populations. Laboratoire Génome, Populations, Interactions, CNRS UMR 5171. 1996–2004. Université de Montpellier II, Montpellier

35. Benzécri JP (1992) Correspondence analysis handbook. Statistics, textbooks and monographs, Vol 225. Marcel Dekker, New York, NY, p 688

36. Kalinowski ST, Manlove KR, Taper ML (2007) ONCOR: a computer program for genetic stock identification. Department of Ecology, Montana State University, Bozeman, MT, http://www.montana.edu/kalinowski/Software/ONCOR.htm

37. Rannala B, Mountain JL (1997) Detecting immigration by using multilocus genotypes. Proc Natl Acad Sci U S A 94(17):9197–9201

38. Drywa A, Poćwierz-Kotus A, Dobosz S, Kent MP, Lien S, Wenne R (2014) Identification of multiple diagnostic SNP loci for differentiation of three salmonid species using SNP-arrays. Mar Genomics 15:5–6. doi:10.1016/j.margen.2014.03.003

39. Drywa A, Poćwierz-Kotus A, Wąs A, Dobosz S, Kent MP, Lien S, Bernaś R, Wenne R (2013) Genotyping of two populations of Southern Baltic sea trout *Salmo trutta m. trutta* using an

Atlantic salmon derived SNP-array. Mar Genomics 9:25–32. doi:10.1016/j.margen. 2012.08.001

40. Poćwierz-Kotus A, Bernaś R, Dębowski P, Kent MP, Lien S, Kesler M, Titov S, Leliuna E, Jespersen H, Drywa A, Wenne R (2014) Genetic differentiation of southeast Baltic populations of sea trout inferred from single nucleotide polymorphisms. Anim Genet 45(1): 96–104. doi:10.1111/age.12095

Chapter 7

The Next-Generation PCR-Based Quantification Method for Ambient Waters: Digital PCR

Yiping Cao, John F. Griffith, and Stephen B. Weisberg

Abstract

Real-time quantitative PCR (qPCR) is increasingly being used for ambient water monitoring, but development of digital polymerase chain reaction (digital PCR) has the potential to further advance the use of molecular techniques in such applications. Digital PCR refines qPCR by partitioning the sample into thousands to millions of miniature reactions that are examined individually for binary endpoint results, with DNA density calculated from the fraction of positives using Poisson statistics. This direct quantification removes the need for standard curves, eliminating the labor and materials associated with creating and running standards with each batch, and removing biases associated with standard variability and mismatching amplification efficiency between standards and samples. Confining reactions and binary endpoint measurements to small partitions also leads to other performance advantages, including reduced susceptibility to inhibition, increased repeatability and reproducibility, and increased capacity to measure multiple targets in one analysis. As such, digital PCR is well suited for ambient water monitoring applications and is particularly advantageous as molecular methods move toward autonomous field application.

Key words Polymerase chain reaction, Beach water quality, Ambient water monitoring, Multiplex, Droplet digital PCR

1 Introduction

Real-time quantitative polymerase chain reaction (qPCR) measurements are increasingly becoming part of ambient water quality monitoring [1–3]. In beach water quality monitoring, qPCR methods have been found to provide comparable results to traditional culture-based methods [4, 5], but with a tremendous speed advantage; whereas culture methods require 18–72 h, qPCR methods can be conducted in less than 2 h, creating the opportunity for same day health warnings [6]. qPCR methods also provide the opportunity for measuring not only the fecal indicator bacteria on which beach health warnings are based but also genetic source identification markers that help identify the fecal sources that need to be abated [7]. Similarly, qPCR measurements of environmental

Sarah J. Bourlat (ed.), *Marine Genomics: Methods and Protocols*, Methods in Molecular Biology, vol. 1452,
DOI 10.1007/978-1-4939-3774-5_7, © Springer Science+Business Media New York 2016

DNA (eDNA) have become a popular molecular surveillance tool among aquatic researchers and managers because it is nondestructive and provides improved sensitivity and efficiency over traditional taxonomic methods that rely on morphological identification of sampled aquatic organisms [8]. Monitoring of cyanobacteria in source waters by qPCR [9] may also provide early warning of harmful cyanobacterial bloom that is of extreme public health concern [10].

Digital PCR is a further refinement in DNA quantification methods [11] that has already found its way into ambient water [12] and beach health monitoring applications [13]. In qPCR, quantification is achieved by monitoring fluorescence accumulation through repeated amplification steps, using the response of a known DNA calibrator to estimate the concentration of an unknown. Digital PCR uses the same primers and probes as qPCR but is based on partitioning the sample into thousands to millions of nanoliter or picoliter reactions (i.e., miniature chambers/wells on a chip for chamber digital PCR or water-in-oil droplets for droplet digital PCR) that are examined individually for fluorescence, with DNA density calculated from the fraction of positive endpoint reactions using Poisson statistics. Confining reactions and binary endpoint measurements to small partitions connotes several potential performance advantages, including increased precision and reduced inhibition [14]. However, digital PCR's biggest advantage is that it allows for direct quantification without the need for standard curves, eliminating the labor, material, and error associated with creating and running standards with each batch. Standard-free quantification is particularly advantageous as molecular methods move down the path of automation [15].

In this chapter, we introduce the fundaments of digital PCR quantification basis and workflow, and elaborate on advantages and limitations of digital PCR over qPCR. We present results for how traditional qPCR and digital PCR compare for a number of analytes for which digital has been developed. We also include a discussion on the suitability for digital PCR implementation in ambient water quality monitoring applications. Note that we use the term digital PCR for general discussion applicable to both droplet and chamber digital PCR but specify droplet digital PCR (ddPCR) or chamber digital PCR for discussion and references specific to either form of digital PCR.

2   Differences in Quantification Approach Used in qPCR and Digital PCR

Fundamental to qPCR quantification is the standard curve. With the addition of fluorescent probe or DNA-binding dye to PCR, bulk reactions are amplified on a thermal cycler equipped with optics that continuously monitor the fluorescence increase in real time, which is proportional to the increase of target DNA in the reaction. The more target DNA a qPCR starts with, the less time (i.e., fewer PCR cycles) needed for fluorescence to accumulate to a measurable threshold. Serial diluted reference material is run to establish a standard curve that depicts this inverse relationship between quantification cycle (Cq, i.e., number of cycles needed to cross the fluorescent threshold) and starting target concentration. Assuming sample and reference DNA amplify at the same speed/efficiency, an unknown sample can be quantified indirectly through interpolating its Cq from the standard curve.

In contrast, digital PCR quantification is achieved by partitioning the sample prior to PCR amplification and applying Poisson statistics on the binary endpoint results from the partitions [13, 16]. The bulk reaction is partitioned into thousands to millions of nanoliter or picoliter reactions inside small chambers on a chip or within water-in-oil droplets prior to PCR amplification. This partitioning process approximates a Poisson distribution and renders the DNA target present in some of the partitions, but absent in others. Consequently, positive PCR amplification only occurs in a portion of partitions and is detected with a fluorescent probe [16] or a DNA-binding dye [17] as in qPCR, except that real-time detection of fluorescence accumulation is no longer necessary. Endpoint detection of PCR amplification is sufficient to score the small-volume partitions positive or negative. The percentage of positive partitions is then used with Poisson statistics to estimate the concentration of target DNA copies. As such, no comparative external standard curves are needed to quantify unknown samples. The basis to digital PCR quantification is therefore not how soon a fluorescent signal is detected (as in qPCR), but whether or not the target amplifies in each small-volume partition. This digital quantification is what gives digital PCR advantages over qPCR. Although the elements unique to digital PCR, such as partitioning and rapid detection of massive numbers of individual partitions, previously presented a high level of technical difficulty [18], advancements in microfluidics and chip manufacturing have enabled automation of these two elements, leading to commercial instruments that make digital PCR easy and accessible [19]. Figure 1 compares the typical qPCR and digital PCR workflow using one representative platform from each technology.

3 Basic Performance Metrics

3.1 Accuracy

qPCR depends on establishment of a standard curve and an assumption that standards and unknown samples amplify at the same efficiency, yielding two opportunities for bias. First, the reliability and consistency of the standards greatly affects qPCR quantification accuracy of the unknown. Variability in standard reference

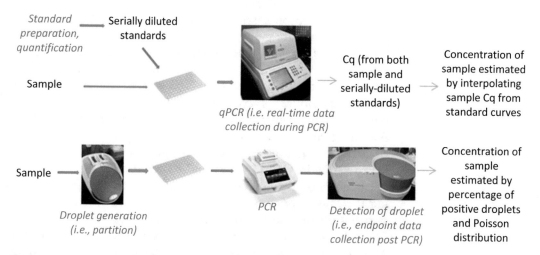

Fig. 1 Workflow comparison of qPCR and digital PCR. Note that a variety of platforms exist for both qPCR and digital PCR. For ease of presentation, a 96-well qPCR platform (CFX96, Bio-Rad Laboratories) and a 96-well droplet digital PCR system (QX100, Bio-Rad Laboratories) are used as examples here

material has been found to be responsible for approximately half a log difference in results between vendors [20] and responsible for as much as a twofold difference between batches within a vendor [21]. As such, lack of access to reliable and consistent standard material has been identified as the biggest obstacle to use of qPCR for recreational water monitoring [20, 22]. In addition, lack of reliable methods for quantification and certification of qPCR standards and the difficulty of maintaining standards' integrity during storage and handling further exacerbate the problem [13].

Second, mismatched amplification efficiency between standard and unknown samples can lead to quantification bias. PCR inhibitory substances that are present in environmental samples, but not in standards, may lower the amplification efficiency and lead to underestimation or false negatives [23]. Even in the absence of inhibition, DNA template type can affect the assumption that the sample and standards share the same amplification efficiency. For example, Whale et al. [24] found that commonly used plasmid DNA standards had a different amplification efficiency than genomic DNA in samples and introduced bias in quantifying samples.

In contrast, the binary nature of digital PCR allows direct quantification of unknown samples without external standards. This direct quantification effectively eliminates the biases associated with variability in standards and amplification efficiency and therefore lends digital PCR greater accuracy [13]. Digital PCR is increasingly being used as reference method to certify qPCR standards, for instance, by the National Measurement Institute in Australia (http://www.measurement.gov.au/Publications/FactSheets/Documents/NMI%2017.pdf) and the National Institute of Science and Technology in USA (https://www-s.

nist.gov/srmors/certificates/2366.pdf?CFID=29867054&CFT
OKEN=7ecd9fcb9d05e13d-93DFC985-EB75-5CA0-
C77CF506D9593C90).

Nevertheless, after correcting for bias in qPCR standards and in the absence of inhibition, qPCR and digital PCR typically provide comparable results. Cao et al. [13] found comparable responses between the two methods when measuring general fecal indicator bacteria (*Enterococcus* spp.) and human-associated fecal marker (HF183) in environmental waters. Nathan et al. [8] also found that ddPCR and qPCR provided similar abundance estimates of cytochrome c oxidase subunit I (COI) genes from round gobies. Building upon the success of previous studies, we have validated a suite of ddPCR assays targeting analytes important for surface water monitoring such as total *Bacteroidales* as general fecal indicator bacteria, cow-, gull-, and additional human-associated fecal markers, and a common pathogen Campylobacter (Tables 1 and 2). All five

Table 1
Primer and probe sequences and references

Target organisms	ddPCR assay	Primer (*F*, forward; *R*, reverse) and probe sequences	Reference
Total *Bacteroidales*	GenBac3 ddPCR	F: GGGGTTCTGAGAGGAAGGT R: CCGTCATCCTTCACGCTACT FAM-CAATATTCCTCACTGCTGCCTCCCGTA-BHQ1	[25]
E. coli and human-associated *Bacteroidales*	EcHF183 duplex ddPCR	F: CAACGAACTGAACTGGCAGA R: CATTACGCTGCGATGGAT FAM-CCCGCCGGGAATGGTGATTAC-BHQ1 F: ATCATGAGTTCACATGTCCG R: CTTCCTCTCAGAACCCCTATCC HEX-CTAATGGAACGCATCCC-MGB	[26, 27]
E. coli and cow-associated *Bacteroidales*	EcCowM2 duplex ddPCR	F: CAACGAACTGAACTGGCAGA R: CATTACGCTGCGATGGAT FAM-CCCGCCGGGAATGGTGATTAC-BHQ1 F: CGGCCAAATACTCCTGATCGT R: GCTTGTTGCGTTCCTTGAGATAAT Hex-AGGCACCTATGTCCTTTACCTCATCAACTACA GACA-BHQ1	[26, 28]
Avian-associated Catellicoccus	LeeSeagull	F: CACGTGCTACAATGGCATAT R: GGCTTCATGCTCTCGAGTT FAM-CAGAGAACAATCCGAACTGGGACA-BHQ1	[29]
Campylobacter	*Campylobacter*	F: CACGTGCTACAATGGCATAT R: GGCTTCATGCTCTCGAGTT FAM-CAGAGAACAATCCGAACTGGGACA-BHQ1	[30]

Each 20 μl reaction setup contains 1× Droplet PCR Supermix (Bio-Rad), 900 nM each primer, 250 nM each probe, and 5 μl of sample DNA. Experimental procedures are the same as the EntHF183 duplex ddPCR assay, described in details elsewhere in both text and video formats [13, 31]

Table 2
Thermal cycling conditions for the five ddPCR assays in Table 1

Assays	Pre-denature (°C, time)	Denature (°C, time)	Annealing (°C, time)	Number of cycles	Extension (°C, time)	ddPCR system
GenBac3, EcHF183, EcCowM2	95 °C, 10 min	94 °C, 30s	60 °C, 1 min	40	98 °C, 10 min	QX100
Campylobacter, LeeSeagull	95 °C, 10 min	94 °C, 30s	60 °C, 1 min	45	98 °C, 10 min	QX100

A CFX96 was used for thermal cycling, with ramping speed adjusted to 2.0 °C s^{-1}

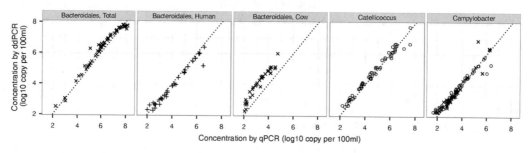

Fig. 2 Comparison of ddPCR and qPCR results for quantifying general fecal indicator bacteria (total *Bacteroidales*), host-associated fecal markers (*Bacteroidales* associated with human and cow fecal material, Catellicoccus associated with gull fecal material), and pathogens (*Campylobacter*). *Symbols* indicate ambient freshwater samples spiked with cow (*x-cross*), gull (*circle*) feces, and sewage (*cross*). The *dotted line* denotes the 1:1 line. *See* Table 1 for primer and probe sequences and references

assays demonstrate high comparability between ddPCR and qPCR results (Fig. 2).

3.2 Repeatability and Reproducibility

A major advantage stemming from the binary nature of digital PCR quantification is improved repeatability and reproducibility over qPCR. Note that repeatability refers to the precision of an assay among replicates of the same sample performed by the same operator, instrument, run, condition, and laboratory, over a short period of time (e.g., short-term precision). Reproducibility refers to the consistency in results among operators, runs, or laboratories (e.g., long-term precision) [32].

Because digital PCR counts the frequency of positives in small-volume partitions, the quantification is not affected by delayed amplification or variability in Cq values, as in the case for qPCR [33]. This leads to higher precision [12–14, 33–36], with coefficients of variation in the same run decreased 37–86% for ddPCR as compared to qPCR [14]. Improvement in repeatability has been found to be most pronounced when target concentrations are low [12, 13, 35]. This high precision improves one's ability to distinguish small differences among samples: ddPCR can detect a

1.25-fold difference, while this goal is only achieved by a great number of replicates ($n = 86$) in qPCR, which can typically detect twofold differences (i.e., one Cq) [16, 37].

As digital PCR quantification is based on binary results, this eliminates variability associated with qPCR standards (e.g., variability in quantification, source, batch, storage, handling, and serial dilution of qPCR standards) that may be the largest contributors to poor reproducibility of qPCR across operators, runs, and laboratories, especially over an extended period of time [22, 38]. For example, Hindson et al. [14] reported a sevenfold increase in day-to-day reproducibility for ddPCR compared to qPCR in microRNA quantification for clinic applications [14]. Similarly, Cao et al. [13] found that run-to-run variability over a month was reduced 2–3 times at log scale by ddPCR (range = 0.15–0.2 $\log_{10}$ copy per μl DNA) compared to qPCR (range = 0.53 and 0.43 $\log_{10}$ copy per μl DNA) for *Enterococcus* spp. and human-associated HF183 fecal marker quantification in recreational water quality applications. Highly reproducible results were also obtained at different times on a chamber digital PCR platform [34] and even between different primer-probe sets targeting the same DNA molecule [13, 34].

3.2.1 Sensitivity

Reports comparing sensitivity between digital PCR and qPCR are less consistent than that for comparison of precision. While some studies reported higher sensitivity [39, 40] of ddPCR, others reported similar [13, 36, 41] or even lower [42] ddPCR sensitivity. These inconsistent findings may be largely attributed to difference in the definition of sensitivity used by these authors and the different ways sensitivity might be compared. Even if the absolute analytical sensitivity (e.g., copy per reaction) is similar between two methods, the nominal analytical sensitivity may differ because of different sample volume or sample quality. For example, ddPCR showed much lower sensitivity for detecting *Cytomegalovirus* than qPCR, but each ddPCR reaction only received a sample volume that was ¼ of that received by each qPCR reaction [42]. With low-quality samples (e.g., samples containing PCR inhibitors), PCR amplification efficiency can be reduced, which reduces qPCR quantification, but affects ddPCR much less due to the binary nature of ddPCR quantification. As a result, higher nominal sensitivity was reported for ddPCR than qPCR in analyzing low-quality samples such as pond water [40] and soil [39].

With well-designed qPCR and digital PCR assays using the same primers and probes, the absolute analytical sensitivities are likely similar and determined by the theoretical detection limit governed by Poisson subsampling. However, digital PCR may have higher nominal sensitivity owing to the binary nature of quantification [39, 40] and the digital PCR partitioning process [16]. While it is difficult for qPCR to detect one copy of mutant DNA in the background of 100,000 copy of wild-type DNA, the partitioning process in ddPCR significantly lowers the difficulty of amplification because the mutant to wild-type ratio in one droplet is drastically increased after the bulk reaction has been partitioned into tens of thousands of droplets.

4 Advanced Performance Metrics

4.1 Tolerance to PCR Inhibition

Increased tolerance to inhibition is another advantage of digital PCR that has been reported across many studies [13, 35, 36, 40, 43–45]. Digital PCR was found to be more tolerant to inhibitors from food and feed samples [35], fecal samples [36], plant material [46], soil [43, 46], environmental waters [13, 40], and effluent from wastewater treatment plants [44, 46], in either the droplet form (most studies) or the chip-based chamber form [43, 45]. Droplet digital PCR quantification was shown to be unaffected by humic acid or organic matter concentrations (spiked into reactions) 1–2 orders of magnitude higher than that tolerated by qPCR [13]. Further, a chip-based chamber digital PCR was shown to provide unaffected quantification at 6% v/v ethanol compared to controls in all nine replicates while qPCR completely failed in six replicates and provided severe underestimation in three replicates [45].

This high tolerance against inhibition is largely attributed to the binary nature of digital PCR. PCR inhibitors often reduce PCR amplification efficiency by interfering with polymerase or the polymerase-DNA machinery, leading to increased Cq values and hence underestimation in qPCR [23]. However, reduced amplification efficiency still yields positive endpoint PCR, albeit with lower fluorescence signals [13] and therefore does not affect digital PCR quantification, which is based on counting the percentage of positive partitions. An additional mechanism that may help combat inhibition in digital PCR is the partitioning of bulk reactions into small volumes because this reduces the total amount of inhibitors available per reaction and/or reduces background DNA concentrations [16], but the benefit from that aspect of partitioning is still in need of further study.

It is important to note that PCR inhibitors function via complex mechanisms which can vary by type and concentration of inhibitors [47] and may not always be alleviated by the binary nature of digital PCR. For example, extremely high concentration of inhibitors can completely shut down the amplification machinery (instead of just reducing efficiency) leading to failure in both qPCR and digital PCR [13, 36]. While a chip-based chamber digital PCR system showed high resistance to the inhibitory effect of ethanol, the same system appeared just as inhibited as qPCR with 25% v/v plasma and even more inhibited than qPCR with 3.5 mM EDTA in the same study [45]. Different digital PCR systems may also differ in tolerance to PCR inhibitors because they use different types of polymerase and reaction buffers that can be differentially susceptible to various inhibitors [23, 48]. Moreover, the binary nature of digital PCR may not be very useful in combating inhibition if inhibition is caused by template sequestration (i.e., inhibitors bind to DNA making it unavailable for amplification) [23].

4.2 Capacity to Multiplex

Another area in which digital PCR has an advantage over qPCR is in the ability to simultaneously amplify and measure multiple targets in the same sample, termed multiplexing. In qPCR, it is difficult to multiplex because simultaneous amplification of multiple targets in one reaction causes competition for reagents between the targets being amplified. Due to differences in primer/probe design and/or differences in target concentrations present in the qPCR bulk reaction, one target gets a head-start in amplification over another target and is more successful in competing for reagents. This differential success in competing for reagents is magnified as PCR progresses, leading to the outperforming target suppressing amplification of the underperforming target, which in turn leads to underestimation of the latter. Therefore, in multiplex qPCR, it is often necessary to painstakingly manipulate primer and probe design and/or concentration to enable multiplexing [49, 50]. Even then, performance of multiplex qPCR is at the mercy of the relative concentrations of the multiplexed targets. A high concentration of one target may completely suppress quantification of the lower concentration target [13, 50].

In contrast, when multiplexing in digital PCR, reagent competition is alleviated. This is due to the partitioning process, in which the "multiplex" bulk reaction is divided into a huge number of miniature reactions containing only one copy of one target or at most a few copies of one or more targets (much less frequent than the one copy scenario due to Poisson distribution governing the partitioning process) [51]. In the case that a miniature reaction contains only one copy of one target, different miniature reactions independently quantify different targets without any adverse competition between targets but enable simultaneous quantification of multiple targets at the bulk reaction level; In the rare case that a miniature reaction contains a few copies of multiple targets, all targets are present at low and similar concentrations (one or two copies at most), significantly reducing the potential for reagent competition.

Two types of digital PCR multiplexing have been reported. The first type is where Taqman probes labeled with different color fluorophores are used to detect different targets [13, 35, 52]. This has been used to simultaneously quantify target and reference genes for genetically modified organisms in food and feed samples [35] and the staphylococcal protein and the methicillin-resistance genes for methicillin-resistance *Staphylococcus aureus* cultures [52] with ddPCR. Another duplex ddPCR assay was also developed to simultaneously quantify general and human-associated fecal contamination in recreational waters [13]. In this case, the duplex ddPCR assay produced nearly identical results as simplex ddPCR assays (Fig. 3), even in the presence of high inhibitor

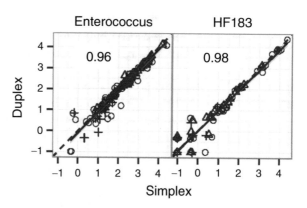

Fig. 3 Comparison of duplex and simplex ddPCR quantification of *Enterococcus* and the HF183 human-fecal marker in fecal (*circles*) and water (freshwater: *triangles*; marine water: *crosses*) samples. Regression lines (*solid lines*), their standard errors (*gray shading*), and corresponding correlation coefficients are as displayed

concentrations [13]. Building on these previous studies, we have developed a large suite of duplex assays for testing environmental waters for fecal contamination and waterborne pathogens, including assays that simultaneously measure general and human- or cow-associated fecal contamination, abundance of generic and pathogenic *Salmonella* and two dominant protozoan pathogens *Giardia* and *Cryptosporidium* (Cao, unpublished data).

The second type of digital PCR multiplexing is multiplexing with a single-color DNA-binding dye, which has been reported for ddPCR [17, 53]. This type of multiplexing is enabled purely by the partitioning process in ddPCR and is not possible with qPCR [17]. Essentially, the fluorescent amplitude (i.e., the accumulative endpoint fluorescence) of DNA-binding dye is proportional to the size of the amplicon (i.e., the length of the amplification target) because a longer amplicon allows more dye molecules to bind, leading to higher fluorescence per amplicon. Since qPCR measures total fluorescence in one bulk reaction where all amplicons are mixed together, qPCR cannot simultaneously quantify two targets that differ in amplicon size but emitting the same wavelength fluorescent signal. The reason it is possible to quantify different size amplicons with the same fluorophore using ddPCR is because the partitioning process causes them to accumulate in different droplets, where fluorescent signals are measured independently. Consequently, the relationship between fluorescence amplitude and amplicon size can be used to distinguish multiple targets that are of different size (or designed to be of different size through manipulating the length of primers) [53]. Because DNA-binding dye is substantially cheaper than customized Taqman probes, such amplicon size-enabled ddPCR multiplexing is preferred by some practitioners. For example, two studies demonstrated proof of concept testing clinical samples [17, 53], which are usually less complex and have less PCR inhibitors than do environmental samples. Whether this form of multiplex is feasible with environmental samples, which often contain inhibitors, is uncertain. This is because inhibition also lowers the fluorescence amplitude [13] just as a small amplicon would, making it difficult to distinguish if a sample has multiple targets or is experiencing inhibition.

4.3 Time to Result

The time to result for digital PCR, although it may differ slightly among the different digital PCR systems, is not appreciably different than that for qPCR. The sampling and preparation steps to capture the DNA are identical between the two, but subsequent analysis contains steps unique to one or the other (Fig. 1). For most commercially available systems, the digital PCR workflow contains two additional steps (Fig. 1), namely, partition before PCR and fluorescence read post PCR, compared to qPCR. These two steps add 2–3 min per sample. However, digital PCR saves time as it eliminates the need to prepare and run (or rerun) standard curves, which could be particularly advantageous when running a small number of samples and for which the ratio of number of standard reactions to number of sample reactions is high. There is also some potential time saving of not having to dilute or purify DNA to overcome inhibition. Overall, time to result consideration will not be a primary reason for adoption of digital PCR.

4.4 Cost

Conflicting reports have been published comparing cost between digital PCR and qPCR. While some researchers reported digital PCR as a less expensive alternative [8, 13, 35], others concluded digital PCR is more expensive than qPCR [12, 36]. The conflicting reports most likely reflect differences in how costs were compared: whether costs were compared per target per sample or per run, whether and how labor costs (waiting vs. hands-on time) were estimated, and whether capital cost is considered. Cost estimates can also differ among different droplet and chamber digital PCR systems due to the different consumables required. Conceptually, though, digital PCR should be more cost-effective than qPCR. First, digital PCR is more resistant to inhibition, and in many circumstances, it may be possible to use crude DNA extracts [13], thus eliminating labor and material cost associated with DNA purification, which is often a significant portion of material and labor cost. Second, the greater flexibility to multiplex in digital PCR than in qPCR offers tremendous opportunity for increasing information gathered per analysis and thus reducing cost [13, 35]. Last, the capacity to run single-color DNA-binding dye-based multiplex assays on droplet-based digital PCR systems can be significantly less costly than typical probe-based multiplex assays [17].

Beyond these theoretical cost advantages, the present cost of digital PCR is higher because it is early in the production cycle for this technology. For instance, the capital cost for a ddPCR system is presently 2–4 times that for a qPCR system as the number of instruments sold is still small, and there are a limited number of

manufacturers. Similarly, many of the supplies are presently produced in quantities appropriate to research applications, which are
more expensive than when developed for mass production as they
are now for qPCR. However, it is difficult to make an accurate comparison of cost at this time since capital and consumable costs for
molecular technologies have been found to decrease quickly with
technology advancement and market growth [54]. Additionally,
the development and commercialization of affordable autonomous
real-time monitoring systems or field portable systems are likely to
reduce technical complexity and cost further [15].

5   Limitations of Digital PCR

As partition and the binary nature of digital PCR leads to many
advantages described above for digital PCR, these same two features also bring limitations unique to digital PCR. Because digital
PCR quantifies based on the proportion of partitions that are positive, digital PCR cannot provide quantification if all partitions are
positive or negative. The dynamic range of digital PCR is therefore
limited by the number of partitions [16]. A dynamic range of five
orders of magnitude may be expected with 10,000–17,000 droplets commonly observed for the QX100 ddPCR system [13, 35,
51]. In comparison, qPCR frequently offers a wider dynamic range
of 6–9 orders of magnitude. While the QX100 ddPCR dynamic
range is generally sufficient for monitoring of fecal contamination
in ambient waters because concentrations of *Enterococcus* spp. and
human-fecal markers rarely exceed the upper qualification limits
[13], dilution of highly concentrated samples may be necessary
when using ddPCR. Nevertheless, for public health management
decisions, a result above upper quantification limit can be as relevant as an exact quantification. Multiple dilutions of the sample
may also be analyzed to provide a combined wide dynamic range,
as commonly done for culture-based methods, which have a nar-
rower dynamic range than digital PCR.

Additionally, the Poisson statistics require uniformity in the
partition. Factors such as viscous DNA template due to high
concentration or extreme length that affect unbiased partitions can
affect accuracy of digital PCR quantification. For example, the
general recommendation for ddPCR is to have <66 ng total
DNA per reaction without pretreatment by restriction enzymes
(Bio-Rad, QX100 and QX200 systems). Dilution or pretreatment
by restriction enzymes should be considered if high biomass is
expected in environmental waters [13]. Dissociation of double-
strand DNA to single-strand DNA due to heating prior to the partition process can lead to up to twofold overestimation by digital
PCR, because one dsDNA molecule can only occupy one partition, while two ssDNA molecules can occupy two partitions [55].
Moreover, tandem distribution of target genes in close proximity

on a DNA template will lead to underestimation of target by ddPCR if these tandem copies remain linked and end up in the same partition [13]. This linkage of targets generally only becomes an issue when the tandem copies are within <50 kb (Bio-Rad, personal communication) because many DNA isolation procedures will fragment DNA such that only tandem copies fairly close to each other on the genome would remain linked [13]. However, assay developers should be mindful in assay design to avoid this linkage issue. For example, one may opt to choose a single copy gene as measurement target or examine the number and distance of multiple operons on the genomes (as done previously; [13] if available.

Lastly, environmental application of reverse transcriptase-digital PCR has been limited to a few reports of reverse transcriptase ddPCR for quantifying RNA viruses [44, 46], and it is uncertain if RT-ddPCR affords to the same extent all advantages of ddPCR. More studies are warranted on both two- and one-step reverse transcriptase-digital PCR.

6   Suitability of Digital PCR for Ambient Water Monitoring

Ambient water monitoring has some unique challenges that digital PCR is uniquely suited to overcome. For instance, ambient water monitoring often involves detecting rare targets in complex environmental matrices. Additionally, ambient waters often contain potentially PCR inhibitory substances and a high background of nontarget nucleic acid pool that can be problematic for qPCR implementation [3, 20]. For example, human pathogens (e.g., bacteria, protozoan, and viral pathogens) are generally present in waters at low titer but generally have a low infectious dose [56]. Consequently, false negatives (i.e., failure to detect rare targets due to inhibition), inability to analyze a higher volume of samples, and/or interference from nontarget DNA are highly undesirable. Similarly, effective biodiversity management requires sensitive early detection of invasive species while they are in low abundances such that control and eradication efforts might be successful and far less expensive than when the invasive population has become highly abundant and has spread [57]. Early warning of potential harmful algal blooms would also benefit greatly from sensitive detection of toxin-producing cyanobacteria before the onset of the blooms [49]. In this regard, digital PCR has demonstrated higher tolerance to inhibition and higher nominal sensitivity [13, 16, 35, 36, 40, 43–45] compared to qPCR and therefore may be well suited to detect low concentration targets in complex ambient water environments. The improved precision of digital PCR over qPCR at low concentration is also particular valuable for ambient water applications [13, 35, 40].

Another important aspect of ambient water monitoring is the great need to discern and/or compare temporal and spatial patterns, but monitoring data can be inherently noisy and being able to distinguish true patterns from methodological variability is challenging. For instance, understanding spatial and temporal patterns of endangered or invasive species is vital to resource management [3]. For qPCR, potentially high run-to-run variability, especially over months to years, can be expected due to the variability in standards preparation, storage and handling and qPCR's intrinsic sensitivity to deviation in amplification efficiency. Such variability creates noise in monitoring data and limits qPCR's ability to identify trends, contributing to reluctance in adopting molecular quantification techniques for routine monitoring [58]. In this regard, the high repeatability and reproducibility afforded by digital PCR within runs, between runs, operators, and laboratories can be a significant advantage [14].

Finally, autonomous real-time monitoring systems are highly sought after because speed is critical to timely water quality notification and remedial action [59–61]. For recreational water quality monitoring, conventional culture-based methods take 18–96 h to achieve results due to the incubation time needed to grow fecal indicator bacteria. This delay allows for public exposure to bad water quality or unnecessary waste of recreational resources while waiting for laboratory results before posting or reopening a beach. Molecular-based methods bypass the culturing step and enable same day notification for better public health protection [6] and have been included as a viable alternative monitoring method in the revised recreational water quality criteria by USEPA [62]. However, such rapid water monitoring has been found to be viable for only a limited number of sites that are relatively close to the laboratory because sample transport adds significantly to the sample-to-result time, making the entire monitoring procedure no longer rapid [6, 60]. Autonomous real-time monitoring systems can remove the sample transport time, and enable fast management response [60]. While many system engineering challenges need to be overcome to arrive at practical and cost-effective autonomous real-time water monitoring systems [59], digital PCR is particularly suited for such systems because it bypasses the challenge of running a standard curve under field conditions. Moreover, because of the binary nature of its quantification, digital PCR only requires endpoint detection of fluorescence after completion of PCR amplification, which eliminates the need for expensive optics necessary for continuous real-time fluorescence detection during amplification. Finally, the droplet form of digital PCR could be particularly advantageous as sample material is encapsulated inside water-in-oil droplets, minimizing sample contact with tubing and other engineering parts inside autonomous systems where effective and complete disinfection can be challenging and sometimes ineffective [60].

Acknowledgment

The authors wish to thank Meredith Raith and Lucy Mao for laboratory assistance in validating the ddPCR assays presented in Table 1 and Jingrang Lu and Josh Steele for discussion in selecting primer/probe for the *Campylobacter* and *Salmonella* ddPCR assays, respectively.

References

1. Boehm AB, Ashbolt NJ, Colford JM, Dunbar LE, Fleming LE, Gold MA, Hansel JA, Hunter PR, Ichida AM, McGee CD, Soller JA, Weisberg SB (2009) A sea change ahead for recreational water quality criteria. J Water Health 7(1):9–20. doi:10.2166/wh.2009.122

2. Bourlat SJ, Borja A, Gilbert J, Taylor MI, Davies N, Weisberg SB, Griffith JF, Lettieri T, Field D, Benzie J, Glockner FO, Rodriguez-Ezpeleta N, Faith DP, Bean TP, Obst M (2013) Genomics in marine monitoring: new opportunities for assessing marine health status. Mar Pollut Bull 74(1):19–31. doi:10.1016/j.marpolbul.2013.05.042

3. Thomsen PF, Willerslev E (2015) Environmental DNA – an emerging tool in conservation for monitoring past and present biodiversity. Biol Conserv 183:4–18. doi:10.1016/j.biocon.2014.11.019

4. Converse RR, Griffith JF, Noble RT, Haugland RA, Schiff KC, Weisberg SB (2012) Correlation between quantitative polymerase chain reaction and culture-based methods for measuring *Enterococcus* over various temporal scales and three California marine beaches. Appl Environ Microbiol 78(4):1237–1242

5. Raith MR, Ebentier DL, Cao Y, Griffith JF, Weisberg SB (2013) Factors affecting the relationship between quantitative polymerase chain reaction (qPCR) and culture-based enumeration of Enterococcus in environmental waters. J Appl Microbiol. doi:10.1111/jam.12383

6. Griffith JF, Weisberg SB (2011) Challenges in implementing new technology for beach water quality monitoring: lessons from a California demonstration project. Mar Techol Soc J 45:65–73

7. Boehm AB, Van De Werfhorst LC, Griffith JF, Holden PA, Jay JA, Shanks OC, Wang D, Weisberg SB (2013) Performance of forty-one microbial source tracking methods: a twenty-seven lab evaluation study. Water Res 47(18):6812–6828

8. Nathan LM, Simmons M, Wegleitner BJ, Jerde CL, Mahon AR (2014) Quantifying environmental DNA signals for aquatic invasive species across multiple detection platforms. Environ Sci Technol 48(21):12800–12806. doi:10.1021/es5034052

9. Zhang W, Lou I, Ung WK, Kong Y, Mok KM (2014) Application of PCR and real-time PCR for monitoring cyanobacteria, Microcystis spp. and Cylindrospermopsis raciborskii in Macau freshwater reservoir. Front Earth Sci 8(2):291–301. doi:10.1007/s11707-013-0409-4

10. Zhang F, Lee J, Liang S, Shum CK (2015) Cyanobacteria blooms and non-alcoholic liver disease: evidence from a county level ecological study in the United States. Environ Health 14:41. doi:10.1186/s12940-015-0026-7

11. Baker M (2011) qPCR: quicker and easier but don't be sloppy. Nat Methods 8(3):207–212. doi:10.1038/nmeth0311-207

12. Doi H, Uchii K, Takahara T, Matsuhashi S, Yamanaka H, Minamoto T (2015) Use of droplet digital PCR for estimation of fish abundance and biomass in environmental DNA surveys. PLoS One 10(3), e0122763. doi:10.1371/journal.pone.0122763

13. Cao Y, Raith MR, Griffith JF (2015) Droplet digital PCR for simultaneous quantification of general and human-associated fecal indicators for water quality assessment. Water Res 70:337–349. doi:10.1016/j.watres.2014.12.008

14. Hindson CM, Chevillet JR, Briggs HA, Gallichotte EN, Ruf IK, Hindson BJ, Vessella RL, Tewari M (2013) Absolute quantification by droplet digital PCR versus analog real-time PCR. Nat Methods 10(10):1003–1005

15. Marx V (2015) PCR heads into the field. Nat Methods 12(5):393–397. doi:10.1038/nmeth.3369

16. Hindson BJ, Ness KD, Masquelier DA, Belgrader P, Heredia NJ, Makarewicz AJ, Bright IJ, Lucero MY, Hiddessen AL (2011) High-throughput droplet digital PCR system for absolute quantitation of DNA copy number. Anal Chem 83:8604–8610

17. McDermott GP, Do D, Litterst CM, Maar D, Hindson CM, Steenblock ER, Legler TC, Jouvenot Y, Marrs SH, Bemis A, Shah P, Wong J, Wang S, Sally D, Javier L, Dinio T, Han C,

Brackbill TP, Hodges SP, Ling Y, Klitgord N, Carman GJ, Berman JR, Koehler RT, Hiddessen AL, Walse P, Bousse L, Tzonev S, Hefner E, Hindson BJ, Cauly TH III, Hamby K, Patel VP, Regan JF, Wyatt PW, Karlin-Neumann GA, Stumbo DP, Lowe AJ (2013) Multiplexed target detection using DNA-binding dye chemistry in droplet digital PCR. Anal Chem 85(23):11619–11627. doi:10.1021/ac403061n

18. Vogelstein B, Kinzler KW (1999) Digital PCR. Proc Natl Acad Sci 96:9236–9241

19. Baker M (2012) Digital PCR hits its stride. Nat Methods 9(6):541–544

20. Cao Y, Sivaganesan M, Kinzelman J, Blackwood AD, Noble RT, Haugland RA, Griffith JF, Weisberg SB (2013) Effect of platform, reference material, and quantification model on enumeration of Enterococcus by quantitative PCR methods. Water Res 47(1):233–241. doi:10.1016/j.watres.2012.09.056

21. Sivaganesan M, Siefring S, Varma M, Haugland RA (2011) MPN estimation of qPCR target sequence recoveries from whole cell calibrator samples. J Microbiol Methods 87(3):343–349. doi:10.1016/j.mimet.2011.09.013

22. Shanks OC, Sivaganesan M, Peed L, Kelty CA, Blackwood AD, Greene MR, Noble RT, Bushon RN, Stelzer EA, Kinzelman J, Anan'eva T, Sinigalliano C, Wanless D, Griffith J, Cao Y, Weisberg S, Harwood VJ, Staley C, Oshima KH, Varma M, Haugland RA (2012) Inter-laboratory general fecal indicator quantitative real-time PCR methods comparison study. Environ Sci Technol 46(2):945–953

23. Cao Y, Griffith JF, Dorevitch S, Weisberg SB (2012) Effectiveness of qPCR permutations, internal controls and dilution as means for minimizing the impact of inhibition while measuring Enterococcus in environmental waters. J Appl Microbiol 113(1):66–75

24. Whale AS, Cowen S, Foy CA, Huggett JF (2013) Methods for applying accurate digital PCR analysis on low copy DNA samples. PLoS One 8(3), e58177

25. U.S. EPA (2010) Method B. Bacteroidales in water by TaqMan® quantitative polymerase chain reaction (qPCR) assay. EPA-822-R-10-003. Office of Water, Washington, DC

26. Chern EC, Siefring S, Paar J, Doolittle M, Haugland RA (2011) Comparison of quantitative PCR assays for Escherichia coli targeting ribosomal RNA and single copy genes. Lett Appl Microbiol 52(3):298–306. doi:10.1111/j.1472-765X.2010.03001.x

27. Green HC, Haugland RA, Varma M, Millen HT, Borchardt MA, Field KG, Walters WA, Knight R, Sivaganesan M, Kelty CA, Shanks OC (2014) Improved HF183 quantitative real-time PCR assay for characterization of human fecal pollution in ambient surface water samples. Appl Environ Microbiol 80(10):3086–3094. doi:10.1128/AEM.04137-13

28. Shanks OC, Atikovic E, Blackwood AD, Lu J, Noble RT, Domingo JS, Seifring S, Sivaganesan M, Haugland RA (2008) Quantitative PCR for detection and enumeration of genetic markers of bovine fecal pollution. Appl Environ Microbiol 74(3):745–752. doi:10.1128/aem.01843-07

29. Lee C, Marion JW, Lee J (2013) Development and application of a quantitative PCR assay targeting Catellicoccus marimammalium for assessing gull-associated fecal contamination at Lake Erie beaches. Sci Total Environ 454–455:1–8. doi:10.1016/j.scitotenv.2013.03.003

30. Lund M, Nordentoft S, Pedersen K, Madsen M (2004) Detection of Campylobacter spp. in chicken fecal samples by real-time PCR. J Clin Microbiol 42(11):5125–5132. doi:10.1128/JCM.42.11.5125-5132.2004

31. Cao Y, Raith MR, Griffith JF (2016) A duplex digital PCR assay for simultaneous quantification of the Enterococcus spp. and the human fecal-associated HF183 marker in waters. J Vis Exp 109, e53611

32. Bustin SA, Benes V, Garson JA, Hellemans J, Huggett J, Kubista M, Mueller R, Nolan T, Pfaffl MW, Shipley GL, Vandesompele J, Wittwer CT (2009) The MIQE guidelines: minimum information for publication of quantitative real-time PCR experiments. Clin Chem 55(4):611–622. doi:10.1373/clinchem.2008.112797

33. Whale AS, Hugget JF, Cowen S, Speirs V, Shaw J, Ellison S, Foy CA, Scott DJ (2012) Comparison of microfluidic digital PCR and conventional quantitative PCR for measuring copy number variation. Nucleic Acid Res 40(11):e82–e89. doi:10.1093/nar/gks1203

34. Sanders R, Huggett JF, Bushell CA, Cowen S, Scott DJ, Foy CA (2011) Evaluation of digital PCR for absolute DNA quantification. Anal Chem 83(17):6474–6484

35. Morisset D, Štebih D, Milavec M, Gruden K, Žel J (2013) Quantitative analysis of food and feed samples with droplet digital PCR. PLoS One 8(5):62583, 62510.61371/journal.pone.0062583

36. Yang R, Paparini A, Monis P, Ryan U (2014) Comparison of next-generation droplet digital PCR (ddPCR) with quantitative PCR (qPCR) for enumeration of Cryptosporidium oocysts in faecal samples. Int J Parasitol 44(14):1105–1113. doi:10.1016/j.ijpara.2014.08.004

37. Norton SE, Lechner JM, Williams T, Fernando MR (2013) A stabilizing reagent prevents cell-free DNA contamination by cellular DNA in

plasma during blood sample storage and shipping as determined by digital PCR. Clin Biochem 46(15):1561–1565. doi:10.1016/j.clinbiochem.2013.06.002

38. Ebentier DL, Hanley KT, Cao Y, Badgley B, Boehm A, Ervin J, Goodwin KD, Gourmelon M, Griffith J, Holden P, Kelty CA, Lozach S, McGee C, Peed L, Raith M, Sadowsky MJ, Scott E, Santodomingo J, Sinigalliano C, Shanks OC, Werfhorst LCVD, Wang D, Wuertz S, Jay J (2013) Evaluation of the repeatability and reproducibility of a suite of PCR-based microbial source tracking methods. Water Res 47(18):6839–6848

39. Kim TG, Jeong SY, Cho KS (2014) Comparison of droplet digital PCR and quantitative real-time PCR for examining population dynamics of bacteria in soil. Appl Microbiol Biotechnol 98(13):6105–6113.   doi:10.1007/s00253-014-5794-4

40. Doi H, Takahara T, Minamoto T, Matsuhashi S, Uchii K, Yamanaka H (2015) Droplet digital polymerase chain reaction (PCR) outperforms real-time PCR in the detection of environmental DNA from an invasive fish species. Environ Sci Technol 49(9):5601–5608. doi:10.1021/acs.est.5b00253

41. Dreo T, Pirc M, Ramsak Z, Pavsic J, Milavec M, Zel J, Gruden K (2014) Optimising droplet digital PCR analysis approaches for detection and quantification of bacteria: a case study of fire blight and potato brown rot. Anal Bioanal Chem 406(26):6513–6528. doi:10.1007/s00216-014-8084-1

42. Hayden RT, Gu Z, Ingersoll J, Abdul-Ali D, Shi L, Pounds S, Caliendo AM (2013) Comparison of droplet digital PCR to real-time PCR for quantitative detection of cytomegalovirus. J Clin Microbiol 51(2):540–546

43. Hoshino T, Inagaki F (2012) Molecular quantification of environmental DNA using microfluidics and digital PCR. Syst Appl Microbiol 35(6):390–395. doi:10.1016/j.syapm.2012.06.006

44. Rački N, Morisset D, Gutierrez-Aguirre I, Ravnikar M (2013) One-step RT-droplet digital PCR: a breakthrough in the quantification of waterborne RNA viruses. Anal Bioanal Chem. doi:10.1007/s00216-013-7476-y

45. Nixon G, Garson JA, Grant P, Nastouli E, Foy CA, Huggett JF (2014) Comparative study of sensitivity, linearity, and resistance to inhibition of digital and nondigital polymerase chain reaction and loop mediated isothermal amplification assays for quantification of human cytomegalovirus. Anal Chem 86(9):4387–4394. doi:10.1021/ac500208w

46. Racki N, Dreo T, Gutierrez-Aguirre I, Blejec A, Ravnikar M (2014) Reverse transcriptase droplet digital PCR shows high resilience to PCR inhibitors from plant, soil and water samples. Plant Methods 10(1):42. doi:10.1186/s13007-014-0042-6

47. Opel KL, Chung D, McCord BR (2010) A study of PCR inhibition mechanisms using real time PCR. J Forensic Sci 55(1):25–33

48. Abu Al-Soud W, Radstrom P (1998) Capacity of nine thermostable DNA polymerases to mediate DNA amplification in the presence of PCR-inhibiting samples. Appl Environ Microbiol 64(10):3748–3753

49. Al-Tebrineh J, Pearson LA, Yasar SA, Neilan BA (2012) A multiplex qPCR targeting hepato- and neurotoxigenic cyanobacteria of global significance. Harmful Algae 15:19–25. doi:10.1016/j.hal.2011.11.001

50. Hoorfar J, Malorny B, Abdulmawjood A, Cook N, Wagner M, Fach P (2004) Practical considerations in design of internal amplification controls for diagnostic PCR assays. J Clin Microbiol 42(5):1863–1868. doi:10.1128/jcm.42.5.1863-1868.2004

51. Huggett JF, Foy CA, Benes V, Emslie K, Garson JA, Haynes R, Hellemans J, Kubista M, Mueller RD, Nolan T, Pfaffl MW, Shipley GL, Vandesompele J, Wittwer CT, Bustin SA (2013) The digital MIQE guidelines: minimum information for publication of quantitative digital PCR experiments. Clin Chem 59(6):892–902

52. Kelley K, Cosman A, Belgrader P, Chapman B, Sullivan DC (2013) Detection of methicillin-resistant Staphylococcus aureus by a duplex droplet digital PCR assay. J Clin Microbiol 51(7):2033–2039. doi:10.1128/JCM.00196-13

53. Miotke L, Lau BT, Rumma RT, Ji HP (2014) High sensitivity detection and quantitation of DNA copy number and single nucleotide variants with single color droplet digital PCR. Anal Chem 86(5):2618–2624. doi:10.1021/ac403843j

54. Hauser L, Seeb JE (2008) Advances in molecular technology and their impact on fisheries genetics. Fish Fish 9(4):473–486. doi:10.1111/j.1467-2979.2008.00306.x

55. Bhat S, McLaughlin JL, Emslie KR (2011) Effect of sustained elevated temperature prior to amplification on template copy number estimation using digital polymerase chain reaction. Analyst 136(4):724–732. doi:10.1039/c0an00484g

56. Jothikumar N, Cromeans TL, Hill VR, Lu X, Sobsey MD, Erdman DD (2005) Quantitative

real-time PCR assays for detection of human adenoviruses and identification of serotypes 40 and 41. Appl Environ Microbiol 71(6):3131–3136. doi:10.1128/AEM.71.6.3131-3136.2005

57. Goldberg CS, Sepulveda A, Ray A, Baumgardt J, Waits LP (2013) Environmental DNA as a new method for early detection of New Zealand mudsnails (Potamopyrgus antipodarum). Freshw Sci 32(3):792–800. doi:10.1899/13-046.1

58. Sagarin R, Carlsson J, Duval M, Freshwater W, Godfrey MH, Litaker W, Muñoz R, Noble R, Schultz T, Wynne B (2009) Bringing molecular tools into environmental resource management: untangling the molecules to policy pathway. PLoS Biol 7(3), e1000069. doi:10.1371/journal.pbio.1000069

59. Scholin CA (2010) What are "ecogenomic sensors?" A review and thoughts for the future. Ocean Sci 6:51–60

60. Yamahara KM, Demir-Hilton E, Preston CM, Marin R 3rd, Pargett D, Roman B, Jensen S, Birch JM, Boehm AB, Scholin CA (2015) Simultaneous monitoring of faecal indicators and harmful algae using an in-situ autonomous sensor. Lett Appl Microbiol 61(2):130–138. doi:10.1111/lam.12432

61. Korostynska O, Mason A, Al-Shamma'a AI (2013) Monitoring pollutants in wastewater: traditional lab based versus modern real-time approaches. In: Mukhopadhyay SC, Mason A (eds) Smart sensors for real-time water quality monitoring, vol 4. Smart sensors, measurement and instrumentation, vol 4. Springer, Berlin, pp 1–24. doi:10.1007/978-3-642-37006-9_1

62. U.S. EPA (2012) Recreational water quality criteria. EPA 820-F-12-058. Office of Water, Washington, DC

Chapter 8

Using Environmental DNA for Invasive Species Surveillance and Monitoring

Andrew R. Mahon and Christopher L. Jerde

Abstract

The method employed for environmental DNA (eDNA) surveillance for detection and monitoring of rare species in aquatic systems has evolved dramatically since its first large-scale applications. Both active (targeted) and passive (total diversity) surveillance methods provide helpful information for management groups, but each has a suite of techniques that necessitate proper equipment training and use. The protocols described in this chapter represent some of the latest iterations in eDNA surveillance being applied in aquatic and marine systems.

Key words eDNA, Noninvasive sampling, Detection, Metagenomics

1 Introduction

Indirect genetic detection of species from environmental samples is an emerging field in natural resource management and conservation biology [1–3]. While the general approach has been used in terrestrial studies for many years, applications of environmental DNA (eDNA) screening in aquatic environments have only recently been appreciated for their insights into the presence of incipient invasive species [4, 5] or threatened and endangered species [6, 7]. The general approach in aquatic systems is to collect a water sample, extract all the DNA from the sample, and then either screen for individual species using targeted, species-specific molecular markers [8] or high-throughput sequencing to reveal communities of species [9–11]. With the limitations in traditional aquatic sampling techniques, such as electrofishing and gill nets where some species are notably undetected due to low abundance or low probability of capture [12], there is growing interest in genetic and genomic applications for improved detection and monitoring of rare species, in particular for nonnative or invasive species [13, 14]. However, the same criticisms applied to traditional aquatic sampling techniques are also applicable to eDNA

Sarah J. Bourlat (ed.), *Marine Genomics: Methods and Protocols*, Methods in Molecular Biology, vol. 1452,
DOI 10.1007/978-1-4939-3774-5_8, © Springer Science+Business Media New York 2016

screening of species presence, and consequently, quantifying the accuracy and reliability of molecular surveillance results is essential to advance natural resource management based on eDNA detection of targeted species and total communities [15, 16].

Most eDNA surveillance studies on aquatic invasive species have focused on developing and implementing active surveillance that targets a single species [8, 17, 18]. Passive surveillance approaches, like high-throughput sequencing (HTS) applications, can potentially detect unexpected invasive species by screening all of the DNA in a given sample [9, 14] and identifying a community of species [10, 11]. In initial uses of eDNA for invasive species surveillance, methods were developed to provide rapid answers for management groups, leaving in-depth development of the tools by the wayside. Thus, the goals of this chapter are to not only describe the methods being implemented for eDNA surveillance of invasive species, but also to provide updates on where the methods in field are evolving and which methods are appropriate for specific situations.

To utilize eDNA as a surveillance platform and to choose a method to apply to the work, one must first consider active surveillance vs. passive surveillance techniques. Active surveillance, the most utilized route for eDNA surveillance to date, involves analyzing samples in a targeted fashion where samples are screened for a single species or group of species. Passive surveillance uses high-throughput sequencing platforms (HTS; i.e., next-generation sequencing methods) to screen for all species in a sample. The overall process for both active and passive eDNA surveillance involves initial sample collection, followed by DNA extraction and subsequent sample analysis (Fig. 1).

2 Materials

2.1 Sample Collection and Filtration

Sample filtration and preservation:

1. Sterile collection containers (250 ml volume or greater).
2. Whatman filter, 25 mm diameter, 5 μm pore size (GE Healthcare).
3. Whatman Swin-Lok filter holder (25 mm) or similar filter holder.
4. Plastic tubing.
5. Vacuum pump (either a hand pump or powered device similar to Pegasus Athena peristaltic pump will suffice).
6. Side-arm collection flask.
7. Plastic tubing.
8. Longmire's lysis buffer solution: 1 M Tris–HCl, pH 8.0, 0.5 M EDTA, pH 8.0, 5 M NaCl, Double-distilled (sterile) water, 25 ml of 20 % SDS per liter. Using a calibrated and decontaminated pipette, add 700 μl of Longmire's preservation buffer to

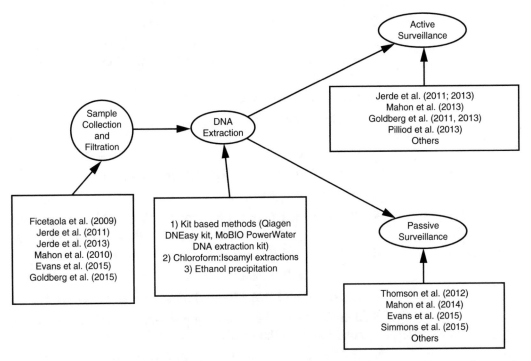

Fig. 1 Schematic flow chart for general eDNA surveillance methods and examples or published references for each associated step

each of the requisite number of 2 ml microcentrifuge tubes (i.e., 2× the number of 2 l water samples).

9. 2 ml microcentrifuge tubes.

2.2 DNA Extraction

1. Water bath (capable of 65 °C).

2. 24:1 chloroform:isoamyl alcohol.

3. Centrifuge for 2 ml tubes capable of $15,000 \times g$.

4. Micropipettes.

5. Ice cold isopropanol.

6. 5 M NaCl.

7. –20 °C freezer.

8. 70% ethanol.

9. TE buffer: 10 mM Tris, bring to pH 8.0 with HCl, 1 mM EDTA.

10. Optional Vacuum Centrifuge (e.g., Eppendorf™ Vacufuge™ Concentrator or equivalent).

2.3 Active Surveillance

1. For quantitative digital droplet Polymerase Chain Reaction (ddPCR): QX200™ AutoDG™ Droplet Digital™ PCR system and all associated consumables related to utilization of this system, available at http://bio-rad.com.

2. Micropipettes and tips for handling samples.

3. Species-specific PCR oligonucleotide primers and hydrolysis probe (project specific, related to intended target organism (s) of interest).

4. Microcentrifuge tubes.

5. Double-distilled (sterile) water.

2.4 Passive Surveillance

1. PCR thermocycler.

2. Micropipettes and tips for processing samples.

3. Microcentrifuge tubes.

4. PCR primers targeting amplicon that is general to the group of organisms under investigation (e.g., fish, invertebrates, etc.).

5. QIAquick Gel Extraction Kit (Qiagen Inc.).

6. Double-distilled (sterile) water.

7. TruSeq Nano DNA Library Preparation kit (Illumina).

8. Illumina MiSeq high-throughput DNA sequencer and associated flow cell (Illumina).

9. Unix-based computer for bioinformatics processing.

3   Methods

3.1 Sample Collection and Filtration

Routine sample collection involved taking a number of water samples from field locations to be screened. Early application of active surveillance using eDNA varied in the amount of water collected. Ficetola et al. used 15 ml samples in ponds [19]. Jerde et al. used two-liter water samples as a part of a broad-scale surveillance program for the invasive bighead and silver Asian carp (*Hypophthalmichthys* sp.) in the Laurentian Great Lakes [5, 17]. Recent work has moved to 250 ml samples being collected and filtered [10, 20]. Samples are collected and filtered in the field.

Using sterile collection containers, 250 ml water samples are collected from field locations and vacuum filtered through the Whatman Swin-lok filter holder onto the 5 µm PCTE filter paper. After filtration, the individual pieces of filter paper are then placed into 2 ml microcentrifuge tubes containing premade Longmire's solution [21]. In this solution, the genetic material collected is stable for at least 150 days at ambient temperature [22].

3.2 DNA Extraction

1. Heat the tube containing Longmire's solution and the collected sample on the PCTE filter at 65 °C in a water bath for 10 min.

2. Briefly cool the sample prior to adding 0.7 ml of 24:1 chloroform:isoamyl alcohol in a fume hood.

3. Mix the samples on a vortexer vertically for 5 min, dissolving the filter papers and lysing any cells in the sample.

4. Centrifuge the samples for 15 min at $15,000 \times g$ at room temperature.

5. Pipette the supernatant (~500 µl) to a new microcentrifuge tube.

6. Precipitate the DNA from the supernatant solution by adding an equal volume of ice-cold isopropanol and a half volume of 5 M NaCl, incubating this solution for ~1 h at –20 °C.

7. Pellet the DNA by centrifuging the sample at $15,000 \times g$ for 15 min at room temperature.

8. Pour off the supernatant and add 150 µl of 70 % ethanol, washing down the inner walls of the tube.

9. Repeat the 70 % ethanol wash and centrifugation.

10. Remove residual ethanol by air drying or use a vacuum centrifuge (45 °C, 5–10 min).

11. Resuspend the DNA by adding 100 µl of TE buffer and vortexing gently. If necessary, heat the solution for 10 min at 55 °C and remix via vortexing gently.

12. DNA extractions can be stored in the refrigerator (~4 °C) or at –20 to –80 °C until downstream analyses can be performed. Repeated freeze–thaw cycles should be avoided.

3.3 Active Surveillance

The goal of eDNA monitoring methods for many studies has been to develop a rapid, accurate, and relatively inexpensive surveillance tool that can be applied to the system in question. The large majority of studies to date have used routine equipment for sample analyses that most standard molecular ecology laboratories have on hand. Largely, active, targeted surveillance has necessitated using a detection platform such as polymerase chain reaction (PCR) for qualitative analyses (presence/absence of target DNA in a given sample). More recent studies have moved to quantitative measures, even beyond traditional qPCR, such as digital droplet PCR (ddPCR) that can calculate concentrations of target species DNA collected in a sample [20, 23–25].

Absolute concentrations of target species DNA can be measured using a BioRad© QX200 Droplet Digital PCR system and primers and hydrolysis probes developed for quantitative PCR (*see* [23], for example, of setup). Hydrolysis probes necessitate tagging, and in our prior work we have utilized a dual-labeled probe with a 5′ 6-FAM fluorescent tag and a 3′ Black Hole Quencher [20, 23], Simmons et al. [20]. The instrument can also utilize EvaGreen fluorescent chemistry, leaving out the need for probes. A routine ddPCR reaction mixture consists of 1000 nM of each primer and probe, 1× BioRad© ddPCR Supermix for probes, 2.5 µl DNA and sterile water for a total reaction volume of 25 µl. The BioRad© QX200 droplet generator partitions the reaction mixture into nanodroplets, combining 20 µl of the reaction mixture with 70 µl of droplet oil. This results in a total sample volume of 40 µl (>20,000 individual nanodroplets) containing sample, primers, probe, and mastermix, which is then transferred to a PCR plate for amplification and then screened and analyzed on the QX200 instrument. For each ddPCR plate run, negative and positive controls are necessary to evaluate potential contamination and success of the reaction chemistry, respectively.

3.4 Passive Surveillance

A number of preparatory steps are needed for using eDNA in passive surveillance, i.e., high-throughput sequencing screenings. Prior to sequencing, DNA extractions from field sites can be pooled by sample location into composite sample(s) [11, 20]. Individual or pooled samples are then PCR amplified using a targeted or universal vertebrate primer set [10, 26, 27]. Amplification and purification procedures vary by amplicon. Our approach described here follows methods developed in Evans et al. [10] for fish community analysis. For metabarcoding studies of marine invertebrates, *see* also Chapters 12 by Fonseca and Lallias, 13 by Bourlat et al., and 14 by Leray et al.

Library preparations are then performed on amplified PCR products for each sample using the Illumina TruSeq Nano DNA Library Preparation Kit, omitting the DNA fragmentation step due to the small, discrete size of the amplicons, typically less than 250 bp. Samples are then loaded onto a MiSeq v2 flow cell in equimolar amounts for sequencing using a 500 cycle (Paired end 250 bp; PE250) v2 reagent kit. Following sequencing, base calling is performed by Illumina Real Time Analysis (RTA) v1.18.54. The output of RTA is demultiplexed and converted to FastQ format with Illumina Bcl2fastq v1.8.4.

3.4.1 Bioinformatic and Statistical Analyses

To analyze the data after MiSeq sequencing, the resulting FastQ files are filtered to remove exact sequence duplicates, singletons, sequences with more than five ambiguous bases, and sequences with less than 100 bp using PRINSEQ v0.20.4 [28]. Custom databases can be generated to screen the resulting data using a script available at http://www.auburn.edu/~santosr/scripts/NCBI_retrieval.prl and NCBI's Genbank database. The NCBI's Basic Local Alignment Search Tool (BLAST) can then be used to analyze sequences at identity thresholds (>98% and with over 100 bp matches and expect values of less than 1e−5).

Evaluation of species distribution as inferred by eDNA detection in georeferenced water samples can be accomplished by using Species Occupancy Models (SOMs) [29, 30]. These models, in general, attempt to provide a probability of species occupancy at a location based on the occurrence record of species coupled to habitat covariates when the detection probability of the species is less than one [31]. These SOMs can incorporate replication at multiple levels (within sample and within locations), account for detection errors, and ultimate quantify incidences of false positives and negatives [32]. However, without SOM connections to the underlying hydrology, which would describe how DNA is transported in a system, occupancy in lotic systems may be limited [16].

4 Quality Assurance and Quality Control (QAQC)

Species distribution modeling has been used for conservation management and planning for many decades [33], but the use of eDNA has posed a number of challenges largely due to the inherently indirect nature of the detection method [15]. What has been coined the 'molecular revolution' for recording of biodiversity and species occupancy [34] is a rapidly evolving approach with changes in collection, extraction, amplification, and screening of DNA (Fig. 1). Each of these steps may introduce unwanted errors in the form of false negatives and false presences [15] that can be largely controlled by improved protocols and procedures [35], quantification of detection errors [30], and assessing the appropriate level of sample replication [32].

4.1 General QAQC

There are multiple QAQC components that are common to all eDNA methods and analysis platforms. One of the most important QAQC components of eDNA studies is instituting protocols that minimize the probability of contamination of eDNA extractions and downstream analyses. This can be achieved through a number of different steps. First, it is important to conduct all DNA extraction and amplifications in a room or location dedicated to low-quantity DNA sources. Concentrated DNA of the eDNA target species, in the form of high concentration DNA extracts and more importantly PCR products, should not be handled or opened in this dedicated space. Researchers also need to restrict the flow of items and individuals between high concentration and low concentration DNA working spaces. To minimize the possibility of contamination among eDNA samples and reagents within the low quantity DNA working space, a number of steps can be taken including the use of filter tips, regular changing of gloves, plus frequent sterilization of pipettes, sample trays, and extraction surfaces. Finally, negative controls should be included in all DNA extractions and PCRs to monitor for contamination events.

4.2 Active Surveillance QAQC

Digital droplet PCR: Multiple research groups have abandoned the traditional endpoint PCR systems to utilize quantitative amplification methods, including quantitative PCR (qPCR) and digital droplet PCR (ddPCR) [9, 14, 36, 37]; and others). These platforms analyze samples for targeted species, either individually or multiplexed (multiple target species at one time), and provide either semiquantitative (qPCR) or total (ddPCR) concentrations (copies of target sequence per microliter) of the targeted DNA fragments from species of interest. This approach and these platforms are reported to be more sensitive [38] and less prone to false positives than traditional endpoint PCR methods [39]. Levels of detection for qPCR and ddPCR have been demonstrated at extremely low levels, in some instances to less than one copy of target DNA per microliter of sample [38–40]. Additionally, even within the quantitative methods, ddPCR may provide substantial advantages over qPCR, particularly because ddPCR does not necessitate production of a standard curve for each sample run, removing a step that both reduces costs of analysis and also lowers the potential for calibration error in the study [23–25]. Additionally, ddPCR has to be a more precise method and has shown reduced susceptibility to reaction inhibitors over traditional qPCR [41].

Quantitative PCR and ddPCR methods require stringent quality assurance procedures, particularly in primer/marker design. When designing the surveillance or monitoring assay, if using a probe-based qPCR and digital droplet PCR methodology, base pair mismatches on both primer and probe, particularly at the 3′ end of the qPCR primers need to be accounted for to avoid false positives [40]. Along with this, false negative problems need to be considered when target DNA is rare and potentially swamped out by nontarget DNA in a sample [40].

The increased sensitivity for qPCR and ddPCR should necessitate additional precautions to help prevent contamination and false positives. This would include additional sterilization of equipment in the laboratory, positive pressure UV capable PCR hoods, procedure room separation, etc., as others have done in the ancient DNA field (*see* Goldberg et al. [35]).

In general, standard qPCR quality control guidelines developed for other methods and procedures should be followed as appropriate (*see* [42]). These include methods to ensure the reliability of results in quantitative eDNA analyses to promote interlaboratory repeatability and to increase experimental transparency [42]. Following the digital guidelines for qPCR, a series of best practice ddPCR guidelines has been developed [41]. These include best practice suggestions ranging from experimental design through ddPCR assay validation [41].

4.3 Passive Surveillance QAQC

HTS analyses of eDNA samples: The advent of high-throughput metagenomic sequencing platforms has the potential to revolutionize the use of DNA for surveillance and monitoring. With these platforms, we have the ability to not only screen eDNA samples for targeted rare species of interest, but we can also screen and analyze samples for overall biodiversity in the system being investigated. Although there are a number of different chemistries and processing methods, high-throughput platforms function by sequencing all fragments of DNA in a sample rather than targeting individual DNA fragments using species-specific amplification.

Additionally, some protocols use a preplatform target enrichment or PCR amplification, providing the ability to target certain groups (e.g., all fish) in a given sample. Depending on the platform utilized, thousands to multiple millions of sequence reads can be generated in a given run, providing depth of coverage of each individual sequence read. Previous eDNA studies utilizing this platform have demonstrated successful application to determine total aquatic biodiversity in real-world systems [10, 11, 20, 43]. To ensure accuracy of matches to target species, particularly if management actions are to be taken based on the data collected, data analyses and stringency of matches to available genetic databases such as NCBI's Genbank should be explicitly stated (e.g., [43]). Consistency of analyses, thresholds for matches to target species, and continued expansion of available genetic barcode-type data within available databases should all be considered when developing the metagenomic assay. Additionally, type of genomic platform utilized should be carefully considered (e.g., Illumina MiSeq or HiSeq or 454, Oxford Nanopore MinION, etc.) as the data each produces differs and can provide different, yet still revealing results.

4.4 Choosing Active vs. Passive Surveillance Methods and Platforms

The standard PCR approach (e.g., [4, 44]) for target eDNA surveillance has the distinct advantage of using technology and techniques found in many molecular genetics labs and can be performed relatively cheaply, assuming a marker exists for the species targeted for surveillance. Progressing up the technological ladder to qPCR, ddPCR, and HTS, the infrastructure necessary to perform the assays on different platforms becomes more costly and with fewer laboratories available to conduct such assays. In many studies, the choice of active vs. passive surveillance methods may be pragmatic. However, it is clear that for at least some platforms, there are issues of detection sensitivity that may drive assay choice. Nathan et al. showed that qPCR and ddPCR were much more sensitive to detecting a target species compared to traditional PCR [23]. Similarly, Doi et al. showed that when eDNA is at very low copy number (<100 per sample) ddPCR outperforms qPCR [25]. A comparison of HTS detection sensitivity to target approaches is an area of ongoing research [20].

While the upfront cost for any platform can be relatively expensive, >$250,000 for some HTS approaches, a per sample cost may also weigh on the decision to choose active or passive surveillance techniques. Nathan et al. estimated a $4.27, $8.87, and $4.02 cost (US$) per sample for PCR, qPCR, and ddPCR platforms, respectively [23]. It should be noted that the uptick in qPCR cost was largely for production of a calibration curve to estimate the amount of DNA in the sample, and with the PCR approach there was no quantification of the amount of DNA.

Ultimately, the choice of using active or passive surveillance will be largely driven by the question needing to be answered [14, 20].

For now, if presence of only one or two species is needed, then it appear PCR, qPCR, or ddPCR platforms are more cost effective, accessible, and reliable. However, if the ecological question of interest is about estimated biodiversity or species richness [10, 11], then HTS to screen and identify suites of species will likely be the best approach. This will particularly be the case as costs for HTS methods, either in house or at commercial facilities, continue to drop and technologies continue to improve [45].

As active and passive approaches to eDNA surveillance advance, data quality will continue to improve and both scientists and management agencies will have the opportunity to more confidently take action to address questions regarding rare species, whether threatened or endangered or invasive, in aquatic environments. These responses can then begin to protect native systems, either through documentation of current biodiversity and potential habitat protection for rare species or instigating early detection and rapid response actions for invasive species. While both active and passive eDNA methods are excellent additions to monitoring science, neither is a 'silver bullet' for surveillance. However, they are both extremely valuable tools and should continue to be developed and supported by scientists and management groups.

References

1. Beja-Pereira A, Oliverira R, Alves PC, Schwartz MK, Luikart G (2009) Advancing ecological understandings through technological transformations in noninvasive genetics. Mol Ecol Resour 9:1279–1301. doi:10.1111/j.1755-0998.2009.02699.x

2. Rees HC, Maddison BC, Middleditch DJ, Patmore JRM, Gough KC (2014) The detection of aquatic animal species using environmental DNA – a review of eDNA as a survey tool in ecology. J Appl Ecol 51:1450–1459. doi:10.1111/1365-2664.12306

3. Bohmann K, Evans A, Gilbert MTP, Carvalho GR, Creer S, Knapp M, Yu DW, de Bruyn M (2014) Environmental DNA for wildlife biology and biodiversity monitoring. Trends Ecol Evol 29:358–367. doi:10.1016/j.tree.2014.04.003

4. Ficetola GF, Miaud C, Pompanon F, Taberlet P (2008) Species detection using environmental DNA from water samples. Biol Lett 4:423–425

5. Jerde CL, Mahon AR, Chadderton WL, Lodge DM (2011) "Sight-unseen" detection of rare aquatic species using environmental DNA. Conserv Lett 4:150–157. doi:10.1111/j.1755-263X.2010.00158.x

6. Goldberg CS, Pilliod DS, Arkle RS, Waits LP (2011) Molecular detection of vertebrates in stream water: a demonstration using rocky mountain tailed frogs and Idaho giant salamanders. PLoS One 6, e22746. doi:10.1371/journal.pone.0022746.s001

7. Goldberg CS, Sepulveda A, Ray A, Baumgardt J, Waits LP (2013) Environmental DNA as a new method for early detection of New Zealand mudsnails (Potamopyrgus antipodarum). Freshw Sci 32:792–800. doi:10.1899/13-046.1.s1

8. Mahon AR, Jerde CL, Galaska M, Bergner JL, Chadderton WL, Lodge DM, Hunter ME, Nico LG (2013) Validation of eDNA surveillance sensitivity for detection of Asian carps in controlled and field experiments. PLoS One 8, e58316. doi:10.1371/journal.pone.0058316.t002

9. Thomsen PF, Kielgast J, Iversen LL, Wiuf C, Rasmussen M, Gilbert MTP, Orlando L, Willerslev E (2012) Monitoring endangered freshwater biodiversity using environmental DNA. Mol Ecol 21:2565–2573. doi:10.1111/j.1365-294X.2011.05418.x

10. Evans NT, Olds BP, Turner CR, Renshaw MA, Li Y, Jerde CL, Mahon AR, Pfrender ME, Lamberti GA, Lodge DM (2016) Quantification of mesocosm fish and amphibian species diversity via eDNA metabarcoding. Mol Ecol Resour 16:29–41. doi:10.1111/1755-0998.12433

11. Mahon AR, Nathan LR, Jerde CL (2014) Meta-genomic surveillance of invasive species in the bait trade. Conserv Genet Resour 6:563–567. doi:10.1007/s12686-014-0213-9

12. Gu W, Swihart R (2004) Absent or undetected? Effects of non-detection of species occurrence on wildlife-habitat models. Biol Conserv 116:195–203. doi:10.1016/S0006-3207(03)00190-3

13. Darling JA, Blum MJ (2007) DNA-based methods for monitoring invasive species: a review and prospectus. Biol Invasions 9:751–765. doi:10.1007/s10530-006-9079-4

14. Lodge DM, Turner CR, Jerde CL, Barnes MA, Chadderton WL, Egan SP, Feder JL, Mahon AR, Pfrender ME (2012) Conservation in a cup of water: estimating biodiversity and population abundance from environmental DNA. Mol Ecol 23:2555–2558

15. Darling JA, Mahon AR (2011) From molecules to management: adopting DNA-based methods for monitoring biological invasions in aquatic environments. Environ Res 111:978–988. doi:10.1016/j.envres.2011.02.001

16. Jerde CL, Mahon AR (2015) Improving confidence in environmental DNA species detection. Mol Ecol Resour 15:461–463. doi:10.1111/1755-0998.12377

17. Jerde CL, Chadderton WL, Mahon AR, Renshaw MA, Corush J, Budny ML, Mysorekar S, Lodge DM (2013) Detection of Asian carp DNA as part of a Great Lakes basin-wide surveillance program. Can J Fish Aquat Sci 70:522–526. doi:10.1139/cjfas-2012-0478

18. Nathan LR, Jerde CL, Budny ML, Mahon AR (2015) The use of environmental DNA in invasive species surveillance of the Great Lakes commercial bait trade. Conserv Biol 29:430–439. doi:10.1111/cobi.12381

19. Ficetola GF, Miaud C, Pompanon F, Taberlet P (2008) Species detection using environmental DNA from water samples. Biol Lett 4:423–425. doi:10.1098/rsbl.2008.0118

20. Simmons M, Tucker A, Chadderton WL, Jerde CL, Mahon AR (2016) Active and passive environmental DNA surveillance of aquatic invasive species. Can J Fish Aquat Sci 73(1):76–83. doi:10.1139/cjfas-2015-0262

21. Renshaw MA, Olds BP, Jerde CL, McVeigh MM, Lodge DM (2014) The room temperature preservation of filtered environmental DNA samples and assimilation into a phenol-chloroform-isoamyl alcohol DNA extraction. Mol Ecol Resour 15:168–176. doi:10.1111/1755-0998.12281

22. Wegleitner BJ, Jerde CL, Tucker A, Chadderton WL, Mahon AR (2015) Long duration, room temperature preservation of filtered eDNA samples. Conserv Genet Resour 7:789–793. doi:10.1007/s12686-015-0483-x

23. Nathan LM, Simmons M, Wegleitner BJ, Jerde CL, Mahon AR (2014) Quantifying environmental DNA signals for aquatic invasive species across multiple detection platforms. Environ Sci Technol 48:12800–12806. doi:10.1021/es5034052

24. Doi H, Uchii K, Takahara T, Matsuhashi S, Yamanaka H, Minamoto T (2015) Use of droplet digital PCR for estimation of fish abundance and biomass in environmental DNA surveys. PLoS One 10, e0122763. doi:10.1371/journal.pone.0122763

25. Doi H, Takahara T, Minamoto T, Matsuhashi S, Uchii K, Yamanaka H (2015) Droplet digital polymerase chain reaction (PCR) outperforms real-time PCR in the detection of environmental DNA from an invasive fish species. Environ Sci Technol 49:150420141853003. doi:10.1021/acs.est.5b00253

26. Kitano T, Umetsu K, Tian W, Osawa M (2007) Two universal primer sets for species identification among vertebrates. Int J Legal Med 121:423–427. doi:10.1007/s00414-006-0113-y

27. Miya M, Sato Y, Fukunaga T, Sado T, Poulsen JY, Sato K, Minamoto T, Yamamoto S, Yamanaka H, Araki H, Kondoh M, Iwasaki W (2015) MiFish, a set of universal PCR primers for metabarcoding environmental DNA from fishes: detection of more than 230 subtropical marine species. R Soc Open Sci 2:150088. doi:10.1016/j.soilbio.2013.05.014

28. Schmieder R, Edwards R (2011) Quality control and preprocessing of metagenomic datasets. Bioinformatics 27:863–864. doi:10.1093/bioinformatics/btr026

29. Schmidt BR, Kéry M, Ursenbacher S (2013) Site occupancy models in the analysis of environmental DNA presence/absence surveys: a case study of an emerging amphibian pathogen. Meth Ecol 4:646–653

30. Hunter ME, Oyler-McCance SJ, Dorazio RM, Fike JA, Smith BJ, Hunter CT, Reed RN, Hart KM (2015) Environmental DNA (eDNA) sampling improves occurrence and detection estimates of invasive Burmese pythons. PLoS One 10, e0121655. doi:10.1371/journal.pone.0121655.s005

31. MacKenzie DI, Nichols JD, Lachman GB, Droege S, ROYLE JA, Langtimm CA (2002) Estimating site occupancy rates when detection probabilities are less than one. Ecology 83:2248–2255

32. Ficetola GF, Pansu J, Bonin A, Coissac E, Giguet-Covex C, De Barba M, GIELLY L,

Lopes CM, Boyer F, Pompanon F, Rayé G, Taberlet P (2015) Replication levels, false presences and the estimation of the presence/absence from eDNA metabarcoding data. Mol Ecol Resour 15:543–556. doi:10.1111/1755-0998.12338

33. Guisan A, Thuiller W (2005) Predicting species distribution: offering more than simple habitat models. Ecol Lett 8:993–1009. doi:10.1111/j.1461-0248.2005.00792.x

34. Handley LL (2015) How will the "molecular revolution"contribute to biological recording? Biol J Linn Soc 115:750–766

35. Goldberg CS, Strickler KM, Pilliod DS (2015) Moving environmental DNA methods from concept to practice for monitoring aquatic macroorganisms. Biol Conserv 183:1–3. doi:10.1016/j.biocon.2014.11.040

36. Takahara T, Minamoto T, Yamanaka H, Doi H, Kawabata Z (2012) Estimation of fish biomass using environmental DNA. PLoS One 7, e35868. doi:10.1371/journal.pone.0035868.t001

37. Pilliod DS, Goldberg CS, Arkle RS, Waits LP, Richardson J (2013) Estimating occupancy and abundance of stream amphibians using environmental DNA from filtered water samples. Can J Fish Aquat Sci 70:1123–1130. doi:10.1139/cjfas-2013-0047

38. Ellison SL, English CA, Burns MJ, Keer JT (2006) Routes to improving the reliability of low level DNA analysis using real-time PCR. BMC Biotechnol 6:33. doi:10.1186/1472-6750-6-33

39. Pinheiro LB, Coleman VA, Hindson CM, Herrmann J, Hindson BJ, Bhat S, Emslie KR (2012) Evaluation of a droplet digital polymerase chain reaction format for DNA copy number quantification. Anal Chem 84:1003–1011. doi:10.1021/ac202578x

40. Wilcox TM, McKelvey KS, Young MK, Jane SF, Lowe WH, Whiteley AR, Schwartz MK (2013) Robust detection of rare species using environmental DNA: the importance of primer specificity. PLoS One 8, e59520. doi:10.1371/journal.pone.0059520.t003

41. Huggett JF, Foy CA, Benes V, Emslie K, Garson JA, Haynes R, Hellemans J, Kubista M, Mueller RD, Nolan T, Pfaffl MW, Shipley GL, Vandesompele J, Wittwer CT, Bustin SA (2013) The digital MIQE guidelines: minimum information for publication of quantitative digital PCR experiments. Clin Chem 59:892–902. doi:10.1373/clinchem.2013.206375

42. Bustin SA, Benes V, Garson JA, Hellemans J, Huggett J, Kubista M, Mueller R, Nolan T, Pfaffl MW, Shipley GL, Vandesompele J, Wittwer CT (2009) The MIQE guidelines: minimum information for publication of quantitative real-time PCR experiments. Clin Chem 55:611–622. doi:10.1373/clinchem.2008.112797

43. Thomsen PF, Kielgast J, Iversen LL, Møller PR, Rasmussen M, Willerslev E (2012) Detection of a diverse marine fish fauna using environmental DNA from seawater samples. PLoS One 7, e41732. doi:10.1371/journal.pone.0041732.t002

44. Mahon AR, Rohly A, Budny ML, Jerde CL, Chadderton WL, Lodge DM (2010) Environmental DNA monitoring and surveillance: standard operating procedures. Report to the United States Army Corps of Engineers, Environmental Laboratories, Cooperative Environmental Studies Unit, Vicksburg, MI. CESU agreement #W912HZ08-02-0014, modification P00007

45. Halanych KM, Mahon AR (2014) Discovering diversity with high-throughput approaches: introduction to a virtual symposium in the biological bulletin. Biol Bull 227:91–92

Chapter 9

Microarrays/DNA Chips for the Detection of Waterborne Pathogens

Filipa F. Vale

Abstract

DNA microarrays are useful for the simultaneous detection of microorganisms in water samples. Specific probes targeting waterborne pathogens are selected with bioinformatics tools, synthesized and spotted onto a DNA array. Here, the construction of a DNA chip for waterborne pathogen detection is described, including the processes of probe in silico selection, synthesis, validation, and data analysis.

Key words DNA chip, Microarray, Waterborne pathogen, Waterborne detection, Molecular method, Water quality, DNA probe, Bacterial detection, Indicator bacteria, Microbial detection

1 Introduction

Microbial water quality monitoring is a field in which novel molecular tools have emerged in order to have rapid, high-throughput, sensitive, and specific detection of a wide spectrum of microbial pathogens that challenge traditional culture-based techniques [1–3].

Microarrays or DNA chips are a technology that allows binding of several nucleic acids (probes) to a surface to detect the presence or determine the relative concentration of complementary nucleic acid sequences (targets) in a mixture through hybridization followed by detection of the hybridization signal. In a way, DNA chips are a scale up of conventional dot blots, in which dozens or hundreds of probes are used to detect the presence of a given nucleic acid [4]. DNA microarrays can also be used to quantify a large number of nucleic acids in a solution, a topic which will not be covered here.

Briefly, DNA microarrays may be used as a diagnostic tool consisting of ordered matrices of DNA sequences spotted on glass slides, which are used for hybridization experiments with fluorescently labeled target genes [5]. This technology, which enables the parallel analysis of many genes in a single reaction, has been applied in the detection of microorganisms in water samples, namely,

Sarah J. Bourlat (ed.), *Marine Genomics: Methods and Protocols*, Methods in Molecular Biology, vol. 1452, DOI 10.1007/978-1-4939-3774-5_9, © Springer Science+Business Media New York 2016

wastewater [6–10] and water intended for human consumption [9, 11]. Moreover, DNA microarrays have been used for the monitoring of toxic microorganisms in marine environments [12, 13].

Pathogen detection microarrays are limited in their ability to detect low-abundance target sequences within complex samples. Therefore, microarray-based pathogen detection generally relies upon target sequence amplification strategies, such as PCR [14], previous culture of the pathogen, or sample volume increase [11].

The performance of a microarray is dependent on the quality of the selected probes. Good probes should present high specificity (they should be completely specific to their respective targets to avoid any cross-hybridization), sensitivity (they should not form stable secondary structures that may interfere with the probes by forming heteroduplexes during hybridization), and homogeneity (they should have similar reaction temperatures) [15]. Moreover, long probes yield better signal intensity than short probes; however, the signal intensity of short probes can be improved by the addition of spacers or by using a higher probe concentration for spotting. Probes optimized for sequence specificity are essential to avoid false-positives due to nonspecific cross-hybridization to highly similar sequences [16]. In fact, if the targets have more than 70–80% global sequence homology to a probe, they can hybridize indiscriminately to that probe. Cross-hybridization also depends on the stringency of the hybridization protocols [16, 17]. Arraying and scanning equipment and their respective software may vary considerably, and thus protocols describing the methods generally do not include instructions on how to operate these equipments. In this chapter, we will present protocols for selection of DNA probes for microorganism detection, DNA chip preparation, target preparation and hybridization, and image acquisition and data analysis.

2 Materials

Prepare all solutions using ultrapure water. Prepare and store all reagents at room temperature (unless indicated otherwise). Diligently follow all waste disposal regulations when disposing of materials. Use gloves in all protocols. Powder-free gloves should be worn while handling the slides.

2.1 DNA Chip Manufacturing

1. CodeLink® slides (Surmodics, USA) or equivalent. Follow the protocol recommended by the manufacturer (note that other reagents are necessary).

2. DNA extracted using Wizard Genomic DNA Purification Kit (Promega Corp., USA), and PCR products purified using QIAquick PCR Purification Kit (Qiagen, Germany), or equivalent.

3. Primers and amine C6 modified primer.

4. Arraying equipment (QArrayMini Personal benchtop microarrayer, Genetix, or equivalent).

2.2 DNA Labeling and Hybridization

2.2.1 DNA Labeling

1. 0.45 μm nitrocellulose filters.

2. DNA extracted using Wizard Genomic DNA Purification Kit (Promega Corp., USA) or equivalent, and PCR products purified using QIAquick PCR Purification Kit (Qiagen, Germany), or equivalent.

3. Nimblegen One-Color DNA labeling kit (Roche, USA), or equivalent.

4. Thermocycler for target amplification.

5. Vacuum concentrator.

2.2.2 DNA Hybridization

1. Hybridization solution: 4× SSC, 0.1 % SDS, 0.1 mg/ml salmon sperm DNA.

2. Incubation chamber, such as Hybriwell incubation chamber (Sigma Aldrich, USA), or equivalent.

3. Slide staining racks for washes.

4. Wash solution 1: 2× SSC, 0.1 % SDS.

5. Wash solution 2: 0.2× SSC.

6. Wash solution 3: 0.1× SSC.

7. Deionized water.

8. Isopropanol.

9. Heat block at 95 °C.

10. Ice.

11. Shaking hybridization oven.

12. Compressed nitrogen.

2.3 Image Acquisition and Data Analysis

1. Microarray scanner (ScanArray Gx, Perkin Elmer, Waltham, MA, USA, or equivalent).

2. Software for microarray image analysis (ScanArray Express Software v. 4.00, Perkin Elmer, or equivalent).

3 Methods

Carry out all procedures at room temperature unless otherwise specified.

3.1 Selection of DNA Probes for Microorganism Detection

1. Select the target microorganisms. For instance, for the drinking water quality test a list of mandatory microorganisms should be compiled (see **Note 1**).

2. Select genomic sequences for ribosomal RNA, toxins, and other conserved sequences that could be specific to a particular

C. jejuni probe sequence:

GCTCTAGGTGCTTGTGTTGCATTTAGTAATGCTAATGCAGCAGAAGGTAAACTTGAGTCTATTAAATCTAAAGGACAATTAATAGTTGGTGTTAAAAATGATGTTCC

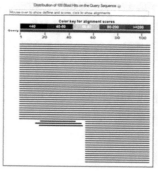

#	Description	Query cover	E value	Ident	Accession
1	Campylobacter jejuni subsp. jejuni F38011, complete genome	1	2E-46	100%	CP006851.1
2	Campylobacter jejuni subsp. jejuni R14, complete genome	1	2E-46	100%	CP005081.1
3	Campylobacter jejuni subsp. jejuni S3, complete genome	1	2E-46	100%	CP001960.1
4	Campylobacter jejuni subsp. doylei 269.97, complete genome	1	2E-46	100%	CP000768.1
5	Campylobacter jejuni RM1221, complete genome	1	2E-46	100%	CP000025.1
(...)					
64	Hymenolepis diminuta genome assembly H_diminuta_Denmark, scaffold HDID_scaffold0000481	0.45	0.076	82%	LM384351.1
(...)					

Fig. 1 BLASTN [18] of *C. jejuni* probe [11] using the NCBI Database "nucleotide collection nr/nt." All significant alignments are produced with *C. jejuni* sequences. The first nonsignificant alignment is shown

microorganism from the NCBI Genbank 'nucleotide collection,' or any other source for organism-specific sequences (EMBL, etc.) (*see* **Note 2**).

3. Prepare a file in FASTA format containing the provisional sequences that may serve as probes.

4. Perform a nucleotide BLAST (BLASTN) [18] for each sequence against the NCBI database "nucleotide collection nr/nt."

5. In the BLAST output, check all sequences presenting a query coverage >70% and a threshold limit (*E*-value) <1e⁻⁶ (*see* Fig. 1).

6. These sequences producing significant alignments should include most of the target microorganism genomes but not other microorganisms' genomes (*see* **Note 3**).

7. Perform a nucleotide BLAST (BLASTN) for each sequence using the NCBI Database "nucleotide collection nr/nt," this time selecting the organism of choice. Select the target organism for each probe and check the "exclude box" in order to observe if any other microorganism produces significant alignments (i.e., with a query coverage >70% and a threshold (*E*-value) >1e⁻⁶). The probe should not produce significant alignments to any other microorganism (Fig. 1).

8. BLASTN each probe using the NCBI Database "nucleotide collection nr/nt" and select, one by one, all microorganisms that may be present in real samples (in this case do not select

the Exclude box). The probe should not produce significant alignment to any of these microorganisms.

9. Select the probes producing significant alignments for the target microorganism only.

10. Download the DNA sequence of the selected probe for several strains of the target microorganism from NCBI or an equivalent database (*see* **Note 4**).

11. Choose a subregion of the gene of the appropriate size for a probe (120–200 bp) showing total, or almost total, identity with the sequences of all the members of each target using the MultAlin tool available at http://multalin.toulouse.inra.fr/multalin/ [19] or the Clustal Omega tool from EBI, available online at http://www.ebi.ac.uk/Tools/msa/clustalo/ [20], or other multialignment site or software.

12. Check for the absence of probe self-folding using the Mfold web server [21], available at http://mfold.rna.albany.edu/?q=mfold/DNA-Folding-Form, or other multialignment site or software.

13. The probes can either be synthetic or PCR amplified from the target microorganism.

14. For synthetic probes, choose the consensus sequence after alignment (*see* Subheading 3.2).

15. Select primers for PCR amplification using Primer3 or equivalent software [22, 23], available at http://bioinfo.ut.ee/primer3-0.4.0/ (*see* Subheading 3.2), or other multialignment site or software.

16. Repeat the same procedure for all probes to be tested on the DNA chip (*see* **Note 5**).

3.2 DNA Chip Manufacturing

Several brands of arraying equipment can be used, for which specific manufacturers' instructions should be followed. However, here are some general aspects to think about when designing a DNA Chip:

1. Use CodeLink® or equivalent slides to spot the probes.

2. Amplify the probe by PCR by single-stranded probe synthesis using a 3′- or 5′-amine C6 modified primer (C6 works as spacer between the slide and the probe) (*see* **Note 6**).

3. Purify the PCR product using standard methods (*see* **Note 7**).

4. Quantify and store the purified probes at −20 °C.

5. Design probe distribution on the microarray and spot the probes using the arraying equipment (*see* **Note 8**).

6. Store the DNA chip at room temperature (or according to manufacturers' instructions) until use. For long-term storage, maintain the slides in a desiccated environment.

**3.3 DNA Labeling
and Hybridization**

1. Extract DNA from all reference microorganisms (obtained from ATCC collection or equivalent) using conventional methods, in order to validate the DNA chip.

2. Collect a minimum sample volume of 1 L of water and transport at 4 °C. Samples should be processed within 48 h.

3. Filter water samples through 0.45 μm nitrocellulose filters (*see* **Note 9**).

4. Extract DNA from the filters using conventional methods for DNA extraction from water (*see* **Note 10**).

5. Store DNA at –20 °C until required.

6. In the case of low abundance targets (low bacterial load in the sample, resulting in a total DNA concentration <0.1 μg after labeling), preamplify the target by PCR using random hexamers as primers. (This step may be included in the target DNA labeling.) (*See* **Note 11**).

7. Purify the PCR product and store at –20 °C.

8. Before labeling, mix the target DNA with the positive control target DNA (only if there is a positive control probe spotted in the microarray).

9. Label the target DNA derived from DNA extraction and/or PCR product purification with Cy3 dye from the Nimblegen One-Color DNA labeling kit (*see* **Note 12**), or equivalent.

10. Quantify the labeled DNA, prepare aliquots of 2 μg, and store at –20 °C in the dark until use.

11. Dry the labeled target DNA in a vacuum concentrator in the dark, or if unavailable, dry at room temperature in the dark.

12. Resuspend the dried labeled DNA in 35 μl of hybridization solution, incubate at 95 °C for 5 min, and quickly cover with ice.

13. Affix the hybridization chamber to the microarray slide.

14. Insert the hybridization mixture into the hole of the DNA chip cover and seal with seal tabs.

15. Repeat the procedure from **steps 13** to **14** as many times as the number of hybridization temperatures to be tested (*see* **Note 13**).

16. Incubate in the dark in a shaking hybridization oven at the selected temperature. Shake at 300 rpm for 16–18 h (*see* **Note 14**).

17. Remove the hybridization chamber and rinse briefly with 4× SSC.

18. Place slides in a rack and wash twice with wash solution 1 at hybridization temperature for 5 min. Discard the solution between washes.

19. Wash with wash solution 2 at room temperature for 1 min. Discard the solution.

20. Wash with wash solution 3 at room temperature for 1 min. Discard the solution.

21. Rinse with deionized water.

22. Rinse with isopropanol.

23. Dry with compressed nitrogen (*see* **Note 15**).

3.4 Image Acquisition and Data Analysis

1. Scan the DNA chip using a microarray scanner with the appropriate laser beam for the fluorophore used in probe labeling.

2. Analyze the scanned images with the software (provided with the microarray scanner) for spot identification and quantification of the fluorescent signal intensities (Fig. 2).

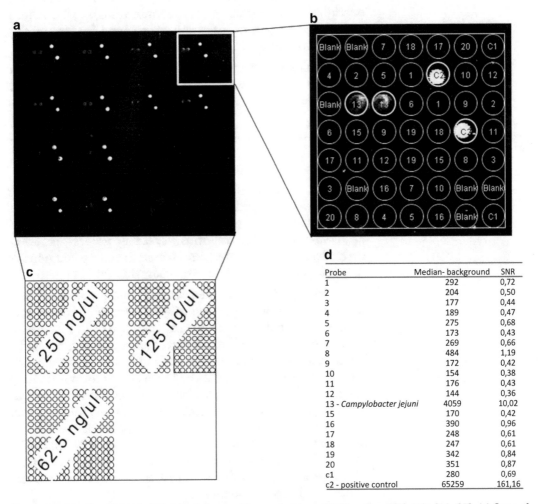

Fig. 2 Hybridization of labeled *C. jejuni* plus positive control target DNA with a DNA chip [11, 25]. (**a**) Scan of the DNA chip. (**b**) Detail of the hybridization results showing positive hybridization for probes 13 (*C. jejuni*) and C2 (positive control), with the probe layout indicated in the grids; (**c**) DNA chip schematics with subarrays layouts, with the localization of probe dilutions of 250, 125, and 62.5 ng/μl; (**d**) SNR determination for all probes, showing two positive identifications (SNR ≥2) for *C. jejuni* and positive control

3. Import the output data of the microarray scanner (usually a csv file) into Excel or equivalent.

4. Consider positive spots presenting a median pixel intensity minus background superior to 400 intensity units and with a signal-to-noise ratio (SNR) ≥ 2 (Fig. 2) (see **Note 16**).

5. Repeat the analysis for all scanned microarrays.

6. Using the DNA microarrays hybridized with the target DNA extracted from pure cultures, determine which spotted microarray concentration and hybridization temperature produces the lowest number of false positives and false negatives (validation step).

7. Use the optimized conditions of probe concentration and hybridization temperature (as determined before) for detecting waterborne pathogens in real samples and for determining the sensitivity of the DNA microarray (see **Note 17**).

8. Validate DNA chip performance by detecting waterborne pathogens in real water samples using another molecular method, such as PCR.

4   Notes

1. Waterborne selection should include microorganisms identified to the species level. Although some of the mandatory organisms screened for water quality testing include specific groups of microorganisms (e.g., coliforms), selecting probes that selectively identify all microorganisms within the group and none of the other microorganisms is particularly difficult [11].

2. To identify species-specific genes, a literature search of genes of that species that are described as species specific, or that have been used in multilocus sequence typing (MLST) schemes or in other molecular methods of detection, can be rather helpful. There is software available for designing the oligonucleotide probes, such as OligoWiz [24]. However, this software usually designs probes of 50 bp, which is shorter than the recommended probe length. Moreover, the cross-hybridization test is done for the entire genome of the species for which the probes are being designed, and not the complete NCBI nucleotide collection. Note that water samples are very complex. This approach can provide an initial set of probes to be tested as described in Subheading 3.1.

3. The number of sequences available in NCBI is constantly growing. For some microorganisms, the number of hits after BLASTN can be very high, not allowing us to quickly understand the specificity of the probe. An example is when the last hit of a BLAST result still presents a near 100% coverage and a very low E-value. In these cases, it is recommended to increase

the maximum number of aligned sequences displayed in the settings before the BLAST analysis.

4. After the BLASTN search, download the sequences of several strains of the target microorganism showing high homology with the probe.

5. Probes should present a similar range of GC content for uniform hybridization, for instance, 35–50% GC.

6. For long DNA probe arrays, double-stranded PCR products may be used, followed by heating at 95 °C for 2 min to allow denaturation and formation of single-stranded DNA probes.

7. Primers remaining in nonpurified PCR reactions can adhere to the slide. In addition, amine contaminants (e.g., ammonia and Tris) in the PCR reaction will decrease the immobilization efficiency.

8. Each probe should be spotted at least in duplicate, preferably even more replicates are recommended. Consider including on the slide blank spots with no probe as well as positive control probes. The positive control may be a synthetic random DNA probe or amplified from a plasmid not found in real samples. Probes should be spotted in random order. Consider including multiple probes for the same target in order to select the best one. Spot several arrays (combinations of probes) presenting different concentrations onto the slide, for example, 62.5, 125, and 250 ng/µl [25].

9. Filtered volume depends on sample turbidity; very turbid samples may require multiple filters (the sample should be filtered until the filter is clogged).

10. DNA extraction from spores and Gram-positive positive bacteria, among others, can be difficult. In addition, the presence of inhibitors in water samples may hinder target DNA labeling. Adapt the DNA extraction protocol to ensure removal of inhibitors and efficacy of DNA extraction [26].

11. For low target concentration samples (DNA concentration after labeling <0.1 µg), a preculture step or increasing the sample volume is an alternative to PCR.

12. For labeling, total DNA is amplified with random hexamers (Nimblegen One-Color DNA labeling kit, Roche, USA). Protocols that do not include amplification may require prior PCR with random hexamers. 1 µg of nonlabeled starting DNA yields an average of 20 µg of labeled DNA, with fragment sizes ranging from 100 to 600 bp [25].

13. The hybridization conditions should first be optimized for the target DNA isolated from pure cultures, and these optimized conditions should then be used for real samples.

14. First test different temperatures, for instance, 42 and 55 °C, but not higher than the recommended temperature (consult

the manufacturer's instructions; for instance, CodeLink slides' maximum recommended hybridization temperature is 55 °C). It is very important that the slides do not dry during incubation, which can be achieved by adding moist paper near the hybridization chamber.

15. The slide should be very clean, without visible seepage zones or fingerprints. Alternatively, use a microarray slide washer and drier.

16. SNR = (signal intensity-background)/standard deviation of background. The background signal refers to local spot background; the standard deviation is calculated across all pixels measured for each array [25, 27]. When probe replicates are present in the microarray, the mean value of replicates should be chosen. Other investigators use SNR >3 to consider the spot positive [9]. Thus, the conditions to consider a spot positive can be optimized for each DNA microarray, providing there are data to support them.

17. To determine the minimum detection level of the DNA microarray, make a series of dilutions of the genomic DNA extracted from pure cultures of a target microorganism and repeat all procedures for DNA labeling and hybridization using the optimized conditions. This will enable determination of the minimum concentration of DNA that can be detected by the DNA chip.

Acknowledgments

F.F.V. is recipient of a postdoctoral fellowship from FCT (SFRH/BPD/95125/2013). The author thanks Patrícia Fonseca for editing the manuscript.

References

1. Vale FF, Silva AM, Granja AT, Vale MJ, Vieira H (2009) Simultaneous detection of microorganisms in water samples for future chip applications: coliform bacteria, non-mandatory bacteria, hepatitis A virus and noroviruses. Phys Status Solidi C 6:2184–2189. doi:10.1002/pssc.200881703

2. Silva AM, Vieira H, Martins N, Granja AT, Vale MJ, Vale FF (2010) Viral and bacterial contamination in recreational waters: a case study in the Lisbon bay area. J Appl Microbiol 108:1023–1031. doi:10.1111/j.1365-2672.2009.04503.x

3. Aw TG, Rose JB (2012) Detection of pathogens in water: from phylochips to qPCR to pyrosequencing. Curr Opin Biotechnol 23:422–430. doi:10.1016/j.copbio.2011.11.016

4. Bumgarner R (2013) Overview of DNA microarrays: types, applications, and their future.

Curr Protoc Mol Biol Chapter 22:Unit 22.1. doi:10.1002/0471142727.mb2201s101

5. Cimarelli L, Singh KS, Mai NT, Dhar BC, Brandi A, Brandi L, Spurio R (2015) Molecular tools for the selective detection of nine diatom species biomarkers of various water quality levels. Int J Environ Res Public Health 12:5485–5504. doi:10.3390/ijerph120505485

6. Maynard C, Berthiaume F, Lemarchand K, Harel J, Payment P, Bayardelle P, Masson L, Brousseau R (2005) Waterborne pathogen detection by use of oligonucleotide-based microarrays. Appl Environ Microbiol 71:8548–8557. doi:10.1128/AEM.71.12.8548-8557.2005

7. Lee DY, Lauder H, Cruwys H, Falletta P, Beaudette LA (2008) Development and application of an oligonucleotide microarray and real-time quantitative PCR for detection of

wastewater bacterial pathogens. Sci Total Environ 398:203–211. doi:10.1016/j. scitotenv.2008.03.004

8. Kelly JJ, Siripong S, McCormack J, Janus LR, Urakawa H, El FS, Noble PA, Sappelsa L, Rittmann BE, Stahl DA (2005) DNA microarray detection of nitrifying bacterial 16S rRNA in wastewater treatment plant samples. Water Res 39:3229–3238. doi:10.1016/j. watres.2005.05.044

9. Miller SM, Tourlousse DM, Stedtfeld RD, Baushke SW, Herzog AB, Wick LM, Rouillard JM, Gulari E, Tiedje JM, Hashsham SA (2008) In situ-synthesized virulence and marker gene biochip for detection of bacterial pathogens in water. Appl Environ Microbiol 74:2200–2209. doi:10.1128/AEM.01962-07

10. Brinkman NE, Francisco R, Nichols TL, Robinson D, Schaefer FW III, Schaudies RP, Villegas EN (2013) Detection of multiple waterborne pathogens using microsequencing arrays. J Appl Microbiol 114:564–573. doi:10.1111/jam.12073

11. Gomes M, Vieira H, Vale FF (2015) Characterization, validation and application of a DNA microarray for the detection of mandatory and other waterborne pathogens. J Biochem 158(5):393–401. doi:10.1093/jb/mvv052

12. Preston CM, Marin R III, Jensen SD, Feldman J, Birch JM, Massion EI, Delong EF, Suzuki M, Wheeler K, Scholin CA (2009) Near real-time, autonomous detection of marine bacterioplankton on a coastal mooring in Monterey Bay, California, using rRNA-targeted DNA probes. Environ Microbiol 11:1168–1180. doi:10.1111/j.1462-2920.2009.01848.x

13. Cariani A, Piano A, Consolandi C, Severgnini M, Castiglioni B, Caredda G, Candela M, Serratore P, De BG, Tinti F (2012) Detection and characterization of pathogenic vibrios in shellfish by a ligation detection reaction-universal array approach. Int J Food Microbiol 153:474–482. doi:10.1016/j.ijfoodmicro

14. Call DR, Borucki MK, Loge FJ (2003) Detection of bacterial pathogens in environmental samples using DNA microarrays. J Microbiol Methods 53:235–243. doi:10.1016/S0167-7012(03)00027-7

15. Kang S-H, Jeong I-S, Choi M-H, Lim H-S (2007) Frontiers in algorithmics. Springer, Berlin, pp 14–25

16. Chou CC, Chen CH, Lee TT, Peck K (2004) Optimization of probe length and the number of probes per gene for optimal microarray analysis of gene expression. Nucleic Acids Res 32, e99. doi:10.1093/nar/gnh099

17. Evertsz EM, Au-Young J, Ruvolo MV, Lim AC, Reynolds MA (2001) Hybridization cross-reactivity within homologous gene families on glass cDNA microarrays. Biotechniques 31:1182–1184–1186

18. Altschul SF, Madden TL, Schaffer AA, Zhang J, Zhang Z, Miller W, Lipman DJ (1997) Gapped BLAST and PSI-BLAST: a new generation of protein database search programs. Nucleic Acids Res 25:3389–3402

19. Corpet F (1988) Multiple sequence alignment with hierarchical clustering. Nucleic Acids Res 16:10881–10890

20. Chenna R, Sugawara H, Koike T, Lopez R, Gibson TJ, Higgins DG, Thompson JD (2003) Multiple sequence alignment with the Clustal series of programs. Nucleic Acids Res 31: 3497–3500

21. Zuker M (2003) Mfold web server for nucleic acid folding and hybridization prediction. Nucleic Acids Res 31:3406–3415

22. Koressaar T, Remm M (2007) Enhancements and modifications of primer design program Primer3. Bioinformatics 23:1289–1291. doi:10.1093/bioinformatics/btm091

23. Untergasser A, Cutcutache I, Koressaar T, Ye J, Faircloth BC, Remm M, Rozen SG (2012) Primer3—new capabilities and interfaces. Nucleic Acids Res 40, e115. doi:10.1093/nar/gks596

24. Wernersson R, Juncker AS, Nielsen HB (2007) Probe selection for DNA microarrays using OligoWiz. Nat Protoc 2:2677–2691. doi:10.1038/nprot.2007.370

25. Martins N, Vale FF, Vieira H (2010) Design and preliminary results of a DNA chip for the detection of microorganisms in water samples. Phys Status Solidi C 7:2751–2754. doi:10.1002/pssc.200983799

26. Mertens K, Freund L, Schmoock G, Hansel C, Melzer F, Elschner MC (2014) Comparative evaluation of eleven commercial DNA extraction kits for real-time PCR detection of *Bacillus anthracis* spores in spiked dairy samples. Int J Food Microbiol 170:29–37. doi:10.1016/j. ijfoodmicro.2013.10.022

27. Yin H, Cao L, Qiu G, Wang D, Kellogg L, Zhou J, Dai Z, Liu X (2007) Development and evaluation of 50-mer oligonucleotide arrays for detecting microbial populations in acid mine drainages and bioleaching systems. J Microbiol Methods 70:165–178. doi:10.1016/j.mimet.2007.04.011

Chapter 10

DNA Barcoding of Marine Metazoans

Dirk Steinke, Sean W.J. Prosser, and Paul D.N. Hebert

Abstract

The accumulation of DNA barcode sequences will provide an increasingly useful and comprehensive library for species identification and discovery of marine metazoans. Here we present a summary of protocols designed to obtain DNA barcodes of marine metazoans from diverse phyla.

Key words DNA barcoding, Metazoa, Primer, Species identification, Protocols

1 Introduction

DNA barcoding uses a short DNA sequence from a standardized position in the genome as a molecular diagnostic for species-level identifications. Because DNA barcode sequences are very short relative to the entire genome, they can be obtained quickly and cheaply. Today's gold standard metazoan barcode is a 648-base pair region at the 5′ end of the mitochondrial COI gene [1]. Because this fragment is flanked by regions of conserved sequences, it is usually easy to amplify and analyze. Many studies have shown that the sequence variability in the barcode region is very low within species while closely related species regularly show divergences of several percent, making it possible to identify species with high confidence. The variability between intraspecific and interspecific genetic distances is termed the 'barcoding gap' [2].

To date about 40,000 species of marine Metazoa have been barcoded, but progress over the last decade has been slow due to the broad taxonomic diversity and the lack of consistently efficient primers [2].

Here we present a comprehensive collection of protocols designed to obtain DNA barcodes of marine metazoans from various phyla (for nonmetazoan taxa see recommended references in **Note 10**). We focus exclusively on 'traditional' Sanger-sequencing-based methods [3] which are highly recommended for building DNA barcode reference libraries of marine life.

Sarah J. Bourlat (ed.), *Marine Genomics: Methods and Protocols*, Methods in Molecular Biology, vol. 1452,
DOI 10.1007/978-1-4939-3774-5_10, © Springer Science+Business Media New York 2016

2   Materials

All solutions should be prepared with ultrapure water and analytical grade reagents. After preparation reagents should be held at room temperature unless indicated otherwise.

2.1   DNA Extraction Reagents

1. CTAB Buffer: 2% CTAB, 100 mM Tris–HCl pH 8.0, 20 mM EDTA pH 8.0, 1.4 mM NaCl.

2. Vertebrate Lysis Buffer: 100 mM NaCl, 50 mM Tris–HCl pH 8.0, 10 mM EDTA pH 8.0, 0.5% SDS.

3. Invertebrate Lysis Buffer: 700 mM GuSCN, 30 mM EDTA pH 8.0, 30 mM Tris–HCl pH 8.0, 0.5% Triton X-100, 5% Tween-20.

4. ProK Solution: 20 mg/mL Proteinase K, 10 mM Tris–HCl pH 7.4, 50% glycerol (v/v).

5. Binding Buffer: 6 M GuSCN, 20 mM EDTA pH 8.0, 10 mM Tris–HCl pH 6.4, 4% Triton X-100.

6. Plant Binding Buffer: 83% Binding Buffer, 17% sterile water.

7. Binding Mix: 50% Binding Buffer, 50% ethanol.

8. Protein Wash Buffer: 26% Binding Buffer, 70% ethanol, 4% sterile water.

9. Wash Buffer: 60% ethanol, 50 mM NaCl, 10 mM Tris–HCl pH 7.4, 0.5 mM EDTA pH 8.0.

10. TNE Buffer: 10 mM Tris-base, 100 mM NaCl, 1 mM EDTA pH 8.0.

11. DTT Solution: 0.39 M dithiothreitol.

12. SDS Solution: 20% SDS.

13. Organic Extraction Buffer: 73% TNE, 10% SDS Solution, 10% DTT Solution, 7% ProK Solution.

14. Phenol–chloroform Solution: 50% phenol, 50% chloroform–isoamyl alcohol (24:1 v/v).

15. 3 M sodium acetate.

16. Sterile water.

17. 100% ethanol.

18. 70% ethanol.

19. Rocking platform and incubator.

20. Silica-membrane-based spin columns.

21. Centrifuge.

22. GHP membrane.

2.2   PCR

1. PCR mix (12.5 µL): 6.25 µL of 10% d-(+)-trehalose dihydrate, 2 µL of sterile water, 1.25 µL of 10× reaction buffer, 0.625 µL of 50 mM $MgCl_2$, 0.125 µL of each 10 µM primer, 0.0625 µL

of 10 mM dNTP, and 0.060 µL of 5 U/µL DNA Polymerase), and 2.0 µL of DNA template.

2. Thermocycler.

2.3 PCR Check

1. Agarose powder.

2. 10× TAE: 48.5 g of Tris-base, 11.4 mL of glacial acetic acid, and 20 mL of 0.5 M EDTA pH 8.0.

3. 1× TAE: 900 mL of water and 100 mL of 10× TAE.

4. 1 % Ethidium bromide.

5. DNA gel electrophoresis equipment.

2.4 Cycle Sequencing

1. 5× Sequencing Buffer: 400 mM Tris–HCl pH 9.0, 10 mM MgCl$_2$.

2. Sequencing Mix: 5.4 µL of 10 % d-(+)-trehalose dihydrate, 1.875 µL of 5× sequencing buffer, 1 µL of 10 µM sequencing primer, 0.875 µL of sterile water, and 0.25 µL of BigDye.

3. Thermocycler

2.5 Sequencing Cleanup

1. Sephadex beads (dry).

2. 0.1 mM EDTA pH 8.0.

3 Methods

3.1 DNA Extraction

See Table 1 for the lysis and DNA extraction protocols most suitable for a particular taxonomic group (see also **Note 1**). Phenol–chloroform extraction is effective for all taxa. Some disadvantages of this method are the toxicity of phenol/chloroform and its lengthy procedure. Moreover, although using commercial kits has widely expanded recently, their high cost limits their use.

3.1.1 CTAB Lysis and Extraction (CTAB)

1. Prepare fresh CTAB lysis buffer by mixing 50 µL of CTAB buffer with 5 µL of ProK solution.

2. Add 50 µL of CTAB lysis buffer to the sample and incubate at 56 °C for 6–18 h on a rocking platform.

3. Add 100 µL of Plant Binding Buffer to each sample and mix by pipetting.

4. Transfer all 150 µL to a silica-membrane-based spin column (see **Note 2**) and centrifuge at $6000 \times g$ for 2 min.

5. Add 180 µL of Binding Mix to the membrane and centrifuge at $6000 \times g$ for 2 min.
   Decant the flow-through from the collection tube.

6. Add 700 µL of Wash Buffer to the membrane and centrifuge at $6000 \times g$ for 4 min.

Table 1
Lysis buffer/DNA extraction and primers used for PCR amplification and sequencing of COI-5P in common marine taxa

Taxonomic group	Lysis/ extraction	PCR forward primer	PCR reverse primer	Sequencing forward primer	Sequencing reverse primer
Annelida: Echiura	Invert	C_LepFolF	SpoonR1	C_LepFolF	SpoonR1
Annelida: Polychaeta[a]	Invert	polyLCO	polyHCO	polyLCO	polyHCO
Brachiopoda	Invert	BrachF1	C_LepFolR	BrachF1	C_LepFolR
Bryozoa	CTAB	C_LepFolF	BryR1	BryR1	C_LepFolR
Chaetognatha	Invert	ChaetF1	ChaetR1	ChaetF1	ChaetR1
Chordata (fish, mammals)[b]	Vert	C_FishF1t1	C_FishR1t1	M13F	M13R
Chordata (mammals, reptiles, fish, amphibians)[b]	Vert	C_VF1LFt1	C_VR1LRt1	M13F	M13R
Chordata (Birds)	Vert	BirdF1	BirdR2	BirdF1	BirdR2
Crustacea (Malacostraca)	Invert	CrustDF1	CrustDR1	CrustDF1	CrustDR1
Crustacea (Maxillopoda, Branchiopoda, Ostracoda)	Invert	ZplankF1_t1	ZplankR1_t1	M13F	M13R
Cnidaria	CTAB	CnidF1	CnidR1	CnidF1	CnidR1
Echinodermata[c]	CTAB	LCOech1aF1	HCO2198	LCOech1aF1	HCO2198
Mollusca: Bivalvia[d]	CTAB	BivF4_t1	BivR1_t1	M13F	M13R
Mollusca: Gastropoda	CTAB	C_GasF1_t1	GasR1_t1	M13F	M13R
Nematoda	Invert	C_NemF1_t1	C_NemR1_t1	M13F	M13R
Nemertea	Invert	RibbonF1	RibbonR1	RibbonF1	RibbonR1
Platyhelminthes (parasitic)	Invert	C_PlatyF1	PlatyR1	C_PlatyF1	PlatyR1
Platyhelminthes (Turbellaria, free-living)	Invert	TurF1	C_LepFolR	TurF1	C_LepFolR
Porifera	CTAB	PorF1	C_LepFolR	PorF1	C_LepFolR
Pycnogonida	Invert	LCO1490_t1	HCO2198_t1	M13F	M13R
Sipuncula	Invert	C_LepFolF	SipR1	C_LepFolF	SipR1
Tunicata	Invert	TunF1	TunR1	TunF1	TunR1
Universal	Ph-Chl	C_LepFolF	C_LepFolR	C_LepFolF	C_LepFolR

[a]See **Note 3**
[b]See **Note 4**
[c]See **Note 6**
[d]See **Note 7**

Decant the flow-through, open and close the column, and centrifuge at $10,000 \times g$ for 4 min.

7. Replace the collection tube with a clean 1.5 mL tube with removed lid and dry at room temperature for 30 min.

8. Add 40 μL of sterile water to the membrane, incubate at room temperature for 1 min, and centrifuge at $10,000 \times g$ for 5 min. Store eluted DNA at 4 °C for short-term storage or at –20 °C for long-term storage.

3.1.2 Vertebrate and Invertebrate Lysis and Extraction (Vert and Invert)

1. Prepare fresh lysis buffer by mixing 50 μL of vertebrate or invertebrate lysis buffer with 5 μL of ProK solution.

2. Add 50 μL of prepared lysis buffer to the sample and incubate at 56 °C for 6–18 h on a rocking platform.

3. Add 100 μL of Binding Mix to each sample and mix by pipetting.

4. Transfer all 150 μL to a silica-membrane-based spin column (see **Note 2**) and centrifuge at $6000 \times g$ for 2 min.

5. Add 180 μL of Protein Wash Buffer to the membrane and centrifuge at $6000 \times g$ for 2 min.

6. Decant the flow-through from the collection tube.

7. Add 700 μL of Wash Buffer to the membrane and centrifuge at $6000 \times g$ for 4 min.

8. Decant the flow-through, open and close the column, and centrifuge at $10,000 \times g$ for 4 min.

9. Replace the collection tube with a clean 1.5 mL tube with removed lid and dry at room temperature for 30 min.

10. Add 40 μL of sterile water to the membrane, incubate at room temperature for 1 min, and centrifuge at $10,000 \times g$ for 5 min. Store eluted DNA at 4 °C for short-term storage or at –20 °C for long-term storage.

3.1.3 Phenol–Chloroform Lysis and Extraction (Ph–Chl)

1. Prepare fresh organic extraction buffer and add 400 μL to the sample.

2. Incubate at 37 °C for a minimum of 1 h (ideally overnight) on a rocking platform.

3. In a fume hood, add 400 μL of phenol–chloroform solution to the sample. Shake to mix. A milky emulsion should form.

4. Centrifuge at $14,000 \times g$ for 5 min.

5. Carefully remove the top aqueous layer (do not take any of the white interphase—leave a little aqueous layer behind if necessary).

6. Add the aqueous phase to a new tube containing 400 μL of phenol:chloroform mixture.

7. Shake to mix and centrifuge at $14,000 \times g$ for 5 min.

8. Carefully remove the top aqueous layer and transfer to a new 1.5 mL tube.

9. Incubate at 65 °C for 45 min to 2 h to evaporate residual chloroform.

10. After evaporation, adjust the total volume to 200 μL with sterile water.

11. Add 20 μL of 3 M sodium acetate and mix.

12. Add 2 volumes (i.e., 440 μL) of cold (–20 °C) 100% ethanol and vortex for 10 s.

13. Incubate at –20 °C overnight.

14. Centrifuge for 20 min at $14,000 \times g$.

15. Carefully remove the supernatant and wash the DNA pellet with 500 μL of cold (–20 °C) 70% ethanol.

16. Centrifuge for 20 min at $14,000 \times g$.

17. Carefully remove the supernatant and wash the DNA pellet with 500 μL of cold (–20 °C) 70% ethanol.

18. Centrifuge for 20 min at $14,000 \times g$.

19. Carefully remove the supernatant and add 20–100 μL of sterile water to the DNA pellet and incubate at 65 °C for 30 min. Pipette or vortex to mix. DNA is ready for use.

3.2 PCR

1. Add 2 μL of DNA to 10.5 μL of PCR mix containing the appropriate primers for the taxa involved (*see* Tables 1 and 2, and also **Note 8**).

2. Pulse centrifuge for 3 s and thermocycle using the following conditions:

(a) 94 °C for 2 min.

(b) 5 cycles of:
- 94 °C for 40 s.
- 45 °C for 40 s.
- 72 °C for 1 min.

(c) 35 cycles of:
- 94 °C for 40 s.
- 51 °C for 40 s.
- 72 °C for 1 min.

(d) 72 °C for 5 min.

3.3 PCR Check

Check PCR success by loading 4 μL of PCR product onto a 2% agarose gel. To make 100 mL of 2% agarose, mix 99 mL of water with 1 mL of 10× TAE and 2 g of agarose powder. Heat the

Table 2
Details of primers and primer cocktails used for amplifying and sequencing COI-5P in common marine taxa

Primer name	Sequence (5′–3′)	Direction	Reference
BirdF1	TTCTCCAACCACAAAGACATTGGCAC	Forward	[10]
BirdR1	ACGTGGGAGATAATTCCAAATCCTG	Reverse	[10]
BivF4_t1	TGTAAAACGACGGCCAGTGKTCWACWAATCATAARGATATTGG	Forward	[11]
BivR1_t1	CAGGAAACAGCTATGACTAMACCTCWGGRTGVCCRAARAACCA	Reverse	[11]
BranchF1	TTATRTCWACWAATCATAARGATATTGG	Forward	This publication
BryR1	TATACTTCKGGDKGHCCAAARAATCA	Reverse	This publication
ChaetF1	TTTCWACWAAYCAYCAAGATATYGG	Forward	This publication
ChaetR1	TAAACTTCWGGATGACCAAARAAYCA	Reverse	This publication
CnidF1	TTTCTACWAAYCATAARGAYATHGG	Forward	This publication
CnidR1	TAAACTTCWGGRTGBCCAAARAAYCA	Reverse	This publication
COIeR1	GCTCGTGTRTCTACRTCCAT	Reverse	[12]
CrustDF1	GGTCWACAAAYCATAAAGAYATTGG	Forward	This publication
CrustDR1	TAAACYTCAGGRTGACCRAARAAYCA	Reverse	This publication
EchinoF1	TTTCAACTAATCATAAGGACATTGG	Forward	[13]
FishF2_t1	TGTAAAACGACGGCCAGTCGACTAATCATAAAGATATCGGCAC	Forward	[14]
FishR2_t1	CAGGAAACAGCTATGACACTTCAGGGTGACCGAAGAATCAGAA	Reverse	[14]
FRld_t1	CAGGAAACAGCTATGACACCTCAGGGTGTCCGAARAAYCARAA	Reverse	[14]
GasF1_t1	TGTAAAACGACGGCCAGTTTTCAACAAACCATAARGATATTGG	Forward	[15]
GasF2_t1	TGTAAAACGACGGCCAGTATTCTACAAACCACAAAGACATCGG	Forward	[15]
GasF3_t1	TGTAAAACGACGGCCAGTTTTCWACWAATCATAAAGATATTGG	Forward	[15]

(continued)

Table 2
(continued)

Primer name	Sequence (5'–3')	Direction	Reference
GasR1_t1	CAGGAAACAGCTATGACACTTCWGGRTGHCCRAARAATCARAA	Reverse	[15]
HCO2198	TAAACTTCAGGGTGACCAAAAAATCA	Reverse	[4]
LCO1490	GGTCAACAAATCATAAAGATATTGG	Forward	[4]
LCOechlaFl	TTTTTTCTACTAAACACAAGGATATTGG	Forward	[16]
LepFl	ATTCAACCAATCATAAAGATATTGG	Forward	[17]
LepFl_t1	TGTAAAACGACGGCCAGTATTCAACCAATCATAAAGATATTGG	Forward	[14]
LepRl	TAAACTTCTGGATGTCCAAAAATCA	Reverse	[17]
LepRl_t1	CAGGAAACAGCTATGACTAAACTTCTGGATGTCCAAAAATCA	Reverse	[14]
M13Fᵃ	TGTAAAACGACGGCCAGT	Reverse	[18]
M13Rᵃ	CAGGAAACAGCTATGAC	Forward	[18]
NemF1_t1	TGTAAAACGACGGCCAGTCRACWGTWAATCAYAARAATATTGG	Forward	[19]
NemF2_t1	TGTAAAACGACGGCCAGTARAGATCTAATCATAAAGATATYGG	Forward	[19]
NemF3_t1	TGTAAAACGACGGCCAGTARAGTTCTAATCATAARGATATTGG	Forward	[19]
NemR1_t1	CAGGAAACAGCTATGACTAAACTTCWGGRTGACCAAAAATCA	Reverse	[19]
NemR2_t1	CAGGAAACAGCTATGACTAWACYTCWGGRTGMCCAAAAAYCA	Reverse	[19]
NemR3_t1	CAGGAAACAGCTATGACTAAACCTCWGGATGACCAAAAAATCA	Reverse	[19]
PlatyF1	TTACTTTGGATCATAAGCGTATAGG	Forward	This publication
PlatyF2	TTACTTTAGATCATAAGCGGGTTGG	Forward	This publication
PlatyR1	TAMACYTCWGGATGACCAAARAAYCA	Reverse	This publication
polyLCO	GAYTATWTTCAACAAATCATAAAGATATTGG	Forward	[20]
polyHCO	TAMACTTCWGGGTGACCAAARAATCA	Reverse	[20]

Primer	Sequence	Direction	Reference
PolyshortCOIR	CCNCCTCCNGCWGGRTCRAARAA	Reverse	[20]
PorF1	TTTCMACWAATCAYAARGAYATWGG	Forward	This publication
RibbonF1	TTTCAACWAATCATAARGATATTGG	Forward	This publication
RibbonR1	TAAACTTCRGGRTGWCCAAARAAYCV	Reverse	This publication
SipR1	TAAACTTCTGGRTGRCCAAARAAYCA	Reverse	This publication
SpoonR1	TATACCTCAGGATGSCCAAARAATCA	Reverse	This publication
TurF1	CTTCTACAAAACATAAGGATATAGG	Forward	This publication
TunF1	TDTCAACDAATCATAARGATATTRG	Forward	This publication
TunR1	TAAACYTCAGGATGTCYAAARAAYCA	Reverse	This publication
VF1_t1	TGTAAAACGACGGCCAGTTCTCAACCACAAAGACATTGG	Forward	[14]
VF1d_t1	TGTAAAACGACGGCCAGTTCTCAACCACAACAARGAYATYGG	Forward	[14]
VF1i_t1	TGTAAAACGACGGCCAGTTCTCAACCACAIAAIGAIATIGG	Forward	[14]
VF2_t1	TGTAAAACGACGGCCAGTTCAACCACAAAGACATTGGCAC	Forward	[14]
VR1d_t1	CAGGAAACAGCTATGACTAGACTTCTGGGTGGCCRAARAAYCA	Reverse	[14]
VR1_t1	CAGGAAACAGCTATGACTAGACTTCTGGGTGGCCAAAGAATCA	Reverse	[14]
VR1i_t1	CAGGAAACAGCTATGACTAGACTTCTGGGTGICCIAAIAAICA	Reverse	[14]
ZplankF1_t1	TGTAAAACGACGGCCAGTTCTASWAATCATAARGATATTGG	Forward	[21]
ZplankR1_t1	CAGGAAACAGCTATGACTTCAGGRTGRCCRAARAATCA	Reverse	[21]

Primer cocktails

C_FishF1t1: VF2_t1 + FishF2_t1 (1:1)

C_FishR1t1: FishR2_t1 + FR1d_t1 (1:1)

C_GasF1_t1: GasF1_t1 + GasF2_t1 + GasF3_t1 (1:1:1)

C_LepFolF: LepF1 + LCO1490 (1:1)

(continued)

Table 2
(continued)

Primer name	Sequence (5′–3′)	Direction	Reference
C_LepFolR: LepR1 + HCO2198 (1:1)			
C_NemF1_t1: NemF1_t1 + NemF2_t1 + NemF3_t1 (1:1:1)			
C_NemR1_t1: NemR1_t1 + NemR2_t1 + NemR3_t1 (1:1:1)			
C_PlatyF1: PlatyF1 + PlatyF2 (1:1)			
C_VF1LFt1: LepF1_t1 + VF1_t1 + VF1d_t1 + VF1i_t1 (1:1:1:3)			
C_VR1LRt1: LepR1_t1 + VR1d_t1 + VR1_t1 + VR1i_t1 (1:1:1:3)			

[a]*See* Note 5

mixture in a microwave until boiling and all agarose has completely dissolved. Allow the solution to cool for 2 min and then add 2 μL of 1 % ethidium bromide and swirl gently to mix. Immediately cast the gel with the appropriate comb inserted. Upon solidifying, submerge the gel in an electrophoresis chamber filled with 1× TAE and load your samples. No ladder is required and electrophoresis needs only to be long enough to visualize the PCR product.

If positive, the PCR product can be sent to a commercial sequencing facility or sequenced in-house (see later).

3.4 Cycle Sequencing

1. Dilute the PCR product by adding 40 μL of sterile water to the product remaining after PCR check.

2. Add 2 μL of the diluted PCR product to 9.5 μL of sequencing mix (see **Note 9**) containing the appropriate sequencing primer (*see* Tables 1 and 2).

3. Pulse centrifuge for 3 s and thermocycle using the following conditions:

   (a) 96 °C for 2 min.

   (b) 30 cycles of:

   - 96 °C for 30 s.
   - 55 °C for 15 s.
   - 60 °C for 4 min.

3.5 Sequencing Cleanup

Sequencing cleanup is performed with Sephadex following the manufacturer's instructions. Briefly:

1. Into a 0.45 μm GHP membrane, measure the appropriate amount of dry Sephadex using the tool provided and hydrate with 300 μL of sterile water for 4 h at room temperature or 18 h at 4 °C.

2. Centrifuge at $750 \times g$ for 3 min to drain water.

3. Add the entire volume of sequencing reaction to the prepared membrane and then add 25 μL of 0.1 mM EDTA pH 8.0.

4. Place the membrane into a clean collection receptacle (tube or plate) and centrifuge at $750 \times g$ for 3 min.

5. The flow-through contains purified product that can now be directly sequenced by Sanger sequencing.

4 Notes

1. The CTAB extraction protocol was initially developed for plants. CTAB selectively precipitates nucleic acids. RNA and DNA form an insoluble complex with CTAB at low salt concentrations (e.g., 0.4 M NaCl) but the CTAB–Nucleic acid

complex becomes soluble at high salt concentration (0.7 M NaCl). Polysaccharides (e.g., from plant cell walls), strong PCR inhibitors, are insoluble at this salt concentration and remain precipitated allowing for their removal. A number of metazoan species are covered in mucus layers (with at times high concentrations of polysaccharides). Therefore, we recommend the use of the CTAB protocol for a number of animal phyla (Table 1).

2. Most of our extraction methods are silica based and involve binding DNA to a glass fiber membrane in the presence of chaotropic salts. There are a variety of glass fiber plates available on the market, but PALL AgroPrep plates (PALL 5051, PALL 5053) have shown the best performance and compatibility with automation.

3. As for polychaetes initial PCR with the primer set polyLCO/ polyHCO (Tables 1 and 2) usually amplifies approximately 70 % of the individuals. Most species of the polychaete families Spionidae, Sabellidae, and Cirratulidae can actually be amplified with the primer cocktail recommended for most vertebrates (C_VF1LFt1/C_VR1LRt1), while members of the family Nephtyidae have been amplified with the pair polyLCO/ PolyshortCOIR (Table 2). Some species of Serpulidae can be amplified with polyLCO/polyHCO using PCR products as template for a second PCR.

4. The combination C_FishF1t1/ C_FishR1t1 works very well for most fish groups. However, some species, especially elasmobranchs, can be better amplified with the alternative chordate pair C_VF1LFt1/C_VR1LRt1. The reverse is true for some mammal species. We recommend the use of the respective second alternative for initial failures.

5. Tailing the primer pair CrustDF1/CrustDR1 with M13F and M13R, respectively, can increase amplification and especially sequencing success for some Malacostraca. It is possible that the conventional primer set is more prone to dimer formation thereby obscuring the first 30–40 base calls at the 5′ terminus.

6. Alternative primer pairs for echinoderms are EchinoF1/ HCO2198 and EchnioF1/COIeRl (Table 2).

7. Some bivalves exhibit a different form of mtDNA transmission called doubly uniparental inheritance. In this case, the animals have two types of mtDNA, a female-transmitted (F-type) and a male-transmitted (M-type), the latter being present only in the male gonads. The primers we suggest are designed to retrieve F-type COI.

8. Several other universal primer combinations have been suggested. Among those are modifications of the classical HCO2198/LCO1490 pair [4], e.g., found in [5, 6], and

other alternatives that target shorter fragments of COI [7]. See also chapters 13 (Bourlat et al.) and 14 (Leray et al.) in this book, which use some of these alternative primers for metabarcoding applications.

9. Our cycle sequencing protocol is optimized for the use of a 1/16 dilution of BigDye v3.1 on an ABI 3730xl DNA Analyzer (Applied Biosystems).

10. DNA barcoding protocols for nonmetazoans have been described for some protists [8] and fungi [9].

Acknowledgements

The protocols summarized here are the result of years of dedicated work by students and staff of the Biodiversity Institute of Ontario. This work was supported by funding from the Government of Canada through Genome Canada and the Ontario Genomics Institute to the International Barcode of Life Project. We also thank the Ontario Ministry of Research and Innovation for funding the Biodiversity Institute of Ontario.

References

1. Hebert PDN, Cywinska A, Ball SL, deWaard JR (2003) Biological identifications through DNA barcodes. Proc R Soc Lond B 270:313–321. doi:10.1098/rspb.2002.2218

2. Bucklin A, Steinke D, Blanco-Bercial L (2011) DNA barcoding of marine metazoans. Ann Rev Mar Sci 3:471–508. doi:10.1146/annurev-marine-120308-080950

3. Sanger F, Nicklen S, Coulson AR (1977) DNA sequencing with chain-terminating inhibitors. Proc Natl Acad Sci U S A 74:5463–5467

4. Folmer OM, Black WH, Lutz R, Vrijenhoek R (1994) DNA primers for amplification of mitochondrial cytochrome c oxidase subunit I from metazoan invertebrates. Mol Mar Biol Biotechnol 3:294–299

5. Geller J, Meyer C, Parker M, Hawk H (2013) Redesign of PCR primers for mitochondrial cytochrome c oxidase subunit I for marine invertebrates and application in all-taxa biotic surveys. Mol Ecol Resour 13:851–861. doi:10.1111/1755-0998.12138

6. Lobo J, Costa PM, Teixeira MAL, Ferreira MSG, Costa MH, Costa FO (2013) Enhanced primers for amplification of DNA barcodes from a broad range of marine metazoans. BMC Ecol 13:34. doi:10.1186/1472-6785-13-34

7. Leray M, Yang JY, Meyer CP, Mills SC, Agudelo N, Vincent R, Boehm JT, Machida RJ

(2013) A new versatile primer set targeting a short fragment of the mitochondrial COI region for metabarcoding metazoan diversity: application for characterizing coral reef fish gut contents. Front Zool 10:34. doi:10.1186/1742-9994-10-34

8. Saunders GW, McDevit DC (2012) Methods for DNA barcoding photosynthetic protists emphasizing the macroalgae and diatoms. Meth Mol Biol (Clifton, NJ) 858:207–222. doi:10.1007/978-1-61779-591-6_10

9. Eberhardt U (2012) Methods for DNA barcoding of fungi. Meth Mol Biol (Clifton, NJ) 858:183–205. doi:10.1007/978-1-61779-591-6_9

10. Hebert PDN, Stoeckle MY, Zemlak TS, Francis CM (2004) Identification of birds through DNA barcodes. PLoS Biol 2(10), e312. doi:10.1371/journal.pbio.0020312

11. Layton KKS, Martel AL, Hebert PDN (2014) Patterns of DNA barcode variation in Canadian marine molluscs. PLoS One 9(4), e95003. doi:10.1371/journal.pone.0095003

12. Arndt A, Marquez C, Lambert P, Smith MJ (1996) Molecular phylogeny of eastern Pacific sea cucumbers (Echinodermata: Holothuroidea) based on mitochondrial DNA sequence. Mol Phylogenet Evol 6:425–437. doi:10.1006/mpev.1996.0091

13. Ward RD, Holmes BH, O'Hara TD (2008) DNA barcoding discriminates echinoderm species. Mol Ecol Resour 8:1202–1211. doi:10.1111/j.1755-0998.2008.02332

14. Ivanova NV, Zemlak TS, Hanner RH, Hebert PDN (2007) Universal primer cocktails for fish DNA barcoding. Mol Ecol Notes 7:544–548. doi:10.1111/j.1471-8286.2007.01748

15. Stein ED, White BP, Mazor RD, Miller PE, Pilgrim EM (2013) Evaluating ethanol-based sample preservation to facilitate use of DNA barcoding in routine freshwater biomonitoring programs using benthic macroinvertebrates. PLoS One 8(1), e51273. doi:10.1371/journal.pone.0051273

16. Corstorphine EA (2010) DNA barcoding of echinoderms: species diversity and patterns of molecular evolution. MSc thesis. University of Guelph, Guelph, ON

17. Hebert PDN, Penton EH, Burns JM, Janzen DH, Hallwachs W (2004) Ten species in one: DNA barcoding reveals cryptic species in the Neotropical skipper butterfly *Astraptes fulgerator*. Proc Natl Acad Sci U S A 101:14812–14817. doi:10.1073/pnas.0406166101

18. Messing J (1983) New M13 vectors for cloning. Methods Enzymol 101:20–78

19. Prosser SWJ, Velarde-Aguilar MG, León-Règagnon V, Hebert PDH (2013) Advancing nematode barcoding: a primer cocktail for the cytochrome *c* oxidase subunit I gene from vertebrate parasitic nematodes. Mol Ecol Resour 13(6):1108–1115. doi:10.1111/1755-0998.12082

20. Carr CM, Hardy SM, Brown TM, Macdonald TA, Hebert PDN (2011) A tri-oceanic perspective: DNA barcoding reveals geographic structure and cryptic diversity in Canadian polychaetes. PLoS One 6(7), e22232. doi:10.1371/journal.pone.0022232

21. Prosser SWJ, Martínez-Arce A, Elías-Gutiérrez M (2013) A new set of primers for COI amplification from freshwater microcrustaceans. Mol Ecol Resour 13(6):1151–1155. doi:10.1111/1755-0998.12132

Chapter 11

DNA Barcoding Marine Biodiversity: Steps from Mere Cataloguing to Giving Reasons for Biological Differences

Mikko Nikinmaa and Miriam Götting

Abstract

DNA barcoding has become a useful tool in many contexts and has opened up a completely new avenue for taxonomy. DNA barcoding has its widest application in biodiversity and ecological research to detect and describe diversity whenever morphological discrimination is difficult or impossible (e.g., in the case of species lacking diagnostic characters, early life stages, or cryptic species). In this chapter, we outline the utility of including physiological parameters as part of species description in publicly available databases that catalog taxonomic information resulting from barcoding projects. Cryptic species or different life stages of a species often differ in their physiological traits. Thus, if physiological aspects were included in species definitions, the presently cryptic species could be distinguished. We furthermore give suggestions for physiological information that should be included in a species description and describe potential applications of DNA barcoding for research with physiological components.

Key words DNA barcoding, Physiology, Cryptic species, Invasive species, Phenotypic plasticity, Speciation

1 Introduction

DNA barcoding has become an indispensable component of research on biological diversity, as witnessed by the fact that in 2012 there was a volume of Methods in Molecular Biology devoted to DNA Barcoding [1]. Although the methodology is only approximately 10 years old, a search at the beginning of 2015 in the Web of Science found several hundred articles that had used DNA barcoding in marine organisms. The aim of the methodology is to characterize species using a short standard DNA sequence [2]. The preferred properties of such a universal DNA sequence are at least the following: first, it is short—in the best case one should be able to amplify it with standard PCR and universal primers without any problems; second, the sequence difference between species is always greater than within species, this is referred to as the 'barcoding gap' [3]; third, the accumulation of mutations occurs at a

Sarah J. Bourlat (ed.), *Marine Genomics: Methods and Protocols*, Methods in Molecular Biology, vol. 1452,
DOI 10.1007/978-1-4939-3774-5_11, © Springer Science+Business Media New York 2016

constant rate, whereby closely related species have a smaller number of sequence differences than distant species; fourth, the sequence starts from the start codon of a gene. In animals, the most commonly used DNA barcoding sequence is the 5′ region of the mitochondrial *Cytochrome C oxidase I* (*CO1, COX1, or COI*), which was the first one published to separate animal species (lepidopterans [4]), because it provides species level resolution in many metazoan groups. Notably, Cytochrome C oxidase is an enzyme involved in aerobic energy production, but any linkage between the function of the protein and molecular taxonomy is currently not known. In fact, it is quite interesting that while there are several hundred articles using DNA barcoding on marine organisms, there is up to now not a single one combining the search terms "DNA barcoding" and "physiology."

The purpose of this chapter is to propose that physiological considerations should play a role in describing species, and in the use of DNA barcoding and additional molecular resources for (molecular) systematics. As there are no earlier resources apart from an opinion paper [5], this chapter cannot give methods ready for use, but will rather give suggestions as to the directions that future endeavors could take.

2 Why Should Physiological Information Be Included in Species Definitions?

DNA barcoding has a wide range of applications, but it has proven to be a powerful tool especially for separating cryptic species, i.e., ones that look alike whereby they cannot be separated by traditional taxonomic means. Cryptic species can have, e.g., different food sources [6], or the abiotic conditions tolerated by the species are different. This possibility is very important for benthic species, as sea bottoms characteristically have different oxygen and sulfide levels. It has been shown that some forms, which can probably be classified as cryptic species, of morphologically the same species have quite different oxygen requirements and sulfide tolerances [7, 8]. It often appears that cryptic species differ in their physiological properties [9]. This actually makes the lack of visual differences between species possible. Because the physiological properties (including timing of reproduction, development and its speed, biotic interactions, and requirements/tolerance of abiotic conditions) separate the species, visual differences are not needed to ensure that the organisms are reproductively isolated. They either cannot occur in the same locality at the time of reproduction or are at different stages of reproductive development. If physiological information in such cases were included in species definition, species which are now defined as cryptic would actually not be such; they would remain visually cryptic but would be distinguishable overall.

There are important reasons why physiologically differing cryptic species should be separated. In estimating human impacts on marine environments, one often uses community diversity as an end point. When a cryptic species pair differs in hypoxia and sulfide tolerance, an increase in the area of anoxic bottom area could remain undetected, if such a species pair (i.e., morphologically one species) were used as a bioindicator of anoxic area. The more sensitive species would be replaced with the species that tolerates hypoxia better with no overall change in the abundance of the morphologically defined species. The importance of knowledge about the tolerances/behavior of the species that are used as bioindicators has also earlier been pointed out [10]. The importance of separating cryptic species becomes even more important as different areas may have seemingly the same species with different proportions of the morphs with different tolerances. In this case, the same human impact can have big differences on the apparent species abundance in different localities. Also, in studies of physiological responses of the species, both the presence of cryptic species in the same locality while having different requirements for abiotic conditions and the occurrence of cryptic species with different environmental requirements in different localities can have significant influence on the interpretation of the results. In the first case, the environmental tolerance seems to be much wider than it actually is. In the latter case, two studies with apparently the same species from different locations yield conflicting results. The reason for this discrepancy may be assigned to, e.g., unstudied contaminants, although the reason is that different morphologically cryptic species have been studied with differences in the physiological features investigated.

3   A Suggestion for Components of a Tree of Life Catalog Entry Including Physiological Component

Table 1 gives a suggestion for different components in any tree of life catalog entry. As Table 2 we have compiled an example of what an entry of a particular species could look like. Currently, the world is filled with species identification books—a brief web search found more than 300 fish guides and more than 200 guides to marine invertebrates and algae. Typically, the guides describe the morphological features of species with the aim that they can be separated from other organisms. In addition, the books usually describe the geographical range, the habitat, and major life history properties of the species. The species identification catalogs are increasingly becoming web based, with at least two major drawbacks. First, the information given, and the different entry categories vary markedly between databases. This increases the difficulty of transferring information from one database to another. Second, often the databases do not include a comprehensive set of links where relevant

Table 1
A suggestion for the layout of information about organisms in media describing biodiversity

1. Species and common name	Given on the basis of traditional taxonomy
2. Morphological characteristics	Description of the characteristics (possibly including illustrations) which define the species
3. DNA barcode	The properties/sequence of DNA used to separate the species from others. Should give a unique identification of the molecular source (e.g., GenBank accession number with link to the database with identification)
4. Classification	Taxonomic lineage
5. Spatial distribution (range)	The geographical distribution of the species
6. Habitat requirements	Description of the types of biotopes where the organism is found
7. General biological characteristics	Preferred food, mode of reproduction, etc.
8. Physiological characteristics	Description of the major characteristics that have most likely contributed to the appearance of the species in its present environment
9. Genes possibly associated with phenotypic variation	Description of the major genes associated with the diversification traits which are probably selected for during adaptation to environment and speciation
10. Links	Internet links to other databases where information on the species is compiled
11. References	The major references pertaining to the above entry categories (maximally 10)

information on the species could also be found. In an ideal world, one could combine all the different databases to a "master" database—a taxonomic counterpart to GenBank. From this "master" database one could/should have links to more specific databases, which would have more specific information on the taxonomic entity. A comprehensive project (www.tolweb.org) already aims to bring together the whole tree of life. This project could be taken as the authoritarian source behind combining taxonomy and genomics (and also other disciplines). In their current form, species pages can have somewhat different structures. In our view, they should be made uniform both in the master and accessory databases. In the master database the lack of a component would inform the reader that this information is missing. This point could be beneficial on two counts: first, if there is information available, but that was not known to the persons compiling the entry, the scientists with relevant information could complete the entry; second, knowledge of the information gaps could direct research on that particular point/species. In accessory databases the lack could also mean that the type of information is not included in the particular database.

Table 2
An example of a species entry to a biodiversity database compiled according to the outline given in Table 1

1. **Species and common name**
   Marenzelleria neglecta Sikorski & Bick, 2004
   Synonyms: *Marenzelleria* type II, *Marenzelleria viridis*, *Marenzelleria* cf. *viridis*
   Common name: Red gilled mud worm

2. **Morphological characteristics**
   Up to 115 mm long, 2.4 mm wide, morphologically difficult to discriminate from the closely related species *M. viridis*, juveniles and larvae are not distinguishable from other species of the genus, can be identified only by the combination of the following characters: length of the nuchal organ is up to setiger 4 and the relation of total number of branchiate setigers to total number of setigers is about ¼ to 1/3 (Sikorski and Bick 2004)

3. **DNA barcode**
   Cytochrome C oxidase subunit I (http://www.ncbi.nlm.nih.gov/nuccore/?term=marenzelleria%20 coi; http://www.boldsystems.org/index.php/TaxBrowser_TaxonPage?taxid=78928)
   Cytochrome b (http://www.ncbi.nlm.nih.gov/nuccore/?term=marenzelleria+cytochrome+b)
   16 s rDNA (http://www.ncbi.nlm.nih.gov/nuccore/?term=marenzelleria+16s)
   18S rDNA (http://www.ncbi.nlm.nih.gov/nuccore/?term=marenzelleria+18s)

4. **Classification**
   Eukaryota; Metazoa; Lophotrochozoa; Annelida; Polychaeta; Scolecida; Spionida; Spionidae;
   Marenzelleria Mesnil, 1896

5. **Spatial distribution (range)**
   GBIF record: http://www.gbif.org/species/
   search?q=marenzelleria&dataset_key=d7dddbf4-2cf0-4f39-9b2a-bb099caae36c#
   Additional information:
   Populations in Europe geographically originate from the East coast of North America
   Species was introduced to the North Sea and Baltic Sea (late 1970s and early 1980s) by ship ballast water
   Inhabits coastal boreal and arctic waters; the southern limit of distribution is approx. 32° latitude

6. **Habitat requirements**
   Muddy and sandy sediments in brackish water estuaries (salinities of 0.5–10 psu), up to 130 m depth

7. **General biological characteristics**
   Life span approx. 3 years, suspension and deposit feeder; inhabits vertical mucus-lined tubes
   Spawning in autumn, sexual reproduction, pelagic larvae (no larval development <5 psu)
   Very abundant, can make up to 90 % of biomass (<40,000 individuals/m^2)
   Hybridizes with *M. viridis*

8. **Physiological characteristics**
   Shows broad tolerance of many abiotic factors (e.g., salinity, hypoxia, temperature, hydrogen sulfide), prefers oligo- to mesohaline habitats, tolerates salinities of 0–30 psu ($LC_{50} < 0.1$ psu in adults, $LC_{50} < 1$ psu in larvae)

9. **Genes associated with phenotypic diversification**
   isocitrate dehydrogenase (idh); malate dehydrogenase (mdh)
   capping protein, gelsolin-like (capg); glyceraldehyde-3-phosphate dehydrogenase (gapdh); adenylate kinase (ak); peroxiredoxin-1 (prdx1); troponin C (tnnc1)

(continued)

Table 2
(continued)

10. Links
http://www.gbif.org/
http://www.marinespecies.org
http://www.ncbi.nlm.nih.gov/
http://www.boldsystems.org/

11. References
Bastrop, R. et al. (1995): Mar. Biol. 121: 509–516
Bastrop, R. et al. (1997): Aquatic Ecology 31: 116–139
Bick, A. (2005): Helgol. Mar. Res. 59, 265–272
Blank, M. et al. (2004): Mar. Ecol. Prog. Ser. 271: 193–205
Blank, M. & Bastrop, R. (2009): Zool. Scr. 38: 313–321
Blank, M. et al. (2012): J. Proteome Res. 11: 897–905
Bochert, R. (1997): Aquatic Ecology 31: 163–175
Schiedek, D. (1997): Aquatic Ecology 31: 199–210
Sikorski, A.V. & Bick, A. (2004): Sarsia 89: 253–275

An important database that certainly needs to be continued is the comprehensive database of the DNA barcoding community (www.barcodeoflife.org) [11], which, importantly, has minimum standards on what features should be included when submitting DNA barcode data. Additional information such as collection sites, collectors, primers used to amplify the barcode, pictures, and maps can be deposited with the barcode sequence data. BOLD is directly linked to the member databases of the International Nucleotide Sequence Database Collaboration (INSDC), DNA Databank of Japan (DDBJ), European Nucleotide Archive (ENA), and Genbank (National Center for Biotechnology Information, NCBI, North America). Data exchange between databases ensures a global synchronization of records.

4   DNA Sequences Can Be Used to Define Species When This Is Difficult on the Basis of Traditional Taxonomy

The discussion earlier points to the fact that in addition to morphological features, physiological features should be included in a species definition. However, this does not abolish the fact that if organisms are visually not distinguishable, it is difficult to separate them. Before the era of DNA barcoding it was virtually impossible to determine if forms inhabiting different environments have DNA sequences that are divergent enough to say that the similar-looking forms are, in fact, different species. In most instances, traditional and molecular taxonomies agree, and as has been suggested, their strengths should be combined [12]. Without connecting the DNA sequence to a living organism, the DNA barcode is not very informative. Thus, to assign biological significance to it, molecular taxonomy can most conveniently be tied to traditional taxonomy. However, there are two major instances when traditional taxonomy can be at odds with DNA barcoding. The first of these is cryptic species. In this case, any reproductive isolation is the result of physiological differences between the morphs, and, consequently, a difference between the species can be seen provided that physiological differences are recorded and included in the definition of species. When speciation is incomplete and the barriers causing reproductive isolation are broken down, interbreeding, producing fertile offspring, may take place. This is probably the case in whitefish (*Coregonus lavaretus*) in which several subspecies/morphs have been described [13–15]. Second, it is possible that two specimens of the same species have very different morphological characteristics. Consequently, if they are separated on the basis of morphology, two species may be described, although separation is not warranted based on their DNA. This situation is conspicuous especially for species which have multiple life stages, e.g., hydrozoans with pelagic and sessile forms. Similarly, how can we discern which pelagic larvae belong to which adults [16]? There are additional examples of morphological dimorphism in fish: e.g., African cichlids, which are characterized by rapid evolution [17], display markedly different coloration patterns, even when they belong to the same species [18].

5 Associating Gene Sequences, Physiological Properties, and Phenotypic Plasticity

The concepts that are important for evaluating the use of DNA sequences to separate species are many and include at least the following. (a) For barcoding, short DNA sequences that show more interspecific than intraspecific variation are used. Sequences are not selected on the basis of their involvement in the speciation process. One can argue that for DNA barcoding it is best if the sequence is inert, whereby the accumulated differences do not result in any change in the function of the gene product. Many point mutations occur without changing the function of the gene product, but some point mutations can result in the alteration of a critical amino acid in the encoded protein. For example, enzymatic activity may change leading to, e.g., different hypoxia tolerances in organisms. The effects of single amino acid changes on protein function are best known for hemoglobins, where there are many instances showing marked alterations of oxygen affinity after only a single amino acid change [19]. (b) Individuals of a species display a range of responses to an environmental change. This individual variation is actually the basis for selection, but most studies report means and standard deviation. Usually a study is thought to be

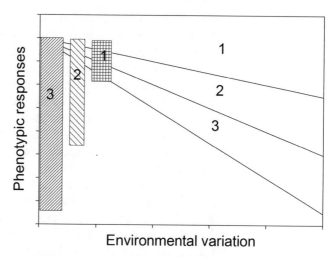

Fig. 1 Phenotypic plasticity of the genotypes in a population can be very different. Three different populations (with different genotypes) are represented here (*1–3*). The possible variation of traits as a function of environment in every population is shown by the *lines* (*1–3*). The trait variation (range of phenotypes corresponding to the trait, shown as the *rectangles*) in the different environmental conditions is smallest for population 1, intermediate for population 2, and greatest for population 3. The larger the variation between individuals in a population is, the more difficult it is to determine if the organisms at the opposite ends of the variation belong to the same or different species

good, if the standard deviation of the response is small. Individual variation should increasingly be taken into account when assessing the responses of populations to environmental impacts [20, 21]. For example, in terms of environmental adaptation, "an outlier" may display a response to an environmental stress which helps it to adapt to the environmental challenge, such as an increase in temperature. Different populations of a species can have different ranges of possible responses (*see* Fig. 1). The phenotypic plasticity which varies between populations of a species makes it harder to define species, especially cryptic ones. However, in this case, DNA sequence can be decisive. One of the strengths of DNA barcoding is that it does not require detailed taxonomic knowhow once the reference library has been established. (c) With the increasing number of fully sequenced genomes, the possibilities of DNA-based taxonomy increase. One can envision that the type and number of markers used for species delimitation will increase manyfold. While the most common marker for DNA barcoding of animals is the 5′ end of *Cytochrome C oxidase 1* (*CO1*) [4, 22], additional genes are occasionally used, if the *CO1* sequence does not enable species delimitation [23]. In plants, a single marker DNA barcoding system has not become feasible, and the discriminating power of any one barcode is smaller than in animals. Among the markers studied, it appears that the combination of the plasmid sequences of *rbcL* and *matK* is the most informative one [24]. Of these, *matK* is rapidly evolving, similarly to the *CO1* of animals. However, in many plants it is difficult to amplify. The easily amplified *rbcL* is thus also used, even though it has poor discriminating power [24]. The situation with plants reflects the ultimate dilemma of species identification using molecular markers: the more markers are available, the more accurate the identification; however, using several markers increases the cost, and this can hinder their use in some laboratories which could carry out research requiring only a single short and universal DNA marker.

Adding physiological information to the picture is complicated due to the fact that any physiological response is seldom the result of the function of only one gene (naturally the genes involved in the physiological responses are usually different from the one(s) used in DNA barcoding). Furthermore, the same physiological response may be obtained even when different genes involved in the pathway respond differently [21]. For example, during heart metabolism in fish, variation among individuals appears to be the result of marked differences in the activities of various enzymes [25]. However, since speciation and changes in the structure of communities can only take place if some function of an organism is affected, we think that such information should be added to taxonomic databases. The limitation of such physiological response information resides in the fact that while it is possible to sequence the whole genome of an organism (genomics) and to determine which genes are transcribed (transcriptomics) and translated to proteins (proteomics) under certain conditions, as well as to evaluate the stability of a protein, it is virtually impossible to determine the activity of the protein even in 'normal' cellular conditions. Whenever we measure enzyme activity in vitro, we are really measuring its maximal activity in the given conditions under unlimited substrate availability. However, in vivo, there are several cellular factors (examples tabulated in Table 3), which may affect phenotypic response through the regulation of existing proteins. Individual variability in these pathways enables rapid regulation and response to environmental changes, whereby responses to disequilibrium conditions use cellular regulation with existing proteins. Gene expression pathways involving transcription–translation cycles cannot be used in acute (minutes to hours) responses because they are much slower (hours to days) [26]. Also, if an organism is able to survive the environmental challenge without having to resort to a changed gene expression, it is done, because modifying gene expression carries an energetic cost.

6 The Use of DNA Barcoding in Research with Physiological Components

6.1 Biomonitoring

Biomonitoring refers to the use of organisms to evaluate the changes caused in an ecosystem by environmental contamination, addressing both exposure to contaminants and biological responses to them. Normally it uses sentinel organisms, bioindicator species,

Table 3
Examples of major cellular pathways which may change rapidly in response to environmental variation, without changing the amounts of gene products produced

Intracellular pH. The activity of virtually all proteins is pH dependent. As an example, many enzymes have histidine imidazole as a part of the active group, and the protonation of imidazole changes in the physiological pH range (6-8). The activity of pH-regulating membrane transporters can be modulated by several cell signaling pathways so that the steady-state intracellular pH varies

Substrate concentrations of enzymes. While the conditions of in vitro enzyme assays generally have substrate concentrations that are adequate to guarantee that maximal rate of catalysis is reached, within the cells of an organism the substrate concentration can be limiting, and, furthermore, highly variable

Osmolality. Small changes in cellular osmolality affect the three-dimensional structure and aggregation of proteins with consecutive effects on their activity. The activity of membrane transporters can change to affect the steady-state osmolality of the cells. Also, changes in the salinity of the medium may affect the osmolality of the cells either transiently or at equilibrium

Concentrations of gaseous signaling molecules, NO, CO, H_2S, and free radicals. After NO was found to be involved in cellular signaling, several other gaseous molecules have been found to carry out similar functions. The concentrations of all of these can be changed rapidly. Similar for all of these is that they or their parent compounds (e.g., nitrite) are contaminants, and can therefore play a role in the toxicological responses of organisms in marine environments

Calcium signaling and molecules of other signaling pathways. Calcium plays a role in the signaling of many cellular responses. Often the signaling systems have very rapid spikes. Thus, calcium signaling can be involved in very rapid cellular responses, as can also other cellular signaling molecules with rapid turnover

The table gives only a few examples, and the main purpose is to show that cellular conditions can rapidly affect a phenotypic response and thereby the capability of individuals in a population to acclimatize to changing conditions. Presently, the relationship between phenotypic plasticity and genotype is poorly known

and measures their (usually biochemical) responses, biomarker responses. Biomarkers can be broadly divided into biomarkers of exposure and biomarkers of effect. There is a very important difference between the two. Biomarkers of exposure indicate that the organism has been exposed to a contaminant, but no change in the physiology (at any level, molecular, cellular, and integrative functions) of the organism is required. Thus, using microarray technology, a technology to study the expression of many genes (or actually the transcription of many genes) at once, one can detect changes in mRNA levels, but one does not know how this mRNA level change is linked to protein functions (=physiology). One has only shown that exposure has occurred, through a biomarker of exposure. Only if the observed change in gene expression (in this case taken to be the same as gene transcription) is reflected in a change in protein activity, one has determined a biomarker of effect. In our opinion one can talk about functional genomics only if a link between the change in gene transcription and gene product (protein) activity has been established [27]. When a biomarker response is followed in biomonitoring studies, correct species identification is the key. DNA barcoding can be used here to check that a single species (and not its cryptic sister species) is studied. Similarly, if the endpoint is a community of species, DNA barcoding must be used to determine if cryptic species with different physiological properties are found in the community.

6.2 Studies of Invasive Species

In the marine environment, many nonindigenous species have either deliberately or mostly accidentally been introduced to new areas. If these species are successful and establish themselves in the new environment, they can become invasive and replace native species. Occasionally nonindigenous species cannot be easily separated from native species by traditional morphology, and in such cases, DNA barcoding can be of immense help by facilitating species determinations. This could be done for the *Artemia* species group, inhabiting hypersaline environments, which has two American and four Old World species which can only be separated from each other by extremely professional taxonomists. The American *Artemia franciscana* has become an invasive species and presently appears to replace its Old World sibling species in many hypersaline environments. Recently, one reason for the invasiveness has become apparent, as the reproduction of *A. franciscana* is less affected by pesticide exposure than that of the Old World *A. parthenogenetica* [28].

Another example is the cryptic introduction of species of the polychaete genus *Marenzelleria* into the Baltic Sea (Northern Europe). Since 1985, *M. neglecta* has been found in high abundances in coastal areas of the Baltic Sea, where it has been accidentally introduced by ship ballast water from the North American Atlantic coast [29, 30]. The broad tolerance of the species toward many abiotic factors has facilitated its successful establishment and rapid spreading in new habitats. Taxonomic discrimination of *M. neglecta* from its sibling species is very difficult and only possible in adult specimens using the combination of several morphological characters [31]. The use of molecular methods has allowed the detection of two other introduced species in this genus, *M. viridis* and *M. arctia* [32]. The distribution of these species in the Baltic Sea is determined by their physiological characteristics. *M. neglecta* is absent from the western Baltic Sea where salinities ≥ 15 psu are observed, because it has, compared to its sibling species *M. viridis*, a lower ability to adapt to salinities ≥ 10 psu and to fluctuating salinities. This is confirmed by lower constitutive activity levels of enzymes involved in the amino acid metabolism, i.e., alanine aminotransferase (GPT), aspartate aminotransferase (AAT), and glutamate dehydrogenase (GDH). The adjustment of intracellular free amino acid concentrations plays an important role in acclimation to salinity changes in polychaetes [33, 34]. The temperature tolerance of *M. neglecta* is higher compared to both cooccurring species [35]. In Table 2 we give an example of a database entry for *M. neglecta*, including molecular, taxonomic, and physiological information.

In the case of invasive species, it is quite obvious why physiological information should be included in species definitions. From the physiological information, current and potential future distribution range of a species can be predicted and areas likely to be invaded can be identified [36, 37]. This is particularly important for species with harmful effects on ecosystems and human health.

6.3 Speciation

DNA barcodes were established to allow species identification on the premise that the within-species variation in the barcode is smaller than between-species variation [22]. With regard to speciation, a major question is, when do populations differ enough, so that reproductive isolation occurs, even if the physical barrier causing separation of the populations is removed? From a physiological perspective, this can mean that tolerance to environmental conditions (both abiotic and biotic) has changed so that the populations cannot utilize exactly the same environment any more. With regard to abiotic conditions such as temperature, this is very relevant to future climate models. Studies on the temperature tolerances of populations and the functional differences of populations which may have tolerance differences have become common [38, 39]. Temperature is relevant in the context of barcoding as the product of the mitochondrial *CO1* gene, the most commonly used DNA barcode in animals, is an enzyme involved in aerobic energy production, and variations in energy production are expected between populations acclimated to different temperatures.

During their isolation, populations may develop completely different diets, and this difference may be maintained even after the barrier causing isolation has been removed. It is, for example, possible that differences in diet have triggered changes in the proportions of certain digestive enzymes, whereby the food optimal for one population may not sustain growth and reproduction in another. It must be noted that this suggestion is purely hypothetical as most studies on population differentiation, speciation, and phylogenetics do not have a physiological component. Even when genomic information is included, most studies do not test if the transcribed gene is actually translated or if posttranscriptional events carry out major regulation of gene expression, although such information is required if it is assumed that the change in gene function is involved in the response. To conclude, combining genomics and physiological measurements could add a new, virtually unexplored dimension to studies on speciation, as ultimately, any extant organism must be physiologically competent in the environment that it is inhabiting.

References

1. Kress WJ, Erickson DL (2012) DNA barcodes: methods and protocols. Methods Mol Biol 858:1–470

2. Evans N, Paulay G (2012) DNA barcoding methods for invertebrates. Methods Mol Biol 858:47–77

3. Bucklin A, Steinke D, Blanco-Bercial L (2011) DNA barcoding of marine metazoa. Ann Rev Mar Sci 3:471–508

4. Hebert P, Cywinska A, Ball S, de Vaard J (2003) Biological identifications through DNA barcodes. Proc R Soc Lond B 270:313–332

5. Nikinmaa M (2014) What is biodiversity? Stepping forward from barcoding to understanding biological differences. Mar Genomics 17:65–67

6. Pentinsaari M, Mutanen M, Kaila L (2014) Cryptic diversity and signs of mitochondrial introgression in the Agrilus viridis species complex (Coleoptera: Buprestidae). Eur J Entomol 111:475–486

7. Gamenick I, Abbiati M, Giere O (1998) Field distribution and sulphide tolerance of Capitella capitata (Annelida : Polychaeta) around shallow wafer hydrothermal vents off Milos (Aegean Sea). A new sibling species? Mar Biol 130:447–453

8. Kruse I, Strasser M, Thiermann F (2004) The role of ecological divergence in speciation between intertidal and subtidal Scoloplos armiger (Polychaeta, Orbiniidae). J Sea Res 51:53–62

9. Nygren A (2014) Cryptic polychaete diversity: a review. Zool Scripta 43:172–183

10. Zettler ML, Proffitt CE, Darr A, Degraer S, Devriese L, Greathead C, Kotta J, Magni P, Martin G, Reiss H, Speybroeck J, Tagliapietra D, Van Hoey G, Ysebaert T (2013) On the myths of indicator species: Issues and further consideration in the use of static concepts for ecological applications. PLoS One 8, e78219

11. Ratnasingham S, Hebert PDN (2007) BOLD: the barcode of life data system (www.barcodinglife.org). Mol Ecol Notes 7:355–364

12. Boero F, Bernardi G (2014) Phenotypic vs genotypic approaches to biodiversity, from conflict to alliance. Mar Genomics 17:63–64

13. Ostbye K, Amundsen PA, Bernatchez L, Klemetsen A, Knudsen R, Kristoffersen R, Naesje TF, Hindar K (2006) Parallel evolution of ecomorphological traits in the European whitefish Coregonus lavaretus (L.) species complex during postglacial times. Mol Ecol 15:3983–4001

14. Siwertsson A, Knudsen R, Praebel K, Adams CE, Newton J, Amundsen PA (2013) Discrete foraging niches promote ecological, phenotypic, and genetic divergence in sympatric whitefish (Coregonus lavaretus). Evol Ecol 27:547–564

15. Praebel K, Knudsen R, Siwertsson A, Karhunen M, Kahilainen KK, Ovaskainen O, Ostbye K, Peruzzi S, Fevolden SE, Amundsen PA (2013) Ecological speciation in postglacial European whitefish: rapid adaptive radiations into the littoral, pelagic, and profundal lake habitats. Ecol Evol 3:4970–4986

16. Miglietta MP, Cunningham CW (2012) Evolution of life cycle, colony morphology, and host specificity in the family Hydractiniidae (Hydrozoa, Cnidaria). Evolution 66:3876–3901

17. Kornfield I, Smith PF (2000) African cichlid fishes: model systems for evolutionary biology. Annu Rev Ecol Syst 31:163–196

18. Bernardi G (2013) Speciation in fishes. Mol Ecol 22:5487–5502

19. Stamatoyannopoulos G, Bellingham AJ, Lenfant C, Finch CA (1971) Abnormal hemoglobins with high and low oxygen affinity. Annu Rev Med 22:221–234

20. Bennett AF (1987) Interindividual variability: an underutilized resource. In: Feder ME, Bennett AF, Burggren WW, Huey RB (eds) New directions in ecological physiology. Cambridge University Press, Cambridge, pp 147–169

21. Nikinmaa M, Waser W (2007) Molecular and cellular studies in evolutionary physiology of natural vertebrate populations: influences of individual variation and genetic components on sampling and measurements. J Exp Biol 210:1847–1857

22. Hajibabaei M, Singer GAC, Hebert PDN, Hickey DA (2007) DNA barcoding: how it complements taxonomy, molecular phylogenetics and population genetics. Trends Genet 23:167–172

23. Kruck NC, Tibbetts IR, Ward RD, Johnson JW, Loh WKW, Ovenden JR (2013) Multigene barcoding to discriminate sibling species within a morphologically difficult fish genus (Sillago). Fish Res 143:39–46

24. Hollingsworth PM, Graham SW, Little DP (2011) Choosing and using a plant DNA barcode. PLoS One 6, e19254

25. Oleksiak MF, Roach JL, Crawford DL (2005) Natural variation in cardiac metabolism and gene expression in Fundulus heteroclitus. Nat Genet 37:67–72

26. Nikinmaa M, McCairns RJS, Nikinmaa MW, Vuori KA, Kanerva M, Leinonen T, Primmer CR, Merila J, Leder EH (2013) Transcription and redox enzyme activities: comparison of equilibrium and disequilibrium levels in the three-spined stickleback. Proc R Soc B 280:20122974

27. Nikinmaa M, Rytkonen KT (2011) Functional genomics in aquatic toxicology—do not forget the function. Aquat Toxicol 105(Suppl):16–24

28. Varo I, Redon S, Garcia-Roger EM, Amat F, Guinot D, Serrano R, Navarro JC (2015) Aquatic pollution may favor the success of the invasive species A. franciscana. Aquat Toxicol 161:208–220

29. Bastrop R, Jurss K, Sturmbauer C (1998) Cryptic species in a marine polychaete and their independent introduction from North America to Europe. Mol Biol Evol 15:97–103

30. Bick A, Burckhardt R (1989) First record of *Marenzelleria viridis* (Polychaeta, Spionida) in the Baltic Sea with a key to the Spiondae of the Baltic Sea. Mitt Zool Mus Berlin 65:237–247

31. Bick A (2005) A new Spionidae (Polychaeta) from North Carolina, and a redescription of Marenzelleria wireni Augener, 1913, from Spitsbergen, with a key for all species of Marenzelleria. Helgoland Mar Res 59: 265–272

32. Bastrop R, Blank M (2006) Multiple invasions – a polychaete genus enters the Baltic Sea. Biol Inv 8:1195–1200

33. Jurss K, Rohner M, Bastrop R (1999) Enzyme activities and allozyme polymorphism in two genetic types (or sibling species) of the genus Marenzelleria (Polychaeta : Spionidae) in Europe. Mar Biol 135:489–496

34. Blank M, Bastrop R, Rohner M, Jurss K (2004) Effect of salinity on spatial distribution and cell volume regulation in two sibling species of Marenzelleria (Polychaeta: Spionidae). Mar Ecol Prog Ser 271:193–205

35. Blank M, Bastrop R, Jurss K (2006) Stress protein response in two sibling species of Marenzelleria (Polychaeta : Spionidae): is there an influence of acclimation salinity? Comp Biochem Physiol B 144:451–462

36. Kearney M, Porter W (2009) Mechanistic niche modelling: combining physiological and spatial data to predict species' ranges. Ecol Lett 12:334–350

37. Woodin SA, Hilbish TJ, Helmuth B, Jones SJ, Wethey DS (2013) Climate change, species distribution models, and physiological performance metrics: predicting when biogeographic models are likely to fail. Ecol Evol 3:3334–3346

38. Eliason EJ, Clark TD, Hague MJ, Hanson LM, Gallagher ZS, Jeffries KM, Gale MK, Patterson DA, Hinch SG, Farrell AP (2011) Differences in thermal tolerance among sockeye salmon populations. Science 332:109–112

39. Portner HO, Farrell AP (2008) Ecology. Physiology and climate change. Science 322: 690–692

Chapter 12

Metabarcoding Marine Sediments: Preparation of Amplicon Libraries

Vera G. Fonseca and Delphine Lallias

Abstract

The accurate assessment of community composition and ultimately species identification is of utmost importance in any ecological and evolutionary study. Advances in sequencing technologies have allowed the unraveling of levels of biodiversity never imagined before when applied to large-scale environmental DNA studies (also termed metabarcoding/metagenetics/metasystematics/environmental barcoding). Here, we describe a detailed protocol to assess eukaryotic biodiversity in marine sediments, identifying key steps that should not be neglected when preparing Next-Generation Sequencing (NGS) amplicon libraries: DNA extraction, multiple PCR amplification of DNA barcode markers with index/ tag-primers, and final Illumina MiSeq sequencing library preparation.

Key words Metabarcoding, Marine eukaryotes, Environmental DNA, High-throughput sequencing, NGS, Molecular biodiversity, Illumina

1 Introduction

High-throughput (HTP) sequencing techniques [1] cover not only entire genomes but can also sequence and identify multiple taxa simultaneously from bulk environmental samples, revolutionizing the study of biodiversity, ecology, and evolution. With the promise of mass sequencing single molecules in real time (SMRT) in the near future, at present HTP techniques are already highly sensitive, fast and, with high capacity DNA sequencing, produce large amounts of data at a low cost. HTP technology has made high-resolution biodiversity assessments possible and its applicability to large-scale environmental DNA barcoding and diversity is now well established [2–11]. The use of HTP Next-Generation Sequencing (NGS) to study environmental community biodiversity starts with an important step, namely, sample processing and preservation. Sampling and preservation strategies are known to greatly bias diversity levels [3, 12–14] not only because an exhaustive representation of the study area is needed to extrapolate

Sarah J. Bourlat (ed.), *Marine Genomics: Methods and Protocols*, Methods in Molecular Biology, vol. 1452, DOI 10.1007/978-1-4939-3774-5_12, © Springer Science+Business Media New York 2016

biodiversity levels as close to reality as possible [15] but also because sample integrity is lost due to poor preservation. Conceptual issues such as choice of gene(s) and/or gene regions used are also very important to consider. The use of several marker genes and/or regions will greatly augment not only biodiversity resolution but also its coverage [7, 8]. Additionally, the use of rapidly evolving genes or intergenic spacer regions might result in the creation of multiple Operational Taxonomic Units (OTUs) for individuals that can be grouped into a single species using other criteria [16]. DNA isolation [17] and PCR conditions [18–20] are among the main drivers of diversity artifacts in large-scale environmental samples. Actually, all steps of the molecular approach can introduce biases or errors [21, 22]. Specifically, during PCR amplification, when incomplete extension occurs, the resulting amplicon reanneals to a foreign DNA strand and is copied to completion in the following PCR cycles, generating chimeric sequences [23, 24]. These chimeras are then hugely amplified during the HTP sequencing step and further analyzed and mistakenly identified as a new species [20, 25–27], thus greatly inflating community diversity estimates. Although not entirely effective, chimera formation can be minimized experimentally by PCR optimization (e.g., reducing the number of PCR cycles and extension time), less template concentration, and shorter amplicon size [28–31]. NGS library preparation consists of PCR amplifying the gene region of interest, incorporating tags for sample identification and incorporating NGS platform-specific adapters for downstream sequencing. Library design is optimal when using a paired-end approach, e.g., using a Molecular Identification Tag (MID) of 5–8 nucleotides targeting both amplicon ends; despite being more costly, this approach represents an effective way to identify chimeras even without a well-annotated reference database. Primer selection for amplicon strategies will be based upon the study target taxa and/ or objectives but currently several gene regions have been identified using the latest software and curated databases to allow a broader taxonomic diversity estimation of the marine realm [32–40]. Lastly, when using an amplicon approach, the PCR samples are sequenced using massively parallel sequencing followed by in silico meta-analysis. Several PCR-based NGS DNA-sequencing technologies are available, based on different chemistries (emulsion PCR for Roche 454 and Ion Torrent, and sequencing by synthesis for Illumina); importantly, comparative studies (e.g., [41]) have shown that the Illumina sequencing platform is associated with a lower error rate, hence its choice in this protocol. With the fast pace of NGS, several bioinformatic pipelines have become available and the challenge lies in choosing the most accurate and appropriate path to take [42–45]. Some hurdles inherent to the meta-analysis of sequences derived from NGS approaches are well recognized, generally focusing on high levels of richness associated with chimeric sequences [19, 20, 46–48] but currently mainly focusing on sequence clustering, quality filtering, and algorithm used [25–27, 48, 49]. The overall steps within such molecular approaches could become even more powerful if combined with a standardized methodology, namely, for sampling, DNA extraction, choice of sequencing platform, gene regions used, and bioinformatic analysis, since this would allow direct comparisons across space and time within large-scale marine biodiversity and ecology studies (Fig. 1).

2 Materials

2.1 DNA Extraction and Precipitation

1. Analytical grade stainless steel 2 mm wire mesh sieves.
2. 100% molecular biology grade Ethanol.
3. 70% Ethanol (molecular biology grade Ethanol diluted with ultra pure water).
4. 3 M NaOAc pH 5.2.
5. PowerMax Soil DNA Isolation Kit (MOBIO).
6. PowerClean Pro DNA Clean-Up Kit (MOBIO).
7. Aluminum foil.
8. Spatula.
9. Balance.
10. Laboratory disinfectant (e.g., Distel Spray).
11. Ultraviolet Crosslinker.
12. Qubit® fluorometer.
13. Qubit® dsDNA BR Assay Kit.
14. Qubit® 0.5 mL assay tubes.

2.2 Library Preparation

1. Q5 Hot Start High-Fidelity 2× MasterMix (New England BioLabs).
2. Ultra pure or PCR grade water.
3. NGS grade PCR1 amplicon primers (Integrated DNA Technologies) (*see* Fig. 2, **Notes 1** and **16**).
4. PCR2 Index primers: Nextera XT index Kit (Illumina) (*see* Fig. 2 and **Note 1**).
5. HT ExoSAP-IT high-throughput PCR product cleanup (Affymetrix).
6. RNase/DNase-free 8-well PCR strip tubes and caps.
7. Barrier/filter pipette tips (10–1000 µL).
8. Single channel pipettes (10–1000 µL).
9. Multichannel pipettes (10 and 100 µL).
10. Thermocycler.

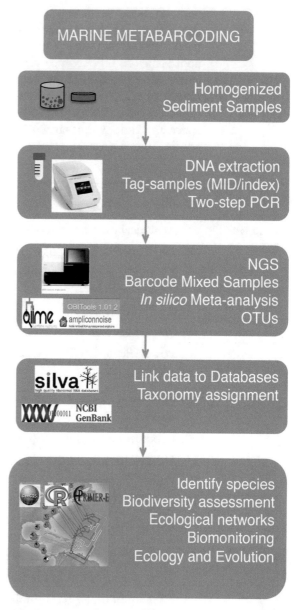

Fig. 1 Overview of environmental marine metabarcoding steps using Next-Generation Sequencing (NGS) approaches. Sediment samples are size fraction homogenized and DNA extracted. All samples can be identified using an 8-nucleotide multiplex identification (MID) tag/index incorporated into the amplicons during PCR amplification. All barcoded mixed samples are massively sequenced using an NGS platform followed by in silico meta-analysis using a bioinformatic pipeline. All data is annotated against public databases, followed by taxonomic assignment and further assessment of biodiversity at the community and ecosystem levels using statistical tools. *OTUs* operational taxonomic units

a

PCR1 Amplicon Primers		
Forward Primer Name	Forward Illumina Adapter/ Linker	**18S Forward Primer**
SSU_FO4	ACACTCTTTCCCTACACGACGCTCTTCCGATCT	GCTTGTCTCAAAGATTAAGCC
Reverse Primer Name	Reverse Illumina Adapter/ Linker	**18S Reverse Primer**
SSU_R22	GTGACTGGAGTTCAGACGTGTGCTCTTCCGATCT	GCCTGCTGCCTTCCTTGGA

b

PCR2 Index Primers			
Forward Index Name	5' Adapter P5	i5 indexes	Forward Linker Adapter
i5_N501	AATGATACGGCGACCACCGAGATCTACAC	TAGATCGC	ACACTCTTTCCCTACACGACGCTC
i5_N502	AATGATACGGCGACCACCGAGATCTACAC	CTCTCTAT	ACACTCTTTCCCTACACGACGCTC
i5_N503	AATGATACGGCGACCACCGAGATCTACAC	TATCCTCT	ACACTCTTTCCCTACACGACGCTC
i5_N504	AATGATACGGCGACCACCGAGATCTACAC	AGAGTAGA	ACACTCTTTCCCTACACGACGCTC
i5_N505	AATGATACGGCGACCACCGAGATCTACAC	GTAAGGAG	ACACTCTTTCCCTACACGACGCTC
i5_N506	AATGATACGGCGACCACCGAGATCTACAC	ACTGCATA	ACACTCTTTCCCTACACGACGCTC
i5_N507	AATGATACGGCGACCACCGAGATCTACAC	AAGGAGTA	ACACTCTTTCCCTACACGACGCTC
i5_N508	AATGATACGGCGACCACCGAGATCTACAC	CTAAGCCT	ACACTCTTTCCCTACACGACGCTC
Reverse Index Name	3' Adapter P7	i7 indexes	Reverse Linker Adapter
i7_N701	CAAGCAGAAGACGGCATACGAGAT	TCGCCTTA	GTGACTGGAGTTCAGACGTGTGCTC
i7_N702	CAAGCAGAAGACGGCATACGAGAT	CTAGTACG	GTGACTGGAGTTCAGACGTGTGCTC
i7_N703	CAAGCAGAAGACGGCATACGAGAT	TTCTGCCT	GTGACTGGAGTTCAGACGTGTGCTC
i7_N704	CAAGCAGAAGACGGCATACGAGAT	GCTCAGGA	GTGACTGGAGTTCAGACGTGTGCTC
i7_N705	CAAGCAGAAGACGGCATACGAGAT	AGGAGTCC	GTGACTGGAGTTCAGACGTGTGCTC
i7_N706	CAAGCAGAAGACGGCATACGAGAT	CATGCCTA	GTGACTGGAGTTCAGACGTGTGCTC
i7_N707	CAAGCAGAAGACGGCATACGAGAT	GTAGAGAG	GTGACTGGAGTTCAGACGTGTGCTC
i7_N708	CAAGCAGAAGACGGCATACGAGAT	CCTCTCTG	GTGACTGGAGTTCAGACGTGTGCTC
i7_N709	CAAGCAGAAGACGGCATACGAGAT	AGCGTAGC	GTGACTGGAGTTCAGACGTGTGCTC
i7_N710	CAAGCAGAAGACGGCATACGAGAT	TAGCAGAC	GTGACTGGAGTTCAGACGTGTGCTC
i7_N711	CAAGCAGAAGACGGCATACGAGAT	TCATAGAC	GTGACTGGAGTTCAGACGTGTGCTC
i7_N712	CAAGCAGAAGACGGCATACGAGAT	TCGCTATA	GTGACTGGAGTTCAGACGTGTGCTC

c

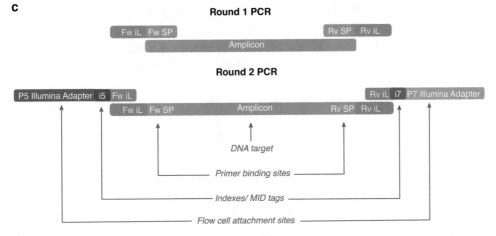

Fig. 2 Overview of the two-step PCR amplification approach for NGS library preparation. First round PCR primer (PCR1) design for the 18S rDNA target region (**a**) and second round PCR (PCR2) index primer design (**b**) are shown. Schematic diagram depicting the arrangement of primers, indexes, and Illumina adapters for PCR1 and PCR2 (**c**). *Fw* forward from the 5′-end, *Rv* reverse from the 3′-end, *SP* specific primer, *iL* Illumina Linker, *i5/i7*: i5/i7 Illumina Indexes or Molecular Identification Tags (MID)

2.3 Amplicon Purification and Quantification

1. Top Vision™ LM GQ Agarose (Fermentas) or equivalent.
2. 100 bp DNA ladder.
3. SafeXtractor tool for DNA fragment extraction from agarose gels (5Prime).
4. QIAquick Gel Extraction Kit (Qiagen).
5. 1.7 ml microcentrifuge tubes.
6. QuBit® Fluorometer.
7. Qubit® dsDNA BR Assay Kit.
8. Qubit® 0.5 mL assay tubes.

3 Methods

3.1 DNA Extraction

1. Homogenize sediment samples by sieving soils on a 2 mm mesh sieve (*see* **Note 2**).
2. Weigh 8–10 g of wet homogenized soil on a clean aluminum foil. These samples can be kept at –80 °C until DNA extraction (*see* **Notes 3** and **4**).
3. Proceed with DNA extraction using the PowerMax Soil DNA isolation kit, following the manufacturer's instructions just up to the DNA elution step. All centrifugation steps are extended an additional 5 min on top of the centrifugation time proposed by the manufacturer.
4. Elute DNA from the spin filter in 4.5 mL of solution C6 (provided by the manufacturer) and leave at room temperature for 30 min (*see* **Note 5**).
5. Collect DNA from the spin filter by centrifuging at $2500 \times g$ for 15 min.
6. Store DNA samples at –20 °C or proceed with the next step.

3.2 DNA Precipitation

1. Add 1/10 volume of 3 M NaOAc to the 4.5 mL DNA eluate.
2. Add 2.5 volumes of 100 % EtOH.
3. Place the samples at –80 °C for 30 min.
4. Centrifuge the samples at $13,000 \times g$ for 35 min at 4 °C.
5. Carefully remove the supernatant (avoiding resuspension of the DNA pellet) and centrifuge again to remove excess EtOH with a pipette.
6. Wash the pellet with fresh cold 70 % EtOH (*see* **Note 6**).
7. Discard the supernatant and centrifuge to remove excess EtOH. Repeat **steps 6** and **7** twice (*see* **Note 7**).
8. Air-dry the pellet for 5–10 min.
9. Resuspend the pellet in 100–300 µL of solution C6 or ultra pure water.

10. Quantify the DNA samples using a fluorometric method (e.g., Qubit® Fluorometer) and dilute all DNA samples to 10 ng/μL (*see* **Notes 8** and **9**).

3.3 Locus-Specific PCR Amplification (PCR1)

1. Prepare all reactions on ice.

2. Set up the following PCR1 reaction mix in a final volume of 15 μL: 7.5 μL Q5 Hot Start High-Fidelity 2× MasterMix, 0.75 μL Amplicon Forward primer SSU_FO4 (10 μM), 0.75 μL Amplicon Reverse primer SSU_R22 (10 μM), 5 μL PCR grade water, 1 μL DNA (10 ng/μL).

3. Set up the following PCR1 conditions: 2 min denaturation at 98 °C, then 15 cycles with 40 s 98 °C, 30 s 57 °C, 30 s 72 °C, and final extension of 5 min at 72 °C.

4. Add a negative control (no template DNA) for all amplification reactions and/or each primer set.

5. Each PCR is performed in triplicate and the use of a multi-channel pipette is advisable when performing several samples simultaneously (*see* **Notes 10** and **11**).

3.4 PCR1 Purification

1. Prepare all reactions on ice (*see* **Note 12**).

2. Set up the following PCR1 purification mix in a final volume of 20 μL: 5 μL HT ExoSAP-IT, 15 μL PCR1.

3. Incubate the reaction at 37 °C for 15 min, followed by 15 min at 80 °C. PCR1 product is now ready for the index PCR step.

3.5 Index PCR (PCR2)

1. This step attaches the indexes/tags and the Illumina sequencing adapters to the locus-specific amplicon (*purified PCR1 product*).

2. Illumina has several index/tag combinations available (i5 and i7) (Fig. 2) that can be used as a single or paired-end approach.

3. Set up the following PCR2 reaction mix in a final volume of 25 μL: 12.5 μL Q5 Hot Start High-Fidelity 2× MasterMix, 1.2 μL Index Forward primer (10 μM), 1.2 μL Index Reverse primer (10 μM), 3.1 μL PCR grade water, 7 μL purified PCR1.

4. Set up the following PCR2 conditions: 2 min denaturation at 98 °C, then 15 cycles with 40 s 98 °C, 40 s 55 °C, 30 s 72 °C, and final extension of 5 min at 72 °C (*see* **Note 13**).

5. Add a negative control (no template DNA) for all amplification reactions and/or each primer set.

3.6 PCR2 Purification

1. Run each PCR2 product including a DNA ladder on a 2 % low melting point agarose gel until the expected index amplicon is clearly isolated from any unspecific amplification fragment and clearly visible at ~550 bp (*see* **Notes 11, 14,** and **15**).

2. Extract each index amplicon product with a new SafeXtractor tool and place the gel band into a 1.7 ml DNAse-/RNAse-free

Eppendorf tube. At this point samples can be kept at –20 °C, otherwise proceed with the next step.

3. Purify the excised gel-band containing the index amplicon with the QIAquick Gel Extraction Kit, following the manufacturer's instructions.

4. Elute the PCR2 amplicon from the spin filter in 20 μL of buffer EB and leave at room temperature for 30 min (*see* **Note 5**).

5. Collect the PCR2 amplicon from the QIAquick column by centrifuging at $10,000 \times g$ for 15 min.

6. Store the PCR2 index samples at –20 °C or proceed with the next step.

3.7 Library Quantification

1. Quantify the PCR2 index samples using a fluorometric method that uses dsDNA-binding dyes (*see* **Note 9**).

2. Dilute the PCR2 index samples to the same concentration using molecular grade water or any EDTA-free elution buffer.

3. Pool equimolar amounts of each PCR2 index sample to a concentration of 3 ng/μL in a final volume 50–60 μL (~100 ng/μL).

4. The pooled amplicon library can now be sent to sequence on an Illumina MiSeq platform using a paired-end sequencing approach (2×300 bp) (*see* **Notes 16** and **17**).

4   Notes

1. The primers used in this protocol target a 450 bp 18S V2 region, selected from Fonseca et al. [6] and Blaxter et al. [50]. The full-length primer sequence for the 18S Amplicon Forward primer (SSU_FO4) is 5′-GCTTGTCTCAAAGATTAAGCC-3′ and for the 18S Amplicon Reverse primer (SSU_R22) 5′-GCCTGCTGCCTTCCTTGGA-3′. For amplification of the locus-specific region, Illumina overhang adapter sequences must be added (during PCR1). The sequence added to the selected locus-specific region is 5′-ACACTCTTTCCCTACACG ACGCTCTTCCGATCT-3′ for the forward Illumina overhang and 5′-GTGACTGGAGTTCAGACGTGTGCTC TTCCGATCT-3′ for the reverse Illumina overhang (Fig. 2). Choices of a specific locus to PCR amplify marine sediment samples for biodiversity purposes are broad but targeting more than one region might prove ideal for a better taxonomic coverage. Other primers targeting the 18S V4–V5 region suggested by Stoeck et al. [38] were also used by the authors but no direct comparisons have yet derived from these studies. A multilocus approach can be performed simultaneously (in the same Illumina run or lane) as long as the amplicon sizes do not differ more than ~50 bp. Hadziavdic et al. [32] also suggest a

comprehensive analysis of several known and alternative 18S rRNA gene regions that can be used for eukaryotic biodiversity appraisals.

2. Sieves must be sterilized in between samples to avoid cross-contamination. They are first cleaned using Distel spray, followed by rinsing with 45 μM filtered distilled water and second by UV sterilizing 5 min on each side of the sieve using a crosslinker.

3. Clean the aluminum foil with Distel Spray (or any other surface decontaminant) before weighing the soil sample or when using any other utensil for this purpose (e.g., disposable polystyrene weighing dishes).

4. DNA extraction of marine meiofauna is usually performed by decanting sediment samples according to Fonseca et al. [51]. However here, we suggest an alternative approach, easier to implement. Although the authors have used both methods, the comparison of biodiversity levels between both approaches has never been tested using the same amount of sediment. Decanting marine sediment samples is quite effective for retaining meiobenthic representatives for metabarcoding/metagenetic approaches [4–6, 10, 14, 51].

5. Make sure that the membrane is well covered in elution buffer to achieve a better DNA yield. Leaving the elution step at room temperature for 30 min also ensures a better recovery/yield of DNA.

6. Ethanol tends to evaporate with time. For the washing steps prepare fresh 70 % EtOH to ensure better results.

7. Removing excess ethanol is crucial, since any residual EtOH will inhibit downstream steps (PCR in particular).

8. To ensure better downstream library and NGS performance, the following steps are recommended before diluting the samples to 10 ng/μL (a) treat DNA with RNase A (DNase- and Protease-free, e.g., Thermo Scientific) and (b) purify the DNA using a column-base method (e.g., PowerClean ProDNA Clean-Up Kit, MOBIO). RNAse treatment is recommended by Illumina to reveal whether degraded samples are derived from gDNA or RNA. Additionally, sediment samples are known to contain humic acid, which is a major PCR-inhibiting compound, highlighting the importance of cleaning/purifying DNA sediment samples before PCR amplification.

9. For accurate DNA and library quantification, fluorometric methods are considered the most reliable and are also recommended by Illumina. Any UV and/or nanodrop quantitation method should be avoided due to the lack of sensitivity and also biased quantification, caused mainly by the presence of

contaminants such as ssDNA, oligos, or RNA that only fluoro-metric approaches can detect. Using the Qubit® dsDNA BR Assay Kit (Promega), only 2 μL of sample is needed in 198 μL of the Qubit working solution.

10. The two-step amplicon PCR strategy used in NGS library preparation will first diminish the probability of secondary structure formation (hairpins and dimers) during PCR due to long primer sets and second it represents a low-cost approach. The latter because there is no need to purchase individual sets of indexed primers for each sample and/or specific gene locus (e.g., it will only require a single set of nonindexed primers to amplify the target region (PCR1) and all index primers (PCR2) can be purchased independently of the target region and multiplexed according to the experimental design; alternatively purified PCR1 products can also be sent directly to a HTP sequencing company).

11. It is important to carry out triplicate PCRs to ensure better taxonomic representation, mainly to try to cover the inherent variability within and between replicated samples. At this point, there is no need to run PCR1 products on an agarose gel due to the low number of PCR cycles. If the user's laboratory is equipped with an Agilent Bioanalyzer, a DNA chip can be used to verify the amplicon size.

12. In between PCR purification steps are crucial to avoid unspe-cific and inefficient amplification in subsequent stages of library preparation due to the formation of dimer and primer–dimer structures. Purification steps after each PCR amplification can be performed using magnetic beads such as AMPure XP, but this also requires a magnetic plate (*see* Chapters 13 by Bourlat et al. and 14 by Leray et al. for further details on DNA purifica-tion using magnetic beads). In this protocol, we use HT ExoSAP-IT enzyme to purify PCR1 amplicons, based on its rapidity for sample processing, and the QIAquick Gel Extraction Kit to purify PCR2 index amplicons, simply to ensure a clean and unique target amplicon selection.

13. Make sure that PCR2 is performed with at least 15 cycles because fewer cycles at this stage will result in incomplete attachment of one of the index adapters to both DNA ampli-con strands (5′ and 3′ ends). Amplicon size check on an Agilent Bioanalyzer at this stage can ensure that complete attachment of the indexes occurred: a single peak with the expected size should be observed.

14. At this point, PCR2 product triplicates can either be run inde-pendently (5 μL) on a 2% agarose gel to confirm successful PCR amplification or they can be pooled and run together (~75 μL total volume) on a 2% low melting point agarose gel.

Running the triplicates independently is recommended to ensure that all three PCR reactions were successful and of same intensity, before pooling.

15. It is also recommended to perform a 30-cycle PCR1 and run it side by side with PCR2 to compare fragment length and thus visually confirm that the Illumina adapters and tags were added to the PCR1 product. This step should be performed only during the optimization phase (e.g., while trying different/new sets of primers).

16. The final paired-end sequence amplicon should have at least ~50 bp of overlapping sequence (e.g., for Illumina 2×300 bp the insert size should be ~550 bp or smaller to ensure overlap). The target gene region should ideally have a melting temperature of 60 °C to avoid 18S secondary structures [20] and for optimal sequencing. The analysis of hairpin and dimer formation on the full amplicon sequence is strongly recommended by using available online tools (e.g., http://www.idtdna.com/analyzer/Applications/OligoAnalyzer/, http://mfold.rna.albany.edu/?q=mfold/DNA-Folding-Form). Illumina recommends that all oligo primer sets are synthetized using TruGrade™ processing (e.g., http://eu.idtdna.com/site) or any similar NGS grade oligo synthesis, not only to ensure 100% quality control and purity but also to avoid cross-talk between barcoded index primer sets.

17. Depending on desired coverage, Illumina allows the pooling of up to 96 libraries (96 possible index combinations) on one MiSeq run. When pooling less than 96 libraries, make sure to use compatible index primers (*see* Illumina guidelines pages 40–41 for low plexity pooling strategies: http://www.liai.org/files/nextera_dna_sample_prep_guide_15027987_b.pdf).

References

1. Metzker ML (2010) Sequencing technologies – the next generation. Nat Rev Genet 11(1):31–46. doi:10.1038/nrg2626

2. Taberlet P, Coissac E, Pompanon F, Brochmann C, Willerslev E (2012) Towards next-generation biodiversity assessment using DNA metabarcoding. Mol Ecol 21(8):2045–2050. doi:10.1111/j.1365-294X.2012.05470.x

3. Bik HM, Porazinska DL, Creer S, Caporaso JG, Knight R, Thomas WK (2012) Sequencing our way towards understanding global eukaryotic biodiversity. Trends Ecol Evol 27(4):233–243. doi:10.1016/j.tree.2011.11.010

4. Lallias D, Hiddink JG, Fonseca VG, Gaspar JM, Sung W, Neill SP, Barnes N, Ferrero T, Hall N, Lambshead PJ, Packer M, Thomas WK, Creer S (2015) Environmental metabarcoding reveals heterogeneous drivers of microbial eukaryote diversity in contrasting estuarine ecosystems. ISME J 9:1208–1221. doi:10.1038/ismej.2014.213

5. Fonseca V, Carvalho G, Nichols B, Quince C, Johnson H, Neill S, Lambshead P, Thomas W, Power D, Creer S (2014) Metagenetic analysis of patterns of distribution and diversity of marine meiobenthic eukaryotes. Glob Ecol Biogeogr 23(11):1293–1302. doi:10.1111/geb.12223

6. Fonseca V, Carvalho G, Sung W, Johnson H, Power D, Neill S, Packer M, Blaxter M, Lambshead P, Thomas W, Creer S (2010) Second-generation environmental sequencing

unmasks marine metazoan biodiversity. Nat Commun 1(7):98. doi:10.1038/ncomms1095

7. Gibson J, Shokralla S, Porter TM, King I, van Konynenburg S, Janzen DH, Hallwachs W, Hajibabaei M (2014) Simultaneous assessment of the macrobiome and microbiome in a bulk sample of tropical arthropods through DNA metasystematics. Proc Natl Acad Sci U S A 111(22):8007–8012. doi:10.1073/pnas.1406468111

8. Shokralla S, Porter TM, Gibson JF, Dobosz R, Janzen DH, Hallwachs W, Golding GB, Hajibabaei M (2015) Massively parallel multiplex DNA sequencing for specimen identification using an Illumina MiSeq platform. Sci Rep 5:9687. doi:10.1038/srep09687

9. Baird DJ, Hajibabaei M (2012) Biomonitoring 2.0: a new paradigm in ecosystem assessment made possible by next-generation DNA sequencing. Mol Ecol 21(8):2039–2044

10. Leray M, Knowlton N (2015) DNA barcoding and metabarcoding of standardized samples reveal patterns of marine benthic diversity. Proc Natl Acad Sci U S A 112(7):2076–2081. doi:10.1073/pnas.1424997112

11. Sogin ML, Morrison HG, Huber JA, Mark Welch D, Huse SM, Neal PR, Arrieta JM, Herndl GJ (2006) Microbial diversity in the deep sea and the underexplored "rare biosphere". Proc Natl Acad Sci U S A 103(32):12115–12120. doi:10.1073/pnas.0605127103

12. Bett BJ, Vanreusel A, Vincx M, Soltwedel T, Pfannkuche O, Lambshead PJD, Gooday AJ, Ferrero T, Dinet A (1994) Sampler bias in the quantitative study of deep-sea meiobenthos. Mar Ecol Prog Ser 104(1-2):197–203

13. Bohmann K, Evans A, Gilbert MT, Carvalho GR, Creer S, Knapp M, Yu DW, de Bruyn M (2014) Environmental DNA for wildlife biology and biodiversity monitoring. Trends Ecol Evol 29(6):358–367. doi:10.1016/j.tree.2014.04.003

14. Creer S, Fonseca V, Porazinska D, Giblin-Davis R, Sung W, Power D, Packer M, Carvalho G, Blaxter M, Lambshead P, Thomas W (2010) Ultrasequencing of the meiofaunal biosphere: practice, pitfalls and promises. Mol Ecol 19:4–20. doi:10.1111/j.1365-294X.2009.04473.x

15. Chao A, Colwell RK, Lin CW, Gotelli NJ (2009) Sufficient sampling for asymptotic minimum species richness estimators. Ecology 90(4):1125–1133

16. O'Mahony EM, Tay WT, Paxton RJ (2007) Multiple rRNA variants in a single spore of the microsporidian Nosema bombi. J Eukaryot Microbiol 54(1):103–109, doi:JEU232 [pii] 10.1111/j.1550-7408.2006.00232.x

17. Medinger R, Nolte V, Pandey RV, Jost S, Ottenwalder B, Schlotterer C, Boenigk J (2010) Diversity in a hidden world: potential and limitation of next-generation sequencing for surveys of molecular diversity of eukaryotic microorganisms. Mol Ecol 19(Suppl 1):32–40. doi:10.1111/j.1365-294X.2009.04478.x

18. Wu JY, Jiang XT, Jiang YX, Lu SY, Zou F, Zhou HW (2010) Effects of polymerase, template dilution and cycle number on PCR based 16 S rRNA diversity analysis using the deep sequencing method. BMC Microbiol 10:255. doi:10.1186/1471-2180-10-255

19. Haas BJ, Gevers D, Earl AM, Feldgarden M, Ward DV, Giannoukos G, Ciulla D, Tabbaa D, Highlander SK, Sodergren E, Methe B, Desantis TZ, Petrosino JF, Knight R, Birren BW (2011) Chimeric 16S rRNA sequence formation and detection in Sanger and 454-pyrosequenced PCR amplicons. Genome Res 21(3):494–504. doi:10.1101/gr.112730.110

20. Fonseca VG, Nichols B, Lallias D, Quince C, Carvalho GR, Power DM, Creer S (2012) Sample richness and genetic diversity as drivers of chimera formation in nSSU metagenetic analyses. Nucleic Acids Res 40(9), e66. doi:10.1093/nar/gks002

21. von Wintzingerode F, Gobel UB, Stackebrandt E (1997) Determination of microbial diversity in environmental samples: pitfalls of PCR-based rRNA analysis. FEMS Microbiol Rev 21(3):213–229

22. Creer S (2010) Second-generation sequencing derived insights into the temporal biodiversity dynamics of freshwater protists. Mol Ecol 19(14):2829–2831. doi:10.1111/j.1365-294X.2010.04670.x

23. Wang GC, Wang Y (1996) The frequency of chimeric molecules as a consequence of PCR co-amplification of 16S rRNA genes from different bacterial species. Microbiology 142:1107–1114

24. Wang GC, Wang Y (1997) Frequency of formation of chimeric molecules as a consequence of PCR coamplification of 16S rRNA genes from mixed bacterial genomes. Appl Environ Microbiol 63(12):4645–4650

25. Huse SM, Welch DM, Morrison HG, Sogin ML (2010) Ironing out the wrinkles in the rare biosphere through improved OTU clustering. Environ Microbiol 12:1889–1898. doi:10.1111/j.1462-2920.2010.02193.x

26. Kunin V, Engelbrektson A, Ochman H, Hugenholtz P (2009) Wrinkles in the rare biosphere: pyrosequencing errors lead to artificial inflation of diversity estimates. Environ Microbiol. doi:10.1111/j.1462-2920.2009.02051.x

27. Quince C, Lanzen A, Curtis TP, Davenport RJ, Hall N, Head IM, Read LF, Sloan WT (2009)

Accurate determination of microbial diversity from 454 pyrosequencing data. Nat Methods 6(9):639–641. doi:10.1038/nmeth.1361

28. Qiu X, Wu L, Huang H, McDonel PE, Palumbo AV, Tiedje JM, Zhou J (2001) Evaluation of PCR-generated chimeras, mutations, and heteroduplexes with 16S rRNA gene-based cloning. Appl Environ Microbiol 67(2):880–887. doi:10.1128/AEM.67.2.880-887.2001

29. Lahr DJ, Katz LA (2009) Reducing the impact of PCR-mediated recombination in molecular evolution and environmental studies using a new-generation high-fidelity DNA polymerase. Biotechniques 47(4):857–866. doi:10.2144/000113219

30. Engelbrektson A, Kunin V, Wrighton KC, Zvenigorodsky N, Chen F, Ochman H, Hugenholtz P (2010) Experimental factors affecting PCR-based estimates of microbial species richness and evenness. ISME J 4(5):642–647, doi:ismej2009153 [pii] 10.1038/ismej.2009.153

31. Schloss PD, Gevers D, Westcott SL (2011) Reducing the effects of PCR amplification and sequencing artifacts on 16S rRNA-based studies. PLoS One 6(12), e27310. doi:10.1371/journal.pone.0027310

32. Hadziavdic K, Lekang K, Lanzen A, Jonassen I, Thompson EM, Troedsson C (2014) Characterization of the 18S rRNA gene for designing universal eukaryote specific primers. PLoS One 9(2), e87624. doi:10.1371/journal.pone.0087624

33. Amaral-Zettler LA, McCliment EA, Ducklow HW, Huse SM (2009) A method for studying protistan diversity using massively parallel sequencing of V9 hypervariable regions of small-subunit ribosomal RNA genes. PLoS One 4(7), e6372. doi:10.1371/journal.pone.0006372

34. Leray M, Yang JY, Meyer CP, Mills SC, Agudelo N, Ranwez V, Boehm JT, Machida RJ (2013) A new versatile primer set targeting a short fragment of the mitochondrial COI region for metabarcoding metazoan diversity: application for characterizing coral reef fish gut contents. Front Zool 10:34. doi:10.1186/1742-9994-10-34

35. Tang CQ, Leasi F, Obertegger U, Kieneke A, Barraclough TG, Fontaneto D (2012) The widely used small subunit 18S rDNA molecule greatly underestimates true diversity in biodiversity surveys of the meiofauna. Proc Natl Acad Sci U S A 109(40):16208–16212. doi:10.1073/pnas.1209160109

36. Epp LS, Boessenkool S, Bellemain EP, Haile J, Esposito A, Riaz T, Erseus C, Gusarov VI, Edwards ME, Johnsen A, Stenoien HK, Hassel K, Kauserud H, Yoccoz NG, Brathen KA, Willerslev E, Taberlet P, Coissac E, Brochmann C (2012) New environmental metabarcodes for analysing soil DNA: potential for studying past and present ecosystems. Mol Ecol 21(8):1821–1833. doi:10.1111/j.1365-294X.2012.05537.x

37. Caporaso JG, Lauber CL, Walters WA, Berg-Lyons D, Huntley J, Fierer N, Owens SM, Betley J, Fraser L, Bauer M, Gormley N, Gilbert JA, Smith G, Knight R (2012) Ultra-high-throughput microbial community analysis on the Illumina HiSeq and MiSeq platforms. ISME J 6(8):1621–1624. doi:10.1038/ismej.2012.8

38. Stoeck T, Bass D, Nebel M, Christen R, Jones MDM, Breiner H-W, Richards TA (2010) Multiple marker parallel tag environmental DNA sequencing reveals a highly complex eukaryotic community in marine anoxic water. Mol Ecol 19:21–31. doi:10.1111/j.1365-294X.2009.04480.x

39. Walters WA, Caporaso JG, Lauber CL, Berg-Lyons D, Fierer N, Knight R (2011) PrimerProspector: de novo design and taxonomic analysis of barcoded polymerase chain reaction primers. Bioinformatics 27(8):1159–1161. doi:10.1093/bioinformatics/btr087

40. Deagle BE, Jarman SN, Coissac E, Pompanon F, Taberlet P (2014) DNA metabarcoding and the cytochrome c oxidase subunit I marker: not a perfect match. Biol Lett 10(9):pii: 20140562. doi:10.1098/rsbl.2014.0562

41. Loman NJ, Misra RV, Dallman TJ, Constantinidou C, Gharbia SE, Wain J, Pallen MJ (2012) Performance comparison of benchtop high-throughput sequencing platforms. Nat Biotechnol 30(5):434–439. doi:10.1038/nbt.2198

42. Schloss PD, Westcott SL, Ryabin T, Hall JR, Hartmann M, Hollister EB, Lesniewski RA, Oakley BB, Parks DH, Robinson CJ, Sahl JW, Stres B, Thallinger GG, Van Horn DJ, Weber CF (2009) Introducing mothur: open-source, platform-independent, community-supported software for describing and comparing microbial communities. Appl Environ Microbiol 75(23):7537–7541. doi:10.1128/AEM.01541-09

43. Caporaso JG, Kuczynski J, Stombaugh J, Bittinger K, Bushman FD, Costello EK, Fierer N, Pena AG, Goodrich JK, Gordon JI, Huttley GA, Kelley ST, Knights D, Koenig JE, Ley RE, Lozupone CA, McDonald D, Muegge BD, Pirrung M, Reeder J, Sevinsky JR, Turnbaugh PJ, Walters WA, Widmann J, Yatsunenko T, Zaneveld J, Knight R (2010) QIIME allows analysis of high-throughput community

sequencing data. Nat Methods 7(5):335–336. doi:10.1038/nmeth.f.303

44. Boyer F, Mercier C, Bonin A, Le Bras Y, Taberlet P, Coissac E (2015) Obitools: a unix-inspired software package for DNA metabarcoding. Mol Ecol Resour. doi:10.1111/1755-0998.12428

45. Bengtsson-Palme J, Hartmann M, Eriksson KM, Pal C, Thorell K, Larsson DG, Nilsson RH (2015) metaxa2: improved identification and taxonomic classification of small and large subunit rRNA in metagenomic data. Mol Ecol Resour. doi:10.1111/1755-0998.12399

46. Huber T, Faulkner G, Hugenholtz P (2004) Bellerophon: a program to detect chimeric sequences in multiple sequence alignments. Bioinformatics 20(14):2317–2319

47. Ashelford KE, Chuzhanova NA, Fry JC, Jones AJ, Weightman AJ (2006) New screening software shows that most recent large 16S rRNA gene clone libraries contain chimeras. Appl Environ Microbiol 72(9):5734–5741. doi:10.1128/AEM.00556-06

48. Quince C, Lanzen A, Davenport RJ, Turnbaugh PJ (2011) Removing noise from pyrosequenced amplicons. BMC Bioinformatics 12(1):38, doi:1471-2105-12-38 [pii] 10.1186/1471-2105-12-38

49. He Y, Caporaso JG, Jiang XT, Sheng HF, Huse SM, Rideout JR, Edgar RC, Kopylova E, Walters WA, Knight R, Zhou HW (2015) Stability of operational taxonomic units: an important but neglected property for analyzing microbial diversity. Microbiome 3:20. doi:10.1186/s40168-015-0081-x

50. Blaxter ML, De Ley P, Garey JR, Liu LX, Scheldeman P, Vierstraete A, Vanfleteren JR, Mackey LY, Dorris M, Frisse LM, Vida JT, Thomas WK (1998) A molecular evolutionary framework for the phylum Nematoda. Nature 392(6671):71–75

51. Fonseca V, Power D, Carvalho G, Lambshead J, Packer M, Creer S (2011) Isolation of marine meiofauna from sandy sediments: from decanting to DNA extraction. Nat Protoc Exchange doi:10.1038/nprot.2010.157

Chapter 13

Preparation of Amplicon Libraries for Metabarcoding of Marine Eukaryotes Using Illumina MiSeq: The Dual-PCR Method

Sarah J. Bourlat, Quiterie Haenel, Jennie Finnman, and Matthieu Leray

Abstract

This protocol details the preparation of multiplexed amplicon libraries for metabarcoding (amplicon-based) studies of microscopic marine eukaryotes. Metabarcoding studies, based on the amplification of a taxonomically informative marker from a collection of organisms or an environmental sample, can be performed to analyze biodiversity patterns or predator–prey interactions. For Metazoa, we use the mitochondrial cytochrome oxidase 1 (CO1) or the small ribosomal subunit (SSU) markers. Here, we describe a strategy for the preparation of multiplexed Illumina MiSeq libraries using a dual-PCR approach for the addition of index and adaptor sequences.

Key words Metabarcoding, Biodiversity, Microscopic eukaryotes, Illumina MiSeq

1 Introduction

The development of high-throughput sequencing technologies offers the possibility to recover DNA information from whole community samples, a technique routinely used for prokaryotes, based on the 16S ribosomal RNA gene [1]. Advances in DNA sequencing and analytical techniques now allow biodiversity assessments from eukaryotes and from various types of environmental samples. Recent studies have shown it possible to study bulk environmental samples dominated by microscopic eukaryotes, such as marine sediments [2, 3], analyze the contents of fish stomachs [4], carry out environmental status assessments for benthic macro-invertebrates [5], or reveal patterns of marine benthic diversity on autonomous reef monitoring structures [6]. The vast majority of metabarcoding studies have so far employed Roche 454 for sequencing due to its long read lengths compared to other technologies [7], but Illumina MiSeq technology is now getting more

Sarah J. Bourlat (ed.), *Marine Genomics: Methods and Protocols*, Methods in Molecular Biology, vol. 1452, DOI 10.1007/978-1-4939-3774-5_13, © Springer Science+Business Media New York 2016

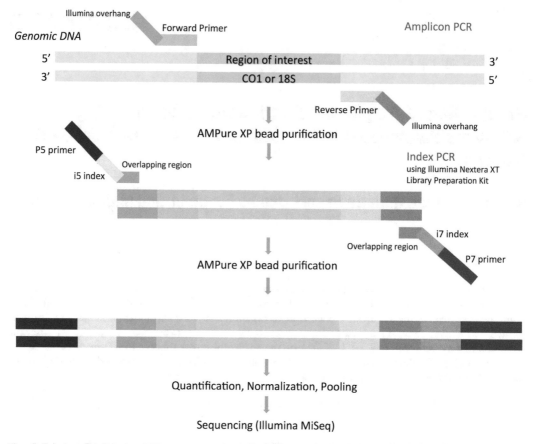

Fig. 1 Schema for Illumina MiSeq library preparation using dual-PCR. The first PCR step uses amplicon-specific primers including Illumina adapter overhangs (amplicon PCR) and the second cycle limited PCR allows the incorporation of Illumina index adapters i5 and i7 (index PCR). Bead purifications are carried out after each step. Quantification, normalization, and pooling are carried out before sequencing on Illumina MiSeq (Figure adapted from [8])

competitive in terms of read length, reaching up to 2×300bp with MiSeq Reagent Kit v3. Marker sequences amplified can have up to 500 bp, including a 100 bp overlap for paired end reads.

This method consists in dual PCR amplification, the first PCR using amplicon-specific primers including an Illumina adapter overhang (referred to here as the amplicon PCR) and a second cycle limited PCR for the incorporation of Illumina index adapters (referred to here as the index PCR) (Fig 1, adapted from [8]).

2 Materials

2.1 DNA Extraction

1. DNA extraction kit. For sediment samples, use the PowerSoil or for larger volumes PowerMax soil DNA isolation kit (MoBio). For tissue samples, use UltraClean tissue and cells DNA isolation (MoBio) or an equivalent kit.

2.2 Amplicon PCR	1. 96-well PCR plates and microseal film.

2. Pfu proofreading polymerase.

3. dNTP mix containing sodium salts of dATP, dCTP, dGTP, and dTTP, each at 10 mM (total concentration 40 mM).

4. Nuclease-free water.

5. Thermocycler.

6. Gel electrophoresis apparatus and reagents.

7. 100 bp DNA ladder.

8. Locus-specific primers with Illumina overhang. Illumina overhang adapter sequences derived from the 16S demonstrated protocol (Illumina) [8] were appended to locus-specific primers for compatibility with Illumina index and sequencing adapters [8]. The universal CO1 primers available for the Metazoa amplify a 658 bp region [9], which is too long for most NGS applications. For the CO1 gene, Illumina overhangs were appended to each of the primer sequences proposed by Leray et al. to amplify a 313 bp fragment, termed the 'mini-barcode' (mlCOIintF-dgHCO2198) [10]. For the reverse CO1 primer, a variation of the primer proposed by Lobo et al. was used, which was shown to enhance amplification of the CO1 region in a wide range of invertebrates [11]. For the SSU region, Illumina overhang adapter sequences were appended to primers modified from Fonseca et al. and yielding a 364 bp fragment (SSU_FO4—SSU_R22) [3]. These primers target a homologous region of the gene and flank a region that is highly divergent, corresponding to the V1–V2 region of the 18S gene. *See* Chapter 12 by Fonseca and Lallias for further details on the SSU_FO4 and SSU_R22 primers.

2.3 Bead Purification

1. Magnetic beads for DNA purification, such as AMPure XP (Agencourt), or equivalent. These are also called SPRI beads for solid-phase reversible immobilization.

2. Magnetic 96-well plate stand.

3. Freshly prepared 80% ethanol.

4. Nuclease-free water.

2.4 Index PCR

1. Nextera XT index Kit, 96 indices, 384 samples for a 96-well plate (Illumina).

2. KAPA HiFi HotStart ready mix or equivalent high-fidelity DNA polymerase mix containing buffer, $MgCl_2$, dNTPs, and polymerase.

2.5 Normalization and Pooling

1. Tapestation (Agilent 2200) with high Sensitivity D1000 ScreenTape.

2. Qubit® 2.0 Fluorometer and Qubit™ dsDNA HS assay kit.

3. Tris-Cl 10 nM buffer, pH 8.5 with 0.1% Tween 20.

2.6 Library Preparation and MiSeq Sequencing

1. MiSeq Instrument (Illumina).

2. MiSeq Reagent Kit v3 (600 cycles).

   - Box 1—MiSeq Reagent Cartridge and Hybridization Buffer (HT1).
   - Box 2—Flow Cell and PR2 Bottle.

3. Heat Block.

4. NaOH stock (1.0 N).

5. Microcentrifuge tubes.

6. PhiX (10 nM).

7. Tween 20.

8. Laboratory grade water.

9. 70% EtOH.

10. Whatman, lens cleaning tissue.

3 Methods

3.1 DNA Extraction

For total DNA extraction from sediment samples, use MoBio's PowerSoil or PowerMax DNA isolation kit, depending on the volume of sediment processed. For DNA extraction from tissue samples, use MoBio's UltraClean tissue and cells DNA isolation kit or an equivalent kit according to the manufacturer's instructions.

3.2 Amplicon PCR

Here, we use locus-specific primers with an Illumina overhang as described in Subheading 2.2. To minimize PCR errors, use Pfu proofreading polymerase. Also, we recommend running three PCR replicates to minimize biases.

1. For a 50 μl reaction volume, use 5 μl Pfu polymerase buffer (10×), 1 μl dNTP mix (final concentration of each dNTP 200 μM), 0.5 μl of each primer at 50 pm/μl, 2 μl DNA template (~10 ng), 0.5 μl Pfu DNA polymerase, and 40.5 μl of nuclease-free water (*see* **Note 1**).

2. Run three PCR replicates (e.g., three independent PCRs for the same sample) using the following cycling conditions: 2 min at 95 °C (1×); 1 min at 95 °C, 45 s at X°C, 1 min at 72 °C (25×); 5 min at 72 °C (1×); hold at 4 °C. Replace X with the adequate annealing temperature for your particular primers (*see* **Note 2**).

3. Run a 1–2% agarose gel to check the size of the amplicons using a DNA ladder. % Agarose depends on the size of your fragment.

4. If any additional bands appear that are not the size of the desired product, increase the annealing temperature of the PCR or perform additional purification steps (*see* **Note 3**).

5. Pool PCR replicates.

3.3 Bead Purification Purify amplicons using magnetic beads and a magnetic stand. Size selection can be achieved using different ratios of beads to sample (*see* **Note 3**). A ratio of bead to sample of 0.8:1 will efficiently purify the amplicons away from primers and primer dimers and allow selection of fragments larger than 200 bp [12].

1. Vortex the beads before use. Add 40 μl beads to 50 μl of PCR product to obtain a ratio of 0.8. Pipette up and down ten times. Incubate a room temperature without shaking for 5 min.

2. Place the plate on the magnetic stand until the supernatant has cleared, at least 3 min.

3. Remove the supernatant with a multichannel pipette if you are using a 96-well plate, making sure not to disturb the beads.

4. With the samples on the magnetic stand, wash the beads by adding 200 μl of freshly prepared 80% ethanol and incubate for 30 s. Carefully remove the supernatant without disturbing the beads.

5. Repeat washing **step 4**.

6. Remove all residual ethanol using a pipette and air dry, leaving the samples on the magnetic stand.

7. Remove the plate from the stand and add 40 μl of nuclease-free water for elution, gently pipetting up and down ten times to resuspend the beads. Incubate the plate at room temperature for 5 min.

8. Place the plate back on the magnetic stand at least 5 min or until the supernatant has cleared. *See* also **Note 4** about bead carryover.

9. Carefully transfer the supernatant to a new plate.

10. Seal the plate and freeze the samples at this point, or proceed with the index PCR.

3.4 Index PCR In this step, barcodes for dual indexing are attached to the purified amplicons containing Illumina overhangs. For indexing, we use the Nextera XT DNA index kit according to the manufacturer's instructions.

1. For a 50 μl reaction volume, use 5 μl of cleaned up PCR amplicons, 5 μl Nextera XT Index Primer i5, 5 μl Nextera XT Index Primer i7, 25 μl 2× KAPA HiFi HotStart ready mix, and 10 μl nuclease-free water.

2. Run the PCR using the following cycling conditions: 3 min at 95 °C (1×); 30 s at 95 °C, 30 s at 55 °C, 30 s at 72 °C (8×); 5 min at 72 °C (1×); hold at 4 °C.

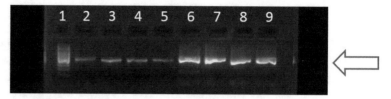

Fig. 2 PCR products run on a 1.5% agarose gel to check the size of the amplicons using a DNA ladder. Well 1: 100 bp DNA ladder; wells 2–5: samples after amplicon PCR and bead purification; wells 6–9: samples after index PCR. The *arrow* shows the desired product at 500 bp

3. Run the product on a 1.5% agarose gel to check the size of the amplicons using a DNA ladder (Fig. 2).

4. If any additional bands appear that are not the size of the desired product, additional purification steps need to be carried out (*see* **Note 3**).

3.5 Bead Purification

Purify the amplicons after the index PCR using magnetic beads and a magnetic stand. Size selection can be achieved using different ratios of beads to sample (*see* **Note 3**). A ratio bead:sample of 0.8:1 effectively purifies amplicons away from primers and primer dimers and allows selection of fragments larger than 200 bp [12]. Follow instructions in Subheading 3.3.

3.6 Library Validation

Verify the average fragment size of the individual samples with Tapestation. Ensure you have the right fragment and that you don't have any additional unwanted peaks (*see* **Notes 4** and **5**). The result should be a Tapestation trace with one main peak of the right size and the upper and lower marker peaks (Fig. 3).

3.7 Library Quantification

1. Measure the concentration of your libraries with Qubit (or some other fluorometric quantification method that uses dsDNA dyes) (*see* **Note 6**).

2. Calculate sample concentration in nM using the following formula. The assumed molecular weight of 1 bp is 660 Da.

$$\frac{(\text{Concentration in ng / } \mu\text{l}) \times 1,000,000}{(660\,\text{g / mol} \times \text{average library size})} = \text{nM}.$$

3.8 Normalization and Pooling

1. Dilute the samples to 50 nM using Tris–Cl 10 nM buffer, pH 8.5 with 0.1% Tween 20.

2. Dilute the samples again to 10 nM using Tris–Cl 10 nM buffer, pH 8.5 with 0.1% Tween 20.

3. Measure sample concentrations on Qubit to check the accuracy of dilution.

4. Correct the concentration of the samples to 10 nM.

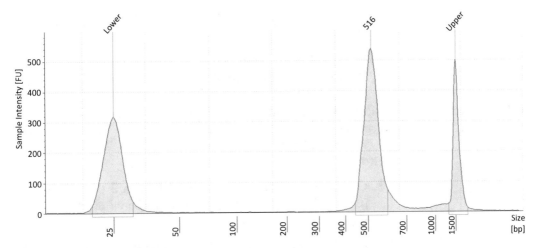

Fig. 3 Tapestation trace after bead purification and pooling

5. Pool the samples, using 2 μl of each sample. Adjust this volume if some of the samples are more or less concentrated than 10 nM.

3.9 Pool Validation

Validate the pool using Qubit and Tapestation. If an unwanted peak is observed at this stage, proceed with additional magnetic bead purification on the pooled samples. Bead purifications should be carried out until all unwanted products are removed (*see* **Note 4**).

1. Run Tapestation to see if the purification was successful.

2. Dilute the pool to 4 nM.

3.10 Library Denaturation

To prepare the DNA for cluster generation and sequencing, the libraries are denatured with NaOH, diluted with hybridization buffer (HT1), and heat denatured. The following steps are done accordingly Illuminas 16S Metagenomic Sequencing Library Preparation protocol [8].

1. Combine 5 μl pool (4 nM) with 5 μl NaOH (0.2 N) in a microcentrifuge tube.

2. Vortex and spin down.

3. Incubate at room temperature for 5 min to make the DNA single stranded.

4. Add 990 μl HT1.

This results in a 20 pM Library in 1 mM NaOH, which can be further diluted to your final concentration. Keep the denatured DNA on ice until you are ready to do the final dilution.

3.11 Dilution of Denatured Library

Dilute the denatured DNA with HT1 to the desired concentration. Illumina recommends starting the first run using a 4 pM loading concentration and to adjust that in following runs (*see* **Note 7**). For this project we diluted the library to 5 pM.

1. Mix 150 μl of your 20 pM denatured DNA with 450 μl pre-chilled HT1 to get 5 pM.

2. Invert and spin down.

3. Place the denatured and diluted DNA on ice.

3.12 Denaturation and Dilution of PhiX Control

PhiX is a balanced and diverse library that can be used as a control in sequencing runs. In this case we spiked in 15 % (*see* **Note 8**).

Follow these steps to denature and dilute PhiX to the same concentration as the amplicon library (5 pM).

1. Combine 2 μl PhiX library (10 nM) with 3 μl Tris (10 mM, pH 8.5) in a microcentrifuge tube to dilute PhiX to 4 nM.

2. Vortex and spin down.

3. Add 5 μl NaOH (0.2 N) to the tube with 5 μl PhiX library (4 nM) to get a 2 nM PhiX library.

4. Vortex and spin down. Incubate at room temperature for 5 min to make the DNA single stranded.

5. Add 990 μl HT1 to dilute PhiX to 20 pM.

6. Mix 150 μl of your 20 pM denatured PhiX with 450 μl pre-chilled HT1 to dilute PhiX to the same loading concentration as your amplicon library (5 pM).

7. Invert and spin down.

8. Place the denatured and diluted PhiX on ice.

3.13 Combining the Library and PhiX Control

This step should be performed directly before loading the library into the MiSeq reagent cartridge.

1. Combine 90 μl PhiX (5 pM) with 510 μl of your library (5 pM) to get a 15 % PhiX spike in.

2. Incubate the combined library and PhiX in a heat block at 96 °C for 2 min.

3. Invert the tube to mix and place it in an ice water bath for 5 min.

3.14 MiSeq Sequencing

The MiSeq Control Software (MCS) guides you through the steps to load the flow cell and reagents. MCS also provides you with an overview of the quality statistics during the run. MCS controls the flow cell stage, fluidics system, and flow cell temperatures, and captures images of clusters on the flow cell during the run. The following steps are done accordingly Illuminas MiSeq System User Guide [14].

1. Prepare the prefilled sequencing reagent cartridge for use (MiSeq Reagent Kit v3, 600c), by thawing it in a water bath with ultrapure water.

2. Wash and dry the flow cell.

3. Load the flow cell.

4. Load the PR2 bottle and empty the waste bottle.

5. Pierce the foil seal in the cartridge where it says "load sample" with a pipette tip and add 600 μl of your denatured and diluted sample.

6. Load the cartridge.

7. After loading the flow cell, buffer and reagent cartridge, MiSeq will search for the correct sample sheet based on the barcode on the cartridge. Review the run parameters in your sample sheet, created with Illumina Experiment Manager (IEM) (*see* **Note 9**). MCS performs the run according to parameters specified in the sample sheet.

8. Review prerun check results.

9. Select 'Start Run' to start sequencing (2 × 300 bp run).

10. Monitor the run from the MCS.

11. Perform a postrun wash when the sequencing run is ready.

4   Notes

1. A smaller reaction volume can also be used if necessary as the triplicate reactions will be later pooled.

2. Cycling conditions should be modified according to the target gene. For example, 48 °C annealing temperature will be best suited if the PCR is carried out with the mlCOIintF-dgHCO2198 primer set. Primer annealing temperature can be calculated as about 5 °C lower than the melting temperature (Tm) of your primers. You can also use a web-based Tm calculator tool. If no product is visible on the gel, lower annealing temperatures can be chosen but this can result in unspecific binding to sequences other than the intended target, visible as additional bands on the gel. Optimal annealing temperatures should result in the highest product yield for the intended amplicon. Regarding number of PCR cycles used, we recommend using the lowest possible number to prevent the introduction of PCR errors. Here we use 25 cycles for the amplicon PCR, but in cases where no PCR product is visible on the gel with 25 cycles, this can be increased to 30 or 35 cycles.

3. Size selection can be carried out by gel purification. An alternative better suited to high-throughput sequencing and low DNA concentrations is to use magnetic beads, as these will give better DNA recovery. Depending on the ratio of beads to sample, different size fragments can be purified [12]. In addition, selection of fragments to the left and right side of the desired fragment range can be carried out. Left side selection is done by binding the larger fragments to the right of the desired range to the beads and eluting the smaller fragments. For right size selection, the larger fragments to the right of the desired range are bound to the beads, and the supernatant containing the smaller fragments is removed to a fresh tube. For more details on this procedure *see* [13].

4. If an unwanted product is seen at 1000 bp, it can be due to bead carryover. To ensure that all magnetic beads are removed

from the sample, an additional purification step can be carried out, by placing the samples on the magnetic stand for 15 min and transferring the supernatant to a new tube.

5. It is not unusual to detect a peak around ~120–130 bp when validating your library. It is important to try to remove this peak (which could be adapter dimer). Adapter dimers will also bind to the flow cell, cluster very efficiently, and represent a high proportion of the total sequencing yield. This will also have an impact on the overall quality of the run, which tends to drop after the adapter dimer. You should be able to successfully remove adapter dimer by carrying out another round of magnetic bead cleanup. If your unwanted peak is much higher in proportion to your library peak, or if you cannot get rid of it by bead purification, a more aggressive selective approach by gel extraction is recommended. Keep in mind that the yield may be compromised when using this method.

6. Because it is very important to get the quantification as correct as possible, it is strongly advised to use a fluorescent dye method such as Qubit or PicoGreen instead of NanoDrop, which is based on UV absorbance. Instruments that use UV absorbance cannot distinguish between DNA, RNA, degraded nucleic acids, and other contaminants. Quantification with fluorescent dyes only detects the molecule of interest, and hence gives the most accurate values.

7. We expect amplicons to have low diversity, this is not an issue in general but with low diversity libraries it is advisable to keep cluster density between 600 and 800 K/mm² (or even lower). It is important to keep this in mind, so you don't overcluster the flowcell, which can lead to run failure. It is better to start with a low loading concentration and adjust it in following runs.

8. Low diversity libraries, such as amplicon libraries, where a large number of the reads have the same sequence, require a PhiX spike in to create a more diverse set of clusters. Illumina recommends a 1% PhiX spike in to all libraries. For low-diversity libraries, the percentage of PhiX depends on the diversity of the library and requires optimization. Between 10 and 20% should be enough.

9. Illumina Experiment Manager (IEM) is an application that helps you with the sample sheet setup of your run parameters for your MiSeq run.

Acknowledgements

This work was supported by Swedish research council grant C0344601 to S.J.B. Financial support to M.L. was provided by the Sant Chair and the Smithsonian Tennenbaum Marine Observatories Network, for which this Contribution No. 4. We would like to thank the Genomics Core Facility platform, at the Sahlgrenska Academy, University of Gothenburg.

References

1. Caporaso JG, Lauber CL, Walters WA, Berg-Lyons D, Lozupone CA, Turnbaugh PJ, Fierer N, Knight R (2011) Global patterns of 16S rRNA diversity at a depth of millions of sequences per sample. Proc Natl Acad Sci U S A 108(Suppl 1):4516–4522. doi:10.1073/pnas.1000080107

2. Bik HM, Porazinska DL, Creer S, Caporaso JG, Knight R, Thomas WK (2012) Sequencing our way towards understanding global eukaryotic biodiversity. Trends Ecol Evol 27:233–234

3. Fonseca VG, Carvalho GR, Sung W, Johnson HF, Power DM, Neill SP, Packer M, Blaxter ML, Lambshead PJD, Thomas WK, Creer S (2010) Second-generation environmental sequencing unmasks marine metazoan biodiversity. Nat Commun 1:98. doi:10.1038/Ncomms1095

4. Leray M, Agudelo N, Mills SC, Meyer CP (2013) Effectiveness of annealing blocking primers versus restriction enzymes for characterization of generalist diets: unexpected prey revealed in the gut contents of two coral reef fish species. PLoS One 8(4), e58076. doi:10.1371/journal.pone.0058076

5. Aylagas E, Borja A, Rodriguez-Ezpeleta N (2014) Environmental status assessment using DNA metabarcoding: towards a genetics based marine biotic index (gAMBI). PLoS One 9(3):e90529. doi:10.1371/journal.pone.0090529

6. Leray M, Knowlton N (2015) DNA barcoding and metabarcoding of standardized samples reveal patterns of marine benthic diversity. Proc Natl Acad Sci U S A 112(7):2076–2081. doi:10.1073/Pnas.1424997112

7. Shokralla S, Spall JL, Gibson JF, Hajibabaei M (2012) Next-generation sequencing technologies for environmental DNA research. Mol Ecol 21(8):1794–1805. doi:10.1111/J.1365-294x.2012.05538.X

8. Illumina (2013) 16S metagenomic sequencing library preparation guide, Part # 15044223 Rev. B. http://www.support.illumina.com/documents/documentation/chemistry_documentation/16s/16s-metagenomic-library-prep-guide-15044223-b.pdf

9. Folmer O, Black M, Hoeh W, Lutz R, Vrijenhoek R (1994) DNA primers for amplification of mitochondrial cytochrome c oxidase subunit I from diverse metazoan invertebrates. Mol Mar Biol Biotechnol 3(5):294–299

10. Leray M, Yang JY, Meyer CP, Mills SC, Agudelo N, Ranwez V, Boehm JT, Machida RJ (2013) A new versatile primer set targeting a short fragment of the mitochondrial COI region for metabarcoding metazoan diversity: application for characterizing coral reef fish gut contents. Front Zool 10:Unsp 34. doi:10.1186/1742-9994-10-34

11. Lobo J, Costa PM, Teixeira MAL, Ferreira MSG, Costa MH, Costa FO (2013) Enhanced primers for amplification of DNA barcodes from a broad range of marine metazoans. BMC Ecol 13:Artn 34. doi:10.1186/1472-6785-13-34

12. CoreGenomics How do SPRI beads work? http://core-genomics.blogspot.co.uk/2012/04/how-do-spri-beads-work.html

13. BeckmanCoulter. http://www.beckmancoulter.com/wsrportal/bibliography?docname=SPRIselect.pdf

14. MiSeq system user guide, part # 15027617 Rev O http://www.support.illumina.com/content/dam/illumina-support/documents/documentation/system_documentation/miseq/miseq-system-guide-15027617-o.pdf

Chapter 14

Preparation of Amplicon Libraries for Metabarcoding of Marine Eukaryotes Using Illumina MiSeq: The Adapter Ligation Method

Matthieu Leray, Quiterie Haenel, and Sarah J. Bourlat

Abstract

Amplicon-based studies of marine microscopic eukaryotes, also referred to as metabarcoding studies, can be performed to analyze patterns of biodiversity or predator–prey interactions targeting the mitochondrial cytochrome oxidase 1 (CO1) or the small ribosomal subunit (SSU) markers. Because high-throughput sequencing (HTS) Illumina platforms provide millions of reads per run, hundreds of samples may be sequenced simultaneously. This protocol details the preparation of multiplexed amplicon libraries for Illumina MiSeq sequencing. We describe a strategy for sample multiplexing using a combination of tailed PCR primers and ligation of indexed adapters.

Key words Metabarcoding, Eukaryotes, Illumina MiSeq, Multiplexing, Tags, TruSeq

1 Introduction

High Throughput Sequencing (HTS) technologies have revolutionized the field of community ecology in recent years. Deep sequencing of PCR amplicons provides cost-effective estimates of species diversity and taxonomic composition from samples that were traditionally sorted by hand [1, 2] and characterized at coarse taxonomic levels [3]. Moreover, community profiles generated using HTS data are independent of taxonomic expertise and therefore more comparable between studies for environmental monitoring and environmental status assessment [4–6]. Because the number of reads produced in a single HTS run is far greater than what is necessary for characterizing most community samples, hundreds of samples may be pooled into a single run to be sequenced simultaneously [7, 8]. Prior to pooling, sequences belonging to each sample must be tagged with a unique identifier to be recognizable in downstream data processing. Several alternative tagging approaches have been used in the literature for sample

Sarah J. Bourlat (ed.), *Marine Genomics: Methods and Protocols*, Methods in Molecular Biology, vol. 1452,
DOI 10.1007/978-1-4939-3774-5_14, © Springer Science+Business Media New York 2016

multiplexing (e.g., the dual PCR method, *see* Chapter 13 by Bourlat et al. and Chapter 12 by Fonseca and Lallias). In this chapter, we present a hierarchical tagging method for sequencing amplicons on the Illumina MiSeq that combines the use of tailed PCR primers followed by the ligation of indexed adapters (*see* Fig. 1). This method uses two sets of tags for maximizing the number of samples pooled in a MiSeq run. The first tag is added to the target fragment during PCR amplification using tailed locus-specific primers. The second tag is added to the product of amplification via ligation in the form of a single-indexed Illumina Y-adapter. An example of the pooling strategy is presented in Fig. 2. Marker sequences amplified using this method may be up to 500 bp using the Illumina V3 reagent kit (2 × 300 bp paired end), including a 100 bp overlap for paired end reads, which is suitable for sequencing fragments of the cytochrome oxidase 1 (CO1) or the small ribosomal subunit (SSU) markers.

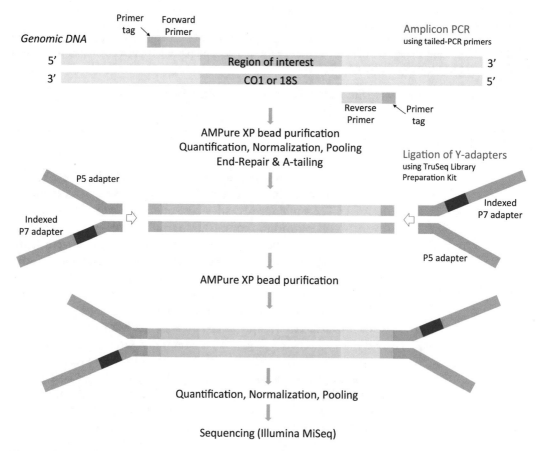

Fig. 1 Scheme for Illumina MiSeq multiplex library preparation using the tailed PCR primers and ligation of single-indexed Y-adapters. The first PCR step uses amplicon-specific primers with a 6-nucleotide tag. The second step uses a ligation to add a single-indexed Y-adapter to pooled PCR amplicons

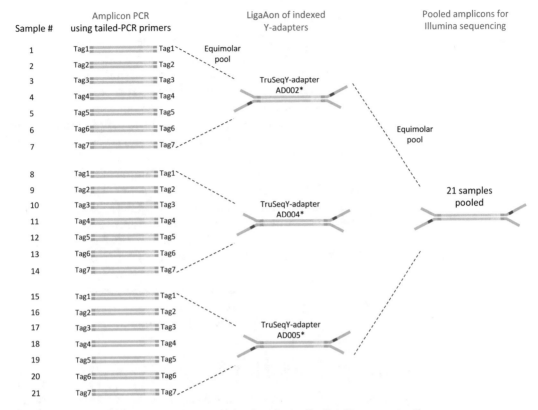

Fig. 2 Illustration of the pooling strategy used for the adaptor ligation library preparation

2 Materials

2.1 DNA Extraction

1. For sediment samples, use the PowerSoil DNA Isolation Kit (MoBio). For tissue samples, use the UltraClean Tissue & Cells DNA Isolation Kit (MoBio) or equivalent. For environmental samples with large biomass (e.g. plankton), use PowerMax Soil DNA Isolation Kit (MoBio).

2. DNA cleanup kit such as PowerClean Pro DNA Clean-Up Kit (MoBio).

2.2 PCR Amplification Using Tailed Locus-Specific PCR

1. 96-well PCR plates and microseal film.

2. 50× Clontech Advantage2 Polymerase Mix (Takara).

3. 10× Clontech Advantage2 PCR buffer (Takara).

4. dntp mix containing sodium salts of dATP, dCTP, dGTP, and dTTP, each at 2.5 mM (total concentration 10 mM).

5. Nuclease-free water.

6. Thermocycler.

7. Gel electrophoresis apparatus and reagents.

8. 100 bp DNA ladder.

9. Tailed locus-specific PCR primers, as detailed below:

For this protocol, we designed six nucleotide tags that are appended to the locus-specific forward and reverse primers (tailed primers) to amplify a 313 bp region of CO1 [9]. Tags differ from each other by at least three nucleotides. A total of 49 primer combinations can be used for sample multiplexing using the seven unique tailed forward and seven unique tailed reverse PCR primers presented below (e.g., sample1, mlCOIint_Tag1—dgHCO_Tag1; sample 2, mlCOIint_Tag1—dgHCO_Tag2; sample 3, mlCOIint_Tag2—dgHCO_Tag1; sample 4, mlCOIint_Tag2—dgHCO_Tag2...). These same tags can be appended to other PCR primers to amplify CO1 (e.g., Lobo_R1, based on [10]) or 18S (e.g., SSU_FO4, SSU_R22, based on [1]). *See* Chapter 13 by Bourlat et al. for further information on the 18S LOBO primers and chapter 12 by Fonseca and Lallias for further information on SSU primer pairs (SSU_FO4 and SSU_R22).

All CO1-specific tailed forward and reverse primers are detailed below:

Primer name	Tailed primer sequence (5′–3′)
mlCOIintF_Tag1	AGACGC**GGWACWGGWTGAACWGTWTAYCCYCC**
mlCOIintF_Tag2	AGTGTA**GGWACWGGWTGAACWGTWTAYCCYCC**
mlCOIintF_Tag3	ACTAGC**GGWACWGGWTGAACWGTWTAYCCYCC**
mlCOIintF_Tag4	ACAGTC**GGWACWGGWTGAACWGTWTAYCCYCC**
mlCOIintF_Tag5	ATCGAC**GGWACWGGWTGAACWGTWTAYCCYCC**
mlCOIintF_Tag6	ATGTCG**GGWACWGGWTGAACWGTWTAYCCYCC**
mlCOIintF_Tag7	ATAGCA**GGWACWGGWTGAACWGTWTAYCCYCC**
dgHCO2198_Tag1	AGACGC**TAAACTTCAGGGTGACCAAARAAYCA**
dgHCO2198_Tag2	AGTGTA**TAAACTTCAGGGTGACCAAARAAYCA**
dgHCO2198_Tag3	ACTAGC**TAAACTTCAGGGTGACCAAARAAYCA**
dgHCO2198_Tag4	ACAGTC**TAAACTTCAGGGTGACCAAARAAYCA**
dgHCO2198_Tag5	ATCGAC**TAAACTTCAGGGTGACCAAARAAYCA**
dgHCO2198_Tag6	ATGTCG **TAAACTTCAGGGTGACCAAARAAYCA**
dgHCO2198_Tag7	ATAGCA**TAAACTTCAGGGTGACCAAARAAYCA**

2.3 Bead Purification

1. Magnetic beads for DNA purification (also called SPRI beads for solid-phase reversible immobilization).

2. Magnetic 96-well plate.

3. Freshly prepared 70 % ethanol.

4. Nuclease-free water or resuspension buffer provided in TruSeq DNA PCR-free LT Library Prep Kit (Illumina).

2.4 Normalization and Pooling	1. Qubit fluorometric quantitation apparatus. 2. Qubit dsDNA HS Assay Kit. 3. Nuclease-free water.
2.5 End Repair	1. End Repair Mix 2 from TruSeq DNA PCR-free LT Library Prep Kit (Illumina). 2. Resuspension Buffer from TruSeq DNA PCR-free LT Library Prep Kit (Illumina). 3. Thermocycler with heated lid.
2.6 A-Tailing	1. A-Tailing Mix from TruSeq DNA PCR-free LT Library Prep Kit (Illumina). 2. Resuspension Buffer from TruSeq DNA PCR-free LT Library Prep Kit (Illumina). 3. Thermocycler with heated lid.
2.7 Ligation of Y-Adapters	1. DNA Adapter Index tubes from TruSeq DNA PCR-free LT Library Prep Kit (Illumina). 2. Ligation Mix from TruSeq DNA PCR-free LT Library Prep Kit (Illumina). 3. Resuspension Buffer from TruSeq DNA PCR-free LT Library Prep Kit (Illumina). 4. Stop Ligation Buffer from TruSeq DNA PCR-free LT Library Prep Kit (Illumina). 5. Thermocycler with heated lid.
2.8 Final Normalization and Pooling Step	1. TapeStation. 2. Qubit fluorometric quantitation apparatus. 3. Qubit dsDNA HS Assay Kit. 4. Tris–Cl 10 nM buffer, pH 8.5 with 0.1% Tween 20.
2.9 Library Validation Using Quantitative PCR	1. ViiA 7 real-time PCR system (Applied Biosystems). 2. KAPA library quantification kit for Illumina platform (ROX low). 3. Tris–Cl 10 nM buffer, pH 8.5 with 0.1% Tween 20. 4. Nuclease-free water.

3 Methods

3.1 DNA Extraction   For total DNA extraction from sediment samples or samples with large biomass, use MoBio's PowerSoil DNA isolation kit according to the manufacturer's instructions. For other sample types, any DNA extraction kit can be used, with an additional DNA purification step to remove inhibitors using MoBio's PowerClean Pro DNA Clean-Up Kit according to the manufacturer's instructions.

3.2 PCR Amplification Using Tailed Locus-Specific PCR

Here, we use locus-specific primers with a 6-nucleotide tag. To minimize PCR errors, use a proofreading polymerase. Also, we recommend running three PCR replicates to minimize biases:

1. For a 20 μl reaction volume, use 2 μl Clontech Advantage2 PCR buffer (10×), 1.4 μl dntp mix (10 mM), 1 μl of each primer (10 μM), 1 μl DNA template (~10 ng), 0.4 μl Clontech Advantage2 Polymerase Mix (50×), and 13.2 μl of nuclease-free water.

2. Run three PCR replicates (e.g., three independent PCR for the same sample) using the following cycling conditions: 5 min at 95 °C (1×); 1 min at 95 °C, 45 s at 48 °C, and 30 s at 72 °C (35×); and 10 min at 72 °C (1×); hold at 4 °C.

3. Run a 1.5% agarose gel to check the size of the amplicons using a DNA ladder.

4. If any additional bands appear that are not the size of the desired product, increase the annealing temperature of the PCR or perform additional purification steps (*see* **Note 1**).

5. Pool PCR replicates.

3.3 Bead Purification

Purify amplicons using magnetic beads and a magnetic stand. Size selection can be achieved using different ratios of beads to sample (*see* **Note 1**). A ratio bead–sample of 1.6:1 will efficiently purify the amplicons away from primers and primer dimers [11]:

1. Vortex the beads before use. Add 80 μl beads to 50 μl of PCR product to obtain a ratio of 1.6. Pipette up and down ten times. Incubate a room temperature without shaking for 5 min.

2. Place the plate on the magnetic stand until the supernatant has cleared, at least 3 min.

3. Remove the supernatant with a multichannel pipette if you are using a 96-well plate, making sure not to disturb the beads.

4. With the samples on the magnetic stand, wash the beads by adding 200 μl of freshly prepared 70% ethanol, and incubate for 30 s. Carefully remove the supernatant, without disturbing the beads.

5. Repeat washing **step 4**.

6. Remove all residual ethanol using a pipette and air dry with the samples on the magnetic stand for 3 min.

7. Remove the plate from the stand and add 40 μl of nuclease-free water for elution, gently pipetting up and down ten times to resuspend the beads. Incubate the plate at room temperature for 5 min.

8. Place the plate back on the magnetic stand at least 5 min or until the supernatant has cleared. *See* also **Note 2** about bead carryover.

9. Carefully transfer the supernatant to a new plate.

3.4 Normalization and Pooling

At this step, equimolar amounts of purified amplicons are pooled, so that each pool contains amplicons generated using different tailed PCR primers (*see* Fig. 2):

1. Check the concentration of the purified amplicons using Qubit.

2. Pool equimolar amounts of each purified amplicon for a final amount of 1 μg in a final volume of 60 μl (add water if necessary).

3.5 End Repair

1. Thaw End Repair Mix 2 and resuspension buffer.

2. Add 40 μl of End Repair Mix 2 to each tube containing 60 μl of pooled PCR amplicon (1 μg) and mix gently by pipetting up and down ten times.

3. Incubate the samples for 30 min at 30 °C in a thermocycler with pre-heated lid.

3.6 Bead Purification

Perform a magnetic bead cleanup (refer to Subheading 3.3) using a ratio of 1:1.6. Add 160 μl of beads to each tube containing 100 μl of end repair mix (*see* **Note 3**). At the end of the cleanup, elute the sample in 20 μl of resuspension buffer and transfer 17.5 μl of the clear supernatant to a new tube. If you don't proceed to the next step immediately, samples can be stored in the –20 °C freezer for up to 7 days.

3.7 A-Tailing

1. Thaw A-Tailing Mix and resuspension buffer.

2. Add 12.5 μl of A-Tailing Mix to each tube containing 17.5 μl of sample and mix gently by pipetting up and down.

3. Incubate the samples for 30 min at 37 °C, followed by 5 min at 70 °C and 5 min at 4 °C in a thermocycler with pre-heated lid.

4. Proceed immediately to the ligation.

3.8 Ligation of Y-Adapters (See Fig. 2)

1. Thaw DNA Adapter Index tubes and stop ligation buffer. Leave Ligation Mix in the freezer until immediately before use and keep on ice once removed from the freezer.

2. Add reagents in the following order to each tube containing 30 μl of end-repaired and A-tailed PCR amplicons – (1) 2.5 μl of resuspension buffer; (2) 2.5 μl of ligation mix; (3) and 2.5 μl of appropriate DNA Adapter Index – and mix gently by pipetting up and down.

3. Incubate the samples for 10 min at 30 °C in a thermocycler with pre-heated lid and then hold at 4 °C.

4. Add 5 μl of stop ligation buffer to each sample and mix gently by pipetting up and down.

3.9 Bead Purifications (Twice)

Perform a magnetic bead cleanup (refer to Subheading 3.3) using a ratio of 1:1 following Illumina TruSeq protocol. Add 42.5 μl of beads to each sample containing 42.5 μl of Adapter mix obtained after Subheading 3.8. At the end of the cleanup, elute the sample in 52.5 µl resuspension buffer and transfer 50 µl of the clear supernatant to a new tube. Perform an additional magnetic bead cleanup (refer to Subheading 3.3) using a ratio of 1:1. At the end of the cleanup, elute the sample in 22.5 µl resuspension buffer and transfer 20 µl of the clear supernatant to a new tube.

3.10 Normalization and Pooling

1. Check fragment sizes of each sample using a TapeStation. One main peak of the right size should be seen in addition to the lower and upper markers.

2. Check sample concentration using Qubit.

3. Dilute each indexed library to 10 ng/µl.

4. Pool 5 µl of each indexed library.

3.11 Library Validation Using Quantitative PCR

1. If the KAPA kit is used for the first time, add the 10× Primer Premix (1 ml) to the bottle of 2× KAPA SYBR FAST qPCR Master Mix and mix well with vortexer.

2. Prepare 1:5000, 1:10,000, and 1:20,000 dilutions of the library using Tris–Cl 10 nM buffer, pH 8.5 with 0.1% Tween 20. It is best to prepare three independent dilutions for each individual dilution (i.e., three independent 1/5000 dilutions). Here is an example on how to prepare dilutions:

Dilution	Library input	10 mM Tris–HCl (µl)
1:50	2 µl of undiluted library	98
1:5000	2 µl of 1/50 dilution	198
1:10,000	10 µl of 1/5000 dilution	10
1:20,000	10 µl of 1/5000 dilution	30

3. Determine the total number of reactions that will be performed for the appropriate number of replicates of each of the following reactions:
   - Three replicates of each of the six DNA standards.
   - Three replicates of each dilution to be assayed.
   - Three replicates of the no template control.

4. Prepare the Master Mix for the total number of reactions. For each 20 µl reaction, add:
   - 12 µl of 2× KAPA SYBR FAST Master Mix.
   - 4 µl of PCR-grade water.

5. Mix and briefly centrifuge the reagent Master Mix.

6. Dispense 16 µl of Master Mix to each well.

7. Add 4 µl of PCR-grade water to each well of the no template control.

8. Add 4 μl of each DNA standard to the appropriate well. Always start with low concentration standard.

9. Add 4 μl of each sample dilution to the appropriate well.

10. Seal the plate, centrifuge, and transfer to the qPCR instrument.

11. Setup experiment on the Applied Biosystems ViiA 7 real-time PCR system according to the manufacturer's instructions. In the menu, select the following options:
    - Fast 96-well block.
    - Standard curve.
    - SYBR mode.
    - Fast.

12. Set the reaction volume to 20 μl.

13. Perform qPCR using the following cycling conditions: 5 min at 95 °C (1×), 30 s at 95 °C, and 45 s at 60 °C (35×).

14. Calculate sample concentration in nM using the KAPA library Quantification Data Analysis Template for Illumina.

15. Dilute the library to 4 nM.

4   Notes

1. Size selection can be carried out by gel purification. An alternative better suited to high-throughput sequencing and low DNA concentrations is to use magnetic beads, as these will give better DNA recovery. Depending on the ratio of beads to sample, different size fragments can be purified [11]. In addition, selection of fragments to the left and right side of the desired fragment range can be carried out. Left side selection is done by binding the larger fragments to the right of the desired range to the beads and eluting the smaller fragments. For right size selection, the larger fragments to the right of the desired range are bound to the beads, and the supernatant containing the smaller fragments is removed to a fresh tube. For more details on this procedure *see* [12].

2. If an unwanted product is seen at 1000 bp, it can be due to bead carryover. To ensure that all magnetic beads are removed from the sample, an additional purification step can be carried out by placing the samples on the magnetic stand for 15 min and transferring the supernatant to a new tube.

3. If bead cleaning is performed in a magnetic plate, beads of the top layer might not efficiently bind to the magnet because of the large volume. To ensure maximum recovery, first pipette off approximately 100 μl of the lower clear layer and wait for an additional 5 min before pipetting the rest of the liquid.

Acknowledgments

Financial support to M.L. was provided by the Sant Chair and the Smithsonian Tennenbaum Marine Observatories Network, for which this is Contribution No. 5. This work was also supported by Swedish research council grant C0344601 to S.J.B.

References

1. Fonseca VG, Carvalho GR, Sung W, Johnson HF, Power DM, Neill SP, Packer M, Blaxter ML, Lambshead PJD, Thomas WK, Creer S (2010) Second-generation environmental sequencing unmasks marine metazoan biodiversity. Nat Commun 1:Artn 98. doi:10.1038/Ncomms1095

2. Ji YQ, Ashton L, Pedley SM, Edwards DP, Tang Y, Nakamura A, Kitching R, Dolman PM, Woodcock P, Edwards FA, Larsen TH, Hsu WW, Benedick S, Hamer KC, Wilcove DS, Bruce C, Wang XY, Levi T, Lott M, Emerson BC, Yu DW (2013) Reliable, verifiable and efficient monitoring of biodiversity via metabarcoding. Ecol Lett 16(10):1245–1257. doi:10.1111/Ele.12162

3. Leray M, Meyer CP, Mills SC (2015) Metabarcoding dietary analysis of coral dwelling predatory fish demonstrates the minor contribution of coral mutualists to their highly partitioned, generalist diet. Peerj 3:Artn e1047. doi:10.7717/peerj.1047

4. Aylagas E, Borja A, Rodriguez-Ezpeleta N (2014) Environmental status assessment using DNA metabarcoding: towards a genetics based marine biotic index (gAMBI). PLoS One 9(3), e90529. doi:10.1371/journal.pone.0090529

5. Leray M, Knowlton N (2015) DNA barcoding and metabarcoding of standardized samples reveal patterns of marine benthic diversity. Proc Natl Acad Sci U S A 112(7):2076–2081. doi:10.1073/Pnas.1424997112

6. Visco JA, Apotheloz-Perret-Gentil L, Cordonier A, Esling P, Pillet L, Pawlowski J (2015) Environmental monitoring: inferring the diatom index from next-generation sequencing data. Environ Sci Technol 49(13):7597–7605. doi:10.1021/es506158m

7. Caporaso JG, Lauber CL, Walters WA, Berg-Lyons D, Huntley J, Fierer N, Owens SM, Betley J, Fraser L, Bauer M, Gormley N, Gilbert JA, Smith G, Knight R (2012) Ultra-high-throughput microbial community analysis on the Illumina HiSeq and MiSeq platforms. ISME J 6(8):1621–1624. doi:10.1038/ismej.2012.8

8. Kozich JJ, Westcott SL, Baxter NT, Highlander SK, Schloss PD (2013) Development of a Dual-Index sequencing strategy and curation pipeline for analyzing amplicon sequence data on the MiSeq Illumina sequencing platform. Appl Environ Microb 79(17):5112–5120. doi:10.1128/AEM.01043-13

9. Leray M, Yang JY, Meyer CP, Mills SC, Agudelo N, Ranwez V, Boehm JT, Machida RJ (2013) A new versatile primer set targeting a short fragment of the mitochondrial COI region for metabarcoding metazoan diversity: application for characterizing coral reef fish gut contents. Frontiers in zoology 10:Unsp 34. doi:10.1186/1742-9994-10-34

10. Lobo J, Costa PM, Teixeira MAL, Ferreira MSG, Costa MH, Costa FO (2013) Enhanced primers for amplification of DNA barcodes from a broad range of marine metazoans. BMC Ecol 13:34. doi:10.1186/1472-6785-13-34

11. CoreGenomics. How do SPRI beads work? http://core-genomics.blogspot.co.uk/2012/04/how-do-spri-beads-work.html

12. BeckmanCoulter. http://www.beckmancoulter.com/wsrportal/bibliography?docname=SPRIselect.pdf

Chapter 15

Visualizing Patterns of Marine Eukaryotic Diversity from Metabarcoding Data Using QIIME

Matthieu Leray and Nancy Knowlton

Abstract

PCR amplification followed by deep sequencing of homologous gene regions is increasingly used to characterize the diversity and taxonomic composition of marine eukaryotic communities. This approach may generate millions of sequences for hundreds of samples simultaneously. Therefore, tools that researchers can use to visualize complex patterns of diversity for these massive datasets are essential. Efforts by microbiologists to understand the Earth and human microbiomes using high-throughput sequencing of the 16S rRNA gene has led to the development of several user-friendly, open-source software packages that can be similarly used to analyze eukaryotic datasets. Quantitative Insights Into Microbial Ecology (QIIME) offers some of the most helpful data visualization tools. Here, we describe functionalities to import OTU tables generated with any molecular marker (e.g., 18S, COI, ITS) and associated metadata into QIIME. We then present a range of analytical tools implemented within QIIME that can be used to obtain insights about patterns of alpha and beta diversity for marine eukaryotes.

Key words Metabarcoding, QIIME, Alpha diversity, Beta diversity, Principal component analysis, Rarefaction

1 Introduction

The world's Oceans harbor an immense diversity of life estimated between 0.3 and 2.2 million species belonging to 31 phyla [1, 2]. Yet, with only about 0.25 million formally described species to date, a considerable portion of that diversity remains either unknown to science or without a formal description. In addition, diagnostic morphological characters used to differentiate species can be very subtle in some invertebrate groups or even absent among microscopic soft-bodied taxa (e.g., nematodes). This taxonomic impediment has dramatically limited our understanding of the way ocean ecosystems function and respond to environmental changes, with most studies focusing on just a few indicator metazoan taxa [3]. The realization that we might not be able to study ocean diversity using morphology alone has led more and more researchers toward DNA approaches to characterize and monitor diversity [4, 5].

Sarah J. Bourlat (ed.), *Marine Genomics: Methods and Protocols*, Methods in Molecular Biology, vol. 1452,
DOI 10.1007/978-1-4939-3774-5_15, © Springer Science+Business Media New York 2016

DNA sequencing expands the taxonomic coverage of ecological studies by providing rapid and reliable species identifiers that do not depend on having taxonomic expertise. Building upon DNA barcode resources and taking advantage of the availability of affordable High-Throughput Sequencing (HTS) technologies, the concept of DNA metabarcoding is now revolutionizing our understanding of patterns of marine diversity. Most commonly, general primer sets are used to mass amplify (via Polymerase Chain Reaction or PCR) a short hypervariable DNA fragment from an collection of organisms mixed together. Reads obtained using an HTS platform are then sorted bioinformatically to delineate Operational Taxonomic Units (OTUs) and provide estimates of richness and community composition [6]. This metabarcoding approach [7] is now widely used, and the scientific community has converged toward using standard DNA markers such as 18S nuclear small subunit (nSSU) ribosomal RNA and the mitochondrial Cytochrome Oxidase c. Subunit I (COI) genes to target a wide taxonomic range of organisms.

The ability to obtain community profiles from hundreds of samples offers the potential for an unprecedented understanding of marine diversity. While powerful analysis tools are essential to handle very large sequence datasets, visualizing patterns of diversity for complex datasets also represents a major challenge. For example, researchers need to be able to see how community profiles vary in relation to each other and in relation to various metadata variables. Quantitative Insights Into Microbial Ecology (QIIME) [8] is one of the most powerful data visualization tools. Like many other sequence data analysis workflows (e.g., Mothur [9]), QIIME was developed to analyze microbial 16S rRNA datasets, but its functionalities can be used to analyze OTU tables obtained with any molecular marker.

QIIME combines many separate programs into a user-friendly software package to perform analysis from the raw data generated by any HTS platform to the graphical representation of the data. Functionalities available within QIIME for sequence processing include sample demultiplexing, OTU picking, phylogenetic analysis, and taxonomic assignments, all of which are also implemented in other software packages (e.g., Mothur [9], CloVR [10], LotuS [11]). On the other hand, QIIME offers some unique interactive graphic tools to explore patterns of diversity in relation to metadata variables (e.g., three-dimensional visualizations with EMPeror [12]). In this chapter, we first describe how to import an OTU table and associated metadata into QIIME. We then present a QIIME tutorial to represent the taxonomic composition (e.g., histograms, heatmaps), plot OTU diversity (alpha diversity), and plot dissimilarities in OTU composition between samples (beta diversity). We illustrate community analysis using amplicon data comparing OTU composition between sessile communities collected on settlement plates in Florida and Virginia (USA). Samples were characterized using HTS of the mitochondrial Cytochrome Oxidase c. Subunit 1 region [5].

2 Materials

2.1 QIIME Packages Available

To avoid installing each program used within QIIME separately, the developing team proposes several full installation packages.

1. The precompiled MacQIIME software package for Mac OS X. The following tutorial assumes that the user is working with MacQIIME. http://www.wernerlab.org/software/macqiime.

2. The QIIME virtual box that can be installed and run on Mac OS X, Windows, and Linux. Instructions are provided in the following link http://qiime.org/install/virtual_box.html.

3. The QIIME virtual machine on Amazon Web Services.

2.2 Getting Ready with MacQIIME 1.9.1

MacQIIME is a precompiled, easy-to-install, and easy-to-use version of QIIME that is maintained by the Werner lab (http://www.wernerlab.org). Version 1.9.1 requires Mac OS X versions 10.7 (Lion) and above.

1. Download the compressed Tar archived MacQIIME file here http://www.wernerlab.org/software/macqiime.

2. Unarchive MacQIIME 1.9.1.
   Open your terminal and type:
   ```
   $ cd ~/Downloads
   $ tar -xvf MacQIIME_1.9.1-20150604_OS10.7.tar
   ```

3. Install MacQIIME 1.9.1.
   ```
   $ cd MacQIIME_1.9.1-20150604_OS10.7
   $ ./install.s
   ```

4. Launch MacQIIME 1.9.1.
   ```
   $ macqiime
   ```

2.3 BIOM Formatted OTU Table (Input File Required)

Regardless of the target gene and the bioinformatics pipeline used for sample demultiplexing, quality filtering, OTU clustering, and taxonomic assignment, the final product of any metabarcoding study is a "sample by observation contingency table" displaying the number of reads per OTU and per sample. The file format traditionally used to represent a raw contingency table is a tab-delimited text file, termed a classic OTU table. A classic OTU table can be easily visualized and manipulated in excel or TextWrangler but it has been deemed an inefficient file format for cross-studies comparison, for transferring data between software packages, and for optimizing the use of disk space [13]. As a result, QIIME now requires classic OTU tables to be converted into Biological Observation Matrix file format (BIOM).

1. Prepare your classic OTU table as shown in Table 1 and save it as a tab-delimited text file called "otu_table.txt" in a directory called "qiime_analysis."

2. Open your terminal and navigate to the directory "qiime_analysis" where the classic OTU table is located.

```
$ cd ~/qiime_analysis
```

3. Assuming that MacQIIME is already open (see earlier), type the following command to convert your classic OTU table to a BIOM formatted table (*see* **Note 1**).

```
$ biom convert -i otu_table.txt -o otu_
table.biom  --process-obs-metadata  taxonomy
--table-type "OTU table" --to-json
```

where the parameter -i is used to specify the input file and the parameter *-o* is used to specify the output file (*see* **Note 2**).

4. Check conversion by summarizing the count information.

```
$ biom summarize-table -i otu_table.biom -o
otu_table_summary_counts.txt --qualitative
```

The number of OTUs per sample is provided. The parameter *--qualitative* should be removed from the script to summarize the number of sequences per sample instead.

5. Filter out singletons.

OTUs represented by a single sequence are often considered less reliable because they may result from sequencing errors. The following command discards all OTUs that are not represented by at least two sequences.

```
$ filter_otus_from_otu_table.py -i otu_table.
biom -o otu_table_nosingleton.biom -n 2
```

2.4 Metadata Mapping File (Input File Required)

The mapping file contains information about each sample present in the OTU table. It can be generated by hand using excel and saved as a tab-delimited text file. Columns "#SampleID," "BarcodeSequence," "LinkerPrimerSequence," and "Description" are mandatory and should be presented in this order. Additional metadata columns may be added between "LinkerPrimerSequence" and "Description" (e.g., Location, Site; Table 2). When QIIME is used for downstream data analysis and visualization only, as is the case in this tutorial, the "BarcodeSequence" and "LinkerPrimerSequence" columns can be left empty (but keep tabs) or with "NA" (Table 2).

QIIME has a functionality to test the validity of a mapping file. -p and –b parameters need to be specified if no Barcode and primer sequences are provided. This command line generates a log file listing potential warnings and errors detected in the mapping file (e.g., invalid characters, duplicated sample ID). In the following command, the parameter *-m* specifies the mapping file labeled "Metadata_map.txt."

```
$ validate_mapping_file.py  -m  Metadata_
map.txt -p -b
```

Table 1
Example of a classic OTU table representing three samples (ML.0136–ML.0138) with a total of 15 OTUs

#OTU ID	ML.0136	ML.0137	ML.0138	taxonomy
171	7900	3809	4328	Root;k__Animalia;p__Bryozoa;c__Gymnolaemata;o__Cheilostomatida;f__Schizoporellidae
768	2201	1864	5967	Root;k__Animalia;p__Cnidaria;c__Hydrozoa;o__Leptothecata;f__Campanulariidae
1031	10,272	5771	3249	Root;k__Animalia;p__Cnidaria;c__Hydrozoa
13	8	1	1	Root;k__Animalia;p__Chordata;c__Ascidiacea;o__Stolidobranchia;f__Styelidae
185	1	3	2	Root;k__Animalia;p__Chordata;c__Ascidiacea;o__Phlebobranchia;f__Ascidiidae
978	9	6	13	Root;k__Animalia;p__Porifera;c__Demospongiae;o__Homosclerophorida;f__Oscarellidae
5	935	1547	2543	Root;k__Animalia;p__Bryozoa;c__Gymnolaemata;o__Cheilostomatida;f__Bugulidae
388	463	595	904	Root;k__Animalia;p__Chordata
971	670	1433	645	Root;k__Animalia;p__Arthropoda
3	555	829	865	Root;k__Animalia;p__Bryozoa;c__Gymnolaemata;o__Cheilostomatida;f__Membraniporidae
589	1397	1449	207	Root;k__Animalia;p__Arthropoda
919	1043	1107	195	Root;k__Animalia;p__Arthropoda;c__Malacostraca;o__Decapoda;f__Panopeidae
517	0	1	0	Root;k__Animalia;p__Porifera;c__Demospongiae;o__Halichondrida
516	3	3	1	Root;k__Animalia;p__Arthropoda;c__Maxillopoda;o__Calanoida
312	3	2	2	Root;k__Animalia;p__Annelida;c__Polychaeta;o__Sabellida;f__Sabellidae

This is a portion of a larger OTU table obtained using high-throughput sequencing of the mitochondrial Cytochrome Oxidase c. Subunit Subunit 1 region [5]. The last column of the table presents taxonomic assignment of each OTU (*see* **Note 3**)

Table 2
Example of a metadata mapping file containing information about 18 samples analyzed in Leray and Knowlton [5]

# Sample ID	Barcode sequence	Linker primer sequence	Location	Site	Description
ML.0136	NA	NA	Virginia	Site1	Virginia.Site1
ML.0137	NA	NA	Virginia	Site1	Virginia.Site1
ML.0138	NA	NA	Virginia	Site1	Virginia.Site1
ML.0139	NA	NA	Virginia	Site3	Virginia.Site3
ML.0140	NA	NA	Virginia	Site3	Virginia.Site3
ML.0141	NA	NA	Virginia	Site3	Virginia.Site3
ML.0142	NA	NA	Virginia	Site2	Virginia.Site2
ML.0143	NA	NA	Virginia	Site2	Virginia.Site2
ML.0144	NA	NA	Virginia	Site2	Virginia.Site2
ML.0145	NA	NA	Florida	Site1	Florida.Site1
ML.0146	NA	NA	Florida	Site1	Florida.Site1
ML.0147	NA	NA	Florida	Site1	Florida.Site1
ML.0148	NA	NA	Florida	Site2	Florida.Site2
ML.0149	NA	NA	Florida	Site2	Florida.Site2
ML.0150	NA	NA	Florida	Site2	Florida.Site2
ML.0151	NA	NA	Florida	Site3	Florida.Site3
ML.0152	NA	NA	Florida	Site3	Florida.Site3
ML.0153	NA	NA	Florida	Site3	Florida.Site3

Each sample represents a community of sessile organisms collected on settlement plates at three sites in Florida and Virginia (*see* **Note 4**)

2.5 Phylogenetic Tree (Input File Optional)

This is used to calculate phylogenetic alpha (e.g., phylogenetic diversity) and beta diversity metrics (e.g., unifrac). The QIIME script "make_phylogeny.py" generates a tree using various methods (default: FastTree). Otherwise a tree can be imported into QIIME as a Newick formatted tree file. In the following tutorial, we do not use phylogenetic alpha and beta metrics.

2.6 Alpha Parameter File (Input File Optional)

A parameter file is used to specify one or a set of values of a parameter within a QIIME script. The parameter file contains the name of the script (i.e., alpha_diversity) followed by the name of the parameter (i.e., metrics), followed by a tab and finally the value of the parameter (i.e., observed_species, chao1). The following line indicates that the observed number of species and chao1 should be used to calculate alpha diversity. It should be saved as a text file (*see* **Note 5** for a list of alpha metrics implemented in QIIME).

alpha_diversity:metrics observed_species,chao1

2.7 Beta Parameter File (Input File Optional)	The beta parameter file specifies the beta metrics to use. The format of the file is similar to the format of the alpha parameter file detailed earlier. It should also be saved as a text file (*see* **Note 6** for a list of beta metrics implemented in QIIME).

beta_diversity:metrics bray_curtis,binary_jaccard

3   Methods

Diversity analyses presented in the following section require four input files placed in the same directory called "qiime_analysis":

- otu_table_nosingleton.biom
- Metadata_map.txt
- alpha_params.txt
- beta_params.txt

See Subheading 2 for details about input file format.

3.1   Rarefy OTU Table

High-throughput sequencing experiments often result in unequal numbers of reads between samples. Differences in sequencing depth affect estimates of alpha and beta diversity because as more sequences are obtained more OTUs are detected. The goal is therefore to scale the number of sequences of the larger samples down to the smallest number of sequences that a sample contains within the dataset. The following QIIME script creates a single OTU table "otu_table_nosingleton_rarefied.biom" that has been subsampled down to 11,982 reads for all samples.

single_rarefaction.py -i otu_table_nosingleton.biom -o otu_table_nosingleton_rarefied.biom -d 11982

3.2   Plot Rank Abundance Curves

Rank abundance curves display OTU richness and evenness. OTU richness in a sample can be viewed as the number of ranks that a curve reaches. OTU evenness corresponds to the slope of the line (Fig. 1). A steep line means that a few OTUs dominate the sample in terms of abundance (low evenness). In the following command line, -*s* is used to specify the name of the sample to plot. '*' means that all samples should be presented on the same plot. We also specify -*a* to use absolute counts and -*x* to represent a linear *x*-axis scale.

plot_rank_abundance_graph.py -i otu_table_nosingleton_rarefied.biom -s '*' -o Rank_abundance_plots.pdf -a -x

3.3   Visualize Taxonomic Composition

Various graphical representations of taxonomic composition are implemented in QIIME. Histograms and heatmaps drawn at various taxonomic levels are particularly useful for interpreting patterns of alpha and beta diversity.

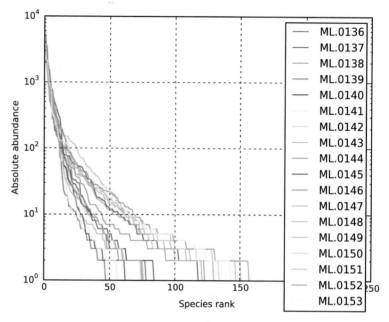

Fig. 1 Rank abundance curves for 18 communities of sessile organisms collected on settlement plates in Virginia (ML.0136 ML.-0144) and Florida (ML.0145-ML .0153). Each community was characterized using HTS of COI amplicons [5]

1. Calculate the relative abundance of taxonomic groups within each sample of the rarefied OTU table. The following script creates one table per taxonomic level (i.e., kingdom, phylum, class). They are later referred to as taxonomy tables.

   ```
   $ summarize_taxa.py -i otu_table_nosingle-
   ton_rarefied.biom  -o  taxa_summary_relative_
   abundance
   ```

2. Generate taxonomy tables with absolute abundance rather than relative abundance using the parameter -*a*

   ```
   $ summarize_taxa.py -i otu_table_nosingle-
   ton_rarefied.biom  -o  taxa_summary_absolute_
   abundance -a
   ```

3. Plot histogram displaying relative sequence abundance within each sample at the phylum (Fig. 2) and class levels. Open the html files to visualize the plots. QIIME also produces each plot in a pdf format.

   ```
   $ plot_taxa_summary.py -i taxa_summary_rel-
   ative_abundance/otu_table_nosingleton_rarefied_
   L3.txt -o taxa_summary_plots/plots_phylum
   $ plot_taxa_summary.py -i taxa_summary_rel-
   ative_abundance/otu_table_nosingleton_rarefied_
   L4.txt -o taxa_summary_plots/plots_class
   ```

4. Plot heatmaps with relative sequence abundance to further explore differences in composition between groups of samples. Like histograms, they can be produced at all taxonomic levels

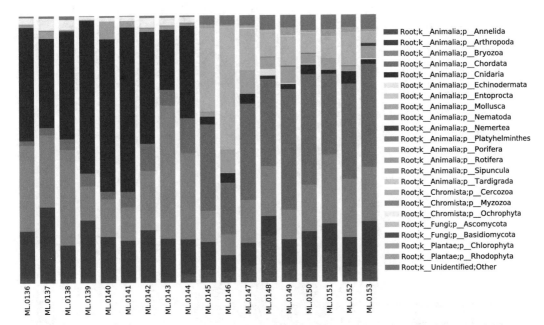

Root;k__Animalia;p__Annelida
Root;k__Animalia;p__Arthropoda
Root;k__Animalia;p__Bryozoa
Root;k__Animalia;p__Chordata
Root;k__Animalia;p__Cnidaria
Root;k__Animalia;p__Echinodermata
Root;k__Animalia;p__Entoprocta
Root;k__Animalia;p__Mollusca
Root;k__Animalia;p__Nematoda
Root;k__Animalia;p__Nemertea
Root;k__Animalia;p__Platyhelminthes
Root;k__Animalia;p__Porifera
Root;k__Animalia;p__Rotifera
Root;k__Animalia;p__Sipuncula
Root;k__Animalia;p__Tardigrada
Root;k__Chromista;p__Cercozoa
Root;k__Chromista;p__Myzozoa
Root;k__Chromista;p__Ochrophyta
Root;k__Fungi;p__Ascomycota
Root;k__Fungi;p__Basidiomycota
Root;k__Plantae;p__Chlorophyta
Root;k__Plantae;p__Rhodophyta
Root;k__Unidentified;Other

Fig. 2 Histogram summarizing the relative number of COI amplicons within each community of sessile organisms collected in Virginia (ML.0136-ML. 0144) and Florida (ML.0145-ML. 0153). Relative abundance is presented at the phylum level. See metadata file for more information about each sample

represented in taxonomy tables (computed by the summarize_taxa.py script). In the following, we specify *--no_log_transform* because the input file contains relative abundances.

```
$ make_otu_heatmap.py -i taxa_summary_rel-
ative_abundance/otu_table_nosingleton_rar-
efied_L3.biom  -o  taxa_summary_plots/plots_
phylum/phylum_heatmap.pdf --no_log_transform
--absolute_abundance
$ make_otu_heatmap.py -i taxa_summary_rel-
ative_abundance/otu_table_nosingleton_rar-
efied_L4.biom  -o  taxa_summary_plots/plots_
class/class_heatmap.pdf  --no_log_transform
--absolute_abundance
```

5. Plot heatmaps with log-transformed absolute sequence abundance at the phylum (Fig. 3) and class levels. Because in most datasets a few OTUs might dominate the sequence counts, transforming the data often helps better visualize differences in taxonomic composition.

```
$ make_otu_heatmap.py -i taxa_summary_abso-
lute_abundance/otu_table_nosingleton_rarefied_
L3.biom  -o  taxa_summary_plots/plots_phylum/
phylum_heatmap_log.pdf --absolute_abundance
$ make_otu_heatmap.py -i taxa_summary_abso-
lute_abundance/otu_table_nosingleton_rarefied_
L4.biom  -o  taxa_summary_plots/plots_class/
class_heatmap_log.pdf --absolute_abundance
```

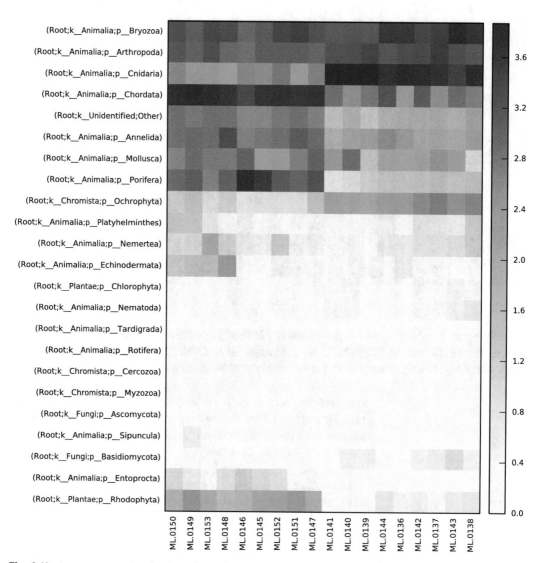

Fig. 3 Heatmap representing log-transformed numbers of COI amplicons within each community of sessile organisms collected in Virginia (ML.0136-ML. 0144) and Florida (ML.0145-ML. 0153)

3.4 Calculate Alpha Diversity

Alpha diversity represents the diversity within each sample (*see* **Note 5** for a list of alpha metrics implemented in QIIME). The following command line creates a table with the observed number of OTUs and Chao1 values for each sample.

```
$ alpha_diversity.py -i otu_table_nosingleton_
rarefied.biom -m observed_otus,chao1 -o alpha_
diversity.txt
```

3.5 Plot Alpha Rarefaction Curves

Unlike species accumulation curves, individual-based rarefaction curves are built using a resampling approach by randomly selecting sequences at increasing levels of accumulation (e.g. 1000, 2000, 3000 reads) until all sequences have been accumulated. Many

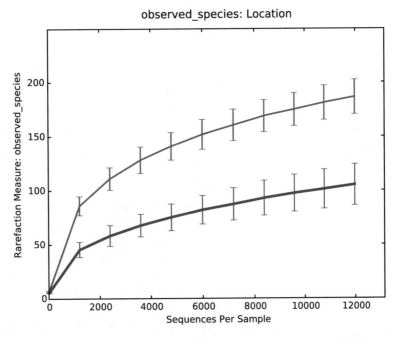

Fig. 4 Alpha rarefaction curves representing the observed number of OTUs as a function of the number of resampled sequences in the OTU table. Curves were averaged per location (red: Florida; blue: Virginia)

resampling iterations are done at each level to calculate the mean and standard deviation of the curve.

1. Plot rarefaction curves using alpha metrics specified in the alpha_params.txt file (*see* Subheading 2.6). An interactive .html output file can be opened with a web browser to visualize curves built with the different alpha metrics. Because a mapping file is also specified, rarefaction curves averaged per groups of samples are also displayed (e.g., Virginia vs. Florida).

   ```
   $ alpha_rarefaction.py -i otu_table_nos-
   ingleton_rarefied.biom -m Metadata_map.txt -o
   alpha_rarefaction -p alpha_params.txt
   ```
   If no alpha parameter file is specified, the default metrics are used, among which PD_whole_tree requires a phylogenetic tree.

2. Plot rarefaction plots in .pdf format (Fig. 4; also *see* **Note 7**).

   ```
   $ make_rarefaction_plots.py -i alpha_rar-
   efaction/alpha_div_collated -o alpha_rarefac-
   tion/pdfs -g pdf -m Metadata_map.txt
   ```

3.6 Calculate Beta Diversity

Beta diversity is a measure of dissimilarity in species composition between samples. QIIME supports both qualitative and quantitative metrics of beta diversity. Qualitative metrics (e.g., binary_jaccard) measure changes in communities driven by presence/absence of OTUs, whereas quantitative metrics (e.g., bray_curtis) measure differences in relative abundance of OTUs between communities.

The following command line calculates distance matrices using the Jaccard and Bray Curtis metrics.

```
$ beta_diversity.py -i otu_table_nosingleton_
rarefied.biom -m binary_jaccard,bray_curtis -o
beta_diversity
```

3.7 Visualize Beta Diversity

In the following section, we provide command lines to represent dissimilarities in OTU composition calculated between samples using both the qualitative Jaccard metric and the quantitative Bray Curtis metric.

1. Plot pairwise distances within and between categories (Fig. 5).

```
$ make_distance_boxplots.py -d beta_diver-
sity/binary_jaccard_otu_table_nosingleton_
rarefied.txt -m Metadata_map.txt -f "Location"
-o beta_boxplot/binary_jaccard
$ make_distance_boxplots.py -d beta_diver-
sity/bray_curtis_otu_table_nosingleton_rar-
efied.txt -m Metadata_map.txt -f "Location"
-o beta_boxplot/bray_curtis
```

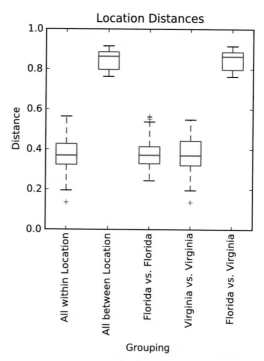

Fig. 5 Boxplot representing Bray Curtis distances within and between locations where sessile communities were collected. These plots show that, based on COI amplicon data, the taxonomic composition of sessile communities is more similar within Florida and Virginia than it is between the two locations

2. Calculate principal coordinate axes.

```
$ principal_coordinates.py -i beta_diver-
sity/binary_jaccard_otu_table_nosingleton_
rarefied.txt -o PC_binary_jaccard.txt
$ principal_coordinates.py -i beta_diver-
sity/bray_curtis_otu_table_nosingleton_rar-
efied.txt -o PC_bray_curtis.txt
```

3. Plot interactive three-dimensional Principal Coordinate Analysis (PCoA) using EMPeror [12] (Fig. 6).

```
$ make_emperor.py -i PC_binary_jaccard.txt
-m Metadata_map.txt -o 3D_PCoA/binary_jaccard/
$ make_emperor.py -i PC_bray_curtis.txt
-m Metadata_map.txt -o 3D_PCoA/bray_curtis/
```

4. Plot two-dimensional PCoA using the Jaccard and Bray Curtis distance matrices.

```
$ make_2d_plots.py -i PC_binary_jaccard.txt
-m Metadata_map.txt -o 2D_PCoA_binary_jaccard
$ make_2d_plots.py -i PC_bray_curtis.txt
-m Metadata_map.txt -o 2D_PCoA_bray_curtis
```

5. Plot hierarchical clustering tree using Unweighted Pair Group Method with Arithmetic mean (UPGMA). The resulting tree can be visualized in FigTree (http:// tree.bio.ed.ac.uk/software/figtree/).

```
$ upgma_cluster.py -i beta_diversity/
binary_jaccard_otu_table_nosingleton_rar-
efied.txt -o UPGMA_binary_jaccard.tre
```

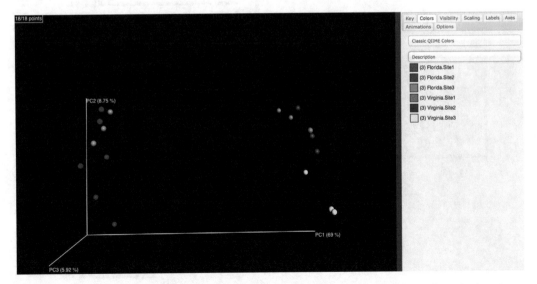

Fig. 6 Three-dimensional PCoA visualized using Emperor in a web browser. Emperor is used to color by category in the metadata mapping file. Here, the PCoA was built using the Bray Curtis distance matrix

```
$ upgma_cluster.py -i beta_diversity/
bray_curtis_otu_table_nosingleton_rarefied.
txt -o UPGMA_bray_curtis.tre
```

3.8 Evaluate Robustness of Beta Diversity Estimates to Sequencing Effort

The reliability of beta diversity estimates is measured by resampling random subsets of the OTU table several times, a process called jackknifing. Beta diversity is then calculated for all independent datasets and compared to the value obtained for the entire dataset.

1. Jackknife the entire dataset and compare beta diversity values. Here, we resample 8986 sequences of each sample (which corresponds to 75% of the smallest sample) to ensure that the smallest sample is also randomly resampled.

```
$ jackknifed_beta_diversity.py -i otu_
table_nosingleton.biom -m Metadata_map.txt -o
beta_jack -e 8986 -p beta_params.txt
```

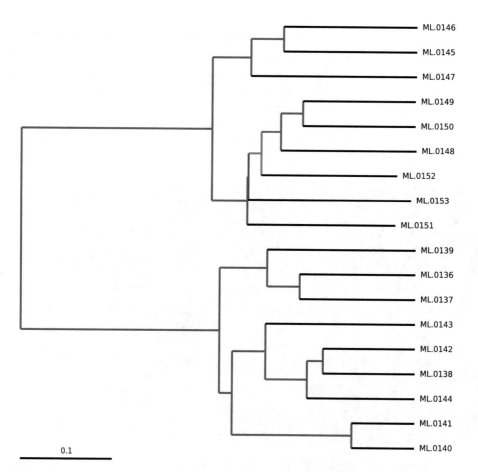

Fig. 7 UPGMA hierarchical clustering tree with branch support calculated using jackknifing. Branch colors represent the level of support: red for 75–100% support; yellow for 50–75% support; green for 25–50% support; blue for < 25% support. Here, the tree shows high level of support for differences in community composition between sessile communities in Virginia (ML.0136–ML.0144) and Florida (ML.0145–ML.0153). It also shows strong support for community structuring at each location

This workflow creates a three-dimensional PCoA with a confidence ellipsoid around each sample. It calculates support values for the UPGMA tree.

2. Support values to UPGMA hierarchical clustering tree (Fig. 7)

```
$  make_bootstrapped_tree.py   -m  beta_jack/
binary_jaccard/upgma_cmp/master_tree.tre  -s
beta_jack/binary_jaccard/upgma_cmp/jack-
knife_support.txt  -o  beta_jack/binary_jac-
card/upgma_cmp/jackknife_named_nodes.pdf
```

```
$  make_bootstrapped_tree.py   -m  beta_jack/
bray_curtis/upgma_cmp/master_tree.tre    -s
beta_jack/bray_curtis/upgma_cmp/jackknife_
support.txt -o beta_jack/bray_curtis/upgma_
cmp/jackknife_named_nodes.pdf
```

3. Plot two-dimensional PCoA with confidence ellipsoid around each sample estimated using jackknifing.

```
$ make_2d_plots.py -i beta_jack/binary_jac-
card/pcoa/ -mMetadata_map.txt -b'Location&&Site'
--ellipsoid_opacity=0.2  -o  beta_jack/binary_
jaccard/pcoa/
```

```
$ make_2d_plots.py -i beta_jack/bray_curtis/
pcoa/ -m Metadata_map.txt -b 'Location&&Site'
--ellipsoid_opacity=0.2     -o     beta_jack/
bray_curtis/pcoa/
```

4. Calculate the mean, median, and standard deviation of the distance matrices previously created by jackknifing the OTU table.

```
$ dissimilarity_mtx_stats.py -i beta_jack/
binary_jaccard/rare_dm/ -o beta_jack/binary_
jaccard/rare_dm/
```

```
$ dissimilarity_mtx_stats.py -i beta_jack/
bray_curtis/rare_dm/ -o beta_jack/bray_cur-
tis/rare_dm/
```

5. Create boxplots to visualize variations in beta distances within and between categories. Here, we specify the category "Location."

```
$  make_distance_boxplots.py  -m  Metadata_
map.txt -o beta_jack/binary_jaccard/distance_
boxplot/ -d beta_jack/binary_jaccard/rare_dm/
means.txt -f Location --save_raw_data
```

```
$  make_distance_boxplots.py  -m  Metadata_
map.txt  -o  beta_jack/bray_curtis/distance_
boxplot/  -d  beta_jack/bray_curtis/rare_dm/
means.txt -f Location --save_raw_data
```

3.9   Test for Differences in Beta Diversity Between Groups of Samples

Several statistical approaches are implemented within QIIME for testing for differences in beta diversity between groups of samples (*see* **Note 8**). Among them, the Permutational Multivariate Analysis of Variance (PERMANOVA) is a nonparametric analog of ANOVA that tests for differences in the position of sets of objects in multivariate space. The parameter *-c* specifies the metadata categories that need to be compared.

```
compare_categories diversity/binary_jaccard_otu_
table_nosingleton_rarefied.txt  -m  Metadata_map.
txt -c Location -o beta_tests/binary_jaccard/-
method  permanova__categories.py  -ibeta_diver-
sity/bray_curtis_otu_table_nosingleton_rarefied.
txt -m Metadata_map.txt -c Location -o beta_tests/
bray_curtis/ --method permanova
```

Notes

1. If file conversion fails and QIIME returns an error message, it is most likely due to the presence of special characters in your classic OTU table that are not supported by the BIOM format. To detect and remove these characters, open your classic OTU table in TextWrangler, and select "Zap Gremlins…" in the "Text" menu.

2. The syntax of QIIME commands is standardized. For example, *-i* is used to specify the input file and *-o* to specify the output file (or directory) in all command lines.

3. Each sample identifier should only contain alphanumeric characters and period (.)

4. Sample identifiers should match between the OTU table and the mapping file.

5. The following alpha metrics are supported in QIIME: ace, berger_parker_d, brillouin_d, chao1, chao1_ci, dominance, doubles, enspie, equitability, esty_ci, fisher_alpha, gini_index, goods_coverage, heip_e, kempton_taylor_q, margalef, mcintosh_d, mcintosh_e, menhinick, michaelis_menten_fit, observed_otus, observed_species, osd, simpson_reciprocal, robbins, shannon, simpson, simpson_e, singles, strong, PD_whole_tree. Further information about each metric can be found at http://scikit-bio.org/docs/latest/generated/skbio.diversity.alpha.html.

6. The following nonphylogenetic beta metrics are supported in Qiime: abund_jaccard, binary_dist_chisq, binary_dist_chord, binary_dist_euclidean, binary_dist_hamming, binary_dist_jaccard, binary_dist_lennon, binary_dist_ochiai, binary_otu_gain, binary_dist_pearson, binary_dist_sorensen_dice, dist_bray_curtis, dist_canberra, dist_chisq, dist_chord, dist_euclidean, dist_gower, dist_hellinger, dist_kulczynski, dist_manhattan, dist_morisita_horn, dist_pearson, dist_soergel, dist_spearman_approx, dist_specprof. Phylogenetic metrics that require a phylogenetic tree are the following: dist_unifrac_G, dist_unifrac_G_full_tree, dist_unweighted_unifrac, dist_unweighted_unifrac_full_tree, dist_weighted_normalized_unifrac, dist_weighted_unifrac.

7. The legend is not displayed on the .pdf files but can be seen in the html file.

8. Statistical methods available in QIIME to test for differences in composition between categories of samples are as follows: ANOSIM, BIO-ENV, Moran's I, MRPP, PERMANOVA, PERMDISP, db-RDA. Further information about each test can be found here http://qiime.org/scripts/compare_categories.html.

Acknowledgments

We thank Sarah Bourlat for inviting this submission. This work was supported by the Sant Chair and the Smithsonian Tennenbaum Marine Observatories Network, for which this is Contribution No. 3.

References

1. Mora C, Tittensor DP, Adl S et al (2011) How many species are there on Earth and in the Ocean? PLoS Biol 9:1001127. doi:10.1371/journal.pbio.1001127

2. Appeltans W, Ahyong ST, Anderson G et al (2012) The magnitude of global marine species diversity. Curr Biol 22:2189–202. doi:10.1016/j.cub.2012.09.036

3. Tittensor DP, Mora C, Jetz W et al (2010) Global patterns and predictors of marine biodiversity across taxa. Nature 466:1098–101. doi:10.1038/nature09329

4. Fonseca VG, Carvalho GR, Sung W et al (2011) Second-generation environmental sequencing unmasks marine metazoan biodiversity. Nat Commun 1:1–8. doi:10.1038/ncomms1095

5. Leray M, Knowlton N (2015) DNA barcoding and metabarcoding of standardized samples reveal patterns of marine benthic diversity. Proc Natl Acad Sci U S A 112:2076–2081. doi:10.1073/pnas.1424997112

6. Leray M, Yang JY, Meyer CP et al (2013) A new versatile primer set targeting a short fragment of the mitochondrial COI region for metabarcoding metazoan diversity: application for characterizing coral reef fish gut contents. Front Zool 10:34. doi:10.1186/1742-9994-10-34

7. Taberlet P, Coissac E, Pompanon F et al (2012) Towards next-generation biodiversity assessment using DNA metabarcoding. Mol Ecol 21:2045–50. doi:10.1111/j.1365-294X.2012.05470.x

8. Caporaso JG, Kuczynski J, Stombaugh J et al (2010) QIIME allows analysis of high-throughput community sequencing data. Nat Methods 7:335–6. doi:10.1038/nmeth.f.303

9. Schloss PD, Westcott SL, Ryabin T et al (2009) Introducing mothur: open-source, platform-independent, community-supported software for describing and comparing microbial communities. Appl Environ Microbiol 75:7537–7541. doi:10.1128/aem.01541-09

10. Angiuoli SV, Matalka M, Gussman A et al (2011) CloVR: a virtual machine for automated and portable sequence analysis from the desktop using cloud computing. BMC Bioinformatics 12:356. doi:10.1186/1471-2105-12-356

11. Hildebrand F, Tadeo R, Voigt A et al (2014) LotuS: an efficient and user-friendly OTU processing pipeline. Microbiome 2:30. doi:10.1186/2049-2618-2-30

12. Vázquez-Baeza Y, Pirrung M, Gonzalez A, Knight R (2013) EMPeror: a tool for visualizing high-throughput microbial community data. Gigascience 2:16. doi:10.1186/2047-217X-2-16

13. McDonald D, Clemente JC, Kuczynski J et al (2012) The Biological Observation Matrix (BIOM) format or: how I learned to stop worrying and love the ome-ome. Gigascience 1:7. doi:10.1186/2047-217X-1-7

Chapter 16

Analysis of Illumina MiSeq Metabarcoding Data: Application to Benthic Indices for Environmental Monitoring

Eva Aylagas and Naiara Rodríguez-Ezpeleta

Abstract

This protocol details the analysis of Illumina MiSeq amplicon libraries derived from marine benthic macroinvertebrate samples and based on two barcodes of the mitochondrial cytochrome oxidase 1 (CO1) gene: a "short region," covered by overlapping forward and reverse reads and a "long region" for which forward and reverse reads do not overlap. Aside from providing guidelines for analyzing both types of amplicons, we show how amplicon reads can be used for the calculation of benthic indices for environmental monitoring.

Key words Marine benthic macroinvertebrates, Amplicon sequencing, CO1, Folmer region, MiSeq

1 Introduction

Metabarcoding, the simultaneous amplification of a standardized DNA fragment specific for a species from the total DNA extracted from an environmental sample, allows the rapid, accurate, and cost-effective identification of the entire taxonomic composition of thousands of samples simultaneously [1]. This is particularly relevant for monitoring programs relying on the application of benthic indices, which are based on indicator species or ecological groups of species classified according to their sensitivity to stress [2]. Implementation of metabarcoding in regular monitoring programs requires both standardized laboratory and data analysis procedures so that results across studies can be compared [3]. Here, we describe the data analysis procedures developed to derive the benthic macroinvertebrate taxonomic composition of an environmental sample from MiSeq amplicon reads such as the ones generated using the protocols described in Chapters 12 (Fonseca and Lallias), 13 (Bourlat et al.), and 14 (Leray et al.). We will focus on barcodes based on two regions of the most commonly used gene for

Sarah J. Bourlat (ed.), *Marine Genomics: Methods and Protocols*, Methods in Molecular Biology, vol. 1452,
DOI 10.1007/978-1-4939-3774-5_16, © Springer Science+Business Media New York 2016

Metazoa, the mitochondrial cytochrome oxidase 1 (CO1) [4]: a "long region" of 658 bp amplified using the LCO1490–HCO2198 [5], dgLCO1490–dgHCO2198 [6], or jgLCO1490–jgHCO2198 [7] primer pairs, and a "short region" of 313 bp amplified using the mlCOIintF [8] forward primer with the HCO2198, dgHCO2198, or jgHCO2198 reverse primers. The analysis for the long region is especially challenging as, unlike in the short region, the reads do not overlap, which requires additional read and database preparation steps. Additionally, we describe the application of Illumina MiSeq amplicon analysis to environmental monitoring based on benthic macroinvertebrate indices. One of the most successful biotic indices used worldwide is AZTI's Marine Biotic Index (AMBI), which uses marine benthic macroinvertebrates as indicators of ecosystem health [9]. Calculation of the currently implemented AMBI is based on abundance-weighted pollution tolerances of the species present in a sample (tolerance expressed categorically as one of five ecological groups—sensitive to pressure, indifferent, tolerant, opportunist of second order, and opportunist of first order). However, estimating abundances from sequence data is difficult due to biological factors such as multicellularity, variation in tissue cell density, inter and intraspecific variations in gene copy number, and technical limitations such as PCR biases (some sequences are amplified more than others) and PCR and sequencing errors [10]. Thus, biodiversity estimation of the species present in a sample using sequencing data should rely on presence/absence metrics [11], such as the p/a AMBI, based on presence/absence of each species and providing biotic index values that are strongly related to the AMBI values [2].

2 Materials

2.1 Sequencing Reads

We assume that 300 bp long forward and reverse sequence reads are provided by the sequencing facility, and demultiplexed based on the barcodes assigned to each sample as described in Chapters 13 (Bourlat et al.) and 14 (Leray et al.). There should be two files per sample in compressed fastq format, usually with extension ".fastq.gz."

2.2 Software

All analyses described in Subheadings 3.1–3.4 are performed on a Unix-based environment. The programs listed as follows need to be previously installed in the system:

1. FastQC [12]: http://www.bioinformatics.babraham.ac.uk/projects/fastqc.

2. Trimmomatic [13]: http://www.usadellab.org/cms/?page=trimmomatic.

3. FLASH [14]: http://ccb.jhu.edu/software/FLASH.

4. mothur [15]: http://www.mothur.org.

5. Cd-hit [16]: http://weizhong-lab.ucsd.edu/cd-hit/.

   For Subheading 3.5, the AMBI software needs to be installed on a Windows environment.

6. AMBI [9]: http://ambi.azti.es.

2.3 Databases

A database that contains the correspondence between each taxon and its barcode is needed for taxonomic assignment. Here, we will use the most complete and curated database for the CO1 marker, the BOLD database. Generating a formatted database with all CO1 barcodes requires the retrieval of aligned sequences and taxonomy files from BOLD (http://www.boldsystems.org) using an existing account (*see* **Note 1**).

1. Aligned sequences are retrieved by searching "Public records" from the "Workbench" section using the option "Let BOLD align my sequences" (*see* **Note 2**).

2. Taxonomy files (in TSV format) are retrieved by using the "Access Published & Released Data" from the taxonomy browser.

3 Methods

Taxonomic assignment of reads is described in Subheading 3.4 and is based on the MiSeq SOP tutorial [17] of mothur. This tutorial starts with the raw reads; however, due to the nature of our data (i.e., non-overlapping forward and reverse reads), the need for a custom database and the fact that this tutorial does not consider quality scores, we have introduced a preprocessing step of the raw data described in Subheadings 3.1 and 3.2 for the CO1 short and long regions, respectively (*see* **Note 3**), and a database preparation step described in Subheading 3.3. In Subheading 3.5, we describe the calculation of benthic indices based on the taxonomic assignment of amplicon reads.

Throughout the methods section, "$" indicates Unix commands run in the terminal window, whereas "mothur>" indicates commands run inside mothur (*see* **Note 4**).

3.1 Preparation of Reads for Analysis of the CO1 "Short Region"

The "short region" amplicons are 313 bp long, meaning that, with 300 bp long MiSeq forward and reverse reads, an overlap of 237 bp is expected.

1. Check the quality of the reads using FastQC:

```
$ fastqc S1_R1.fastq.gz S1_R2.fastq.gz
```

   This will generate a .fastqc.html file for each forward and reverse file that can be visualized in any web browser. The plots generated contain relevant information on the library preparation process and sequence quality (see the FastQC documentation for more information). If everything looks as expected, continue to the next step (*see* **Note 5**).

2. Remove primer sequences (the first 26 bases of the forward and reverse reads, *see* **Note 6**) using Trimmomatic:

```
$ trimmomatic SE -phred33 -trimlog S1_R1.logfile
S1_R1.fastq.gz S1_R1_crop.fastq.gz HEADCROP:26
$ trimmomatic SE -phred33 -trimlog
S1_R2.logfile S1_R2.fastq.gz S1_R2_crop.fastq.
gz HEADCROP:26
```

This will result in two output files, S1_R1_crop.fastq and S1_R2_crop.fastq, that contain the forward and reverse reads without the primer sequence.

3. Merge the forward and reverse reads with a minimum and maximum required overlap length between two reads of 217 and 257 bp, respectively (*see* **Note 7**):

```
$ flash S1_R1_crop.fastq.gz S1_R2_crop.fastq.
gz -M 257 -m 217 -o S1 -z
```

This will generate five output files: S1.hist and S1.histogram that contain numeric and visual histograms of merged read lengths, S1.extendedFrags.fastq.gz that contains the merged reads, and S1.notCombined_1.fastq.gz and S1.notCombined_2.fastq.gz that contain the forward and reverse reads that were not merged, respectively.

4. Remove reads that have an average quality (Phred score) below 25 using the SLIDINGWINDOW option in Trimmomatic and choosing as window length the total length of the amplicon (*see* **Note 8**):

```
$ trimmomatic SE -phred33 -trimlog
S1_extendedFrags_trimmed.logfile  S1.extended-
Frags.fastq.gz
S1_ready.fastq.gz SLIDINGWINDOW:313:25
```

This will generate an output file (S1_ready.fastq.gz) that contains only the reads with an average Phred score above 25.

5. Uncompress the S1_ready.fastq.gz file and transform it into a fasta file using mothur:

```
$ gunzip S1_ready.fastq.gz
$ mothur "#fastq.info(fastq=S1_ready.fastq)"
```

This will generate the S1_ready.fasta file that will be used as the input for Subheading 3.4.

3.2 Preparation of Reads for Analysis of the CO1 "Long Region"

The "long region" amplicons are 658 bp long, meaning that with 300 bp long MiSeq forward and reverse reads, a nonsequenced gap of 109 bp is expected.

1. Check the quality of the reads using FastQC:

```
$ fastqc S1_R1.fastq.gz S1_R2.fastq.gz
```

This will generate a .fastqc.html file for each forward and reverse file that can be visualized in any web browser. The plots generated contain relevant information on the library preparation process and sequence quality (see the FastQC documentation for more information). If everything looks as expected, continue to the next steps, but note at which position the reads have an average quality below 25 (*see* **Note 9**).

2. Trim the forward and reverse reads at the position where the average quality is below 25 (*see* **Note 8**) (260 and 200 for the forward and reverse reads in this example):

```
$ trimmomatic SE -phred33 -trimlog S1_R1.logfile
S1_R1.fastq.gz S1_R1_cut.fastq.gz CROP:260
$ trimmomatic SE -phred33 -trimlog S1_R2.logfile
S1_R2.fastq.gz S1_R2_cut.fastq.gz CROP:200
```

Note that, after this trimming step, the nonsequenced gap gets longer (249 bp in this example)

3. Remove primer sequences (the first 25 and 26 bases of the forward and reverse reads, respectively; *see* **Note 6**) using Trimmomatic:

```
$ trimmomatic SE -phred33 -trimlog S1_R1_cut.
logfile
S1_R1_cut.fastq.gz S1_R1_crop.fastq.gz HEADCROP:25
$ trimmomatic SE -phred33 -trimlog S1_R2_cut.
logfile
S1_R2_cut.fastq.gz S1_R2_crop.fastq.gz HEADCROP:26
```

This will result in two output files: S1_R1_crop.fastq and S1_R2_crop.fastq.

4. Uncompress the S1_R1_crop.fastq.gz and S1_R2_crop.fastq.gz files:

```
$ gunzip *_crop.fastq.gz
```

This will generate S1_R1_crop.fastq and S1_R2_crop.fastq files.

5. Transform the S1_R1_crop.fastq and S1_R2_crop.fastq files into fasta files and reverse-complement the reverse reads:

```
$ mothur "#fastq.info(fastq=S1_R1_crop.fastq)"
$ mothur "#fastq.info(fastq=S1_R2_crop.fastq)"
$ mothur "#reverse.seqs(fasta=S1_R2_crop.fasta)"
```

6. Paste the forward (S1_R1_crop.fasta) and reverse-complemented reverse reads (S1_R2_crop.rc.fasta) generated in the previous step to create an artificial barcode consisting of the trimmed forward and reverse reads. Because the forward and reverse files are in the same order, a simple paste command can be used.

```
$ paste -d '\0' S1_R1_crop.fasta S1_R2_crop.
rc.fasta | cut -d '>' -f1,2 > S1_ready.fasta
```

This will generate the S1_ready.fasta file that will be the input for Subheading 3.4. In this example, the barcode is 409 bp read long, which corresponds to the "long region" that lacks a 249 bp long internal fragment.

3.3 Database Preparation

We start with the files described in Subheading 2.3 that are required to generate the database: the aligned sequences (with .fasta extension) and the taxonomy (with .txt extension).

1. Remove identical sequences from the alignment file and keep one as a representative sequence in order to reduce the size of the database:

```
$ cd-hit -i BOLDdb.fasta -o BOLDdb_clean.fasta
-c 1 M2000
```

2. Trim the sequences down to the 658 bp Folmer CO1 fragment (retain the sequence between positions 38 and 714) using a sequence alignment editor (e.g., Bioedit [18]).

3. Keep the header with the sequence identifier preceded by ">":

```
$ cut -d '|' -f1 BOLDdb_clean.fasta > BOLDrefdb.
fasta
```

4. From the taxonomy file, keep only the columns and lines needed and convert to mothur file format (Fig. 1):

```
$ grep -v 'processid' BOLDtaxonomy.txt | cut
-f1,9,11,13,15,19,21 | sed 's/\t/;/g' | cut
-d ';' -f1 > BOLDtaxonomy1.txt
```

```
$ grep -v 'processid' BOLDtaxonomy.txt | cut
-f1,9,11,13,15,19,21 | sed 's/\t/;/g' | cut -d
';' -f2- | sed 's/ /_/g' | sed 's/$/;/g'>
BOLDtaxonomy2.txt
```

```
$ paste BOLDtaxonomy1.txt BOLDtaxonomy2.txt
> BOLDtax.txt
```

GBAN1430-06	Metazoa;Annelida;Polychaeta;Terebellida;Pectinariidae;Pectinaria;Pectinaria_koreni;
GBAN2075-09	Metazoa;Annelida;Polychaeta;Phyllodocida;Nereididae;Hediste;Hediste_diversicolor;
BCAS090-14	Metazoa;Annelida;Polychaeta;Terebellida;Ampharetidae;Auchenoplax;Auchenoplax_crinita;
GBCMD2886-09	Metazoa;Arthropoda;Malacostraca;Decapoda;Portunidae;Carcinus;Carcinus_maenas;
GBML0020-06	Metazoa;Mollusca;Scaphopoda;Dentaliida;Dentaliidae;Antalis;Antalis_entalis;
NBMOL004-11	Metazoa;Mollusca;Gastropoda;Littorinimorpha;Littorinidae;Littorina;Littorina_littorea;
BCAS104-15	Metazoa;Echinodermata;Ophiuroidea;Ophiurida;Ophiuridae;Ophiura;Ophiura_texturata;

Fig. 1 An extract of the BOLDreftax.txt file used for the taxonomic assignment of reads. The taxonomy file is a two column text file where the first column is the sequence identifier and the second a string of taxonomic information separated by semicolons

5. Retain only the identifiers contained in the reference CO1 alignment (*see* **Note 10**):

```
$ grep '>' BOLDrefdb.fasta | cut -d '>' -f2
> identifiers.txt
$ fgrep -f identifiers.txt BOLDtax.txt >
BOLDreftax.txt
```

If using the CO1 "long region", continue with this step:

6. Remove the 249 bp gap fragment from the BOLDrefdb.fasta file (from positions 246 to 498) using a sequence alignment editor to construct the BOLDgaprefdb.fasta database (*see* **Note 11**).

3.4 Taxonomic Assignment of Amplicon Reads

We assume that we start with quality trimmed and merged reads for the CO1 "short region" (Subheading 3.1) or CO1 "long region" (Subheading 3.2) and that we have an appropriately for-matted database (Subheading 3.3). Usually, Subheadings 3.1 and 3.2 have generated files for more than one sample (probably hundreds), which need to be merged into a single file (let us assume here we only have three samples: S1, S2, and S3). The commands used in this section and their input and output file requirements are carefully explained in the mothur manual.

1. Merge the .fasta files generated in steps 3.1 or 3.2 for each sample and create a group file to assign sequences to a specific sample; for simplicity, rename the group file to a shorter name:

```
$ cat S1_ready.fasta S2_ready.fasta S3_ready.
fasta > all.fasta
$ mothur "#make.group(fasta=S1_ready.fasta-
S2_ready.fasta-S3_ready.fasta,
groups=S1-S2-S3)"
$ mv S1_ready.S2_ready.S3_ready.groups all.
groups
```

2. Discard sequences with at least one ambiguous base (*see* **Note 12**), retain only unique reads (*see* **Note 13**) and count the number of sequences per group:

```
mothur> screen.seqs(fasta=all.fasta, group=all.
groups, maxambig=0, processors=8)
mothur> unique.seqs(fasta=all.good.fasta)
mothur>     count.seqs(name=all.good.names,
group=all.good.groups)
```

3. Align the sequences (here, the COI "short region" is used as an example) to the corresponding CO1 reference database using the Needleman–Wunsch global alignment algorithm. Retain sequences that align inside the barcode region (*see* **Note 14**) and are longer than a given threshold (*see* **Note 15**). In order to obtain a cleaner alignment, regions of the alignment with no data and resulting redundancies are removed:

```
mothur> align.seqs(fasta=all.good.unique.fasta,
reference=BOLDrefdb.fasta, processors=8, flip=T)
```

```
mothur>     screen.seqs(fasta=all.good.unique.
align,    count=all.good.count_table,    min-
length=200, start=420, end=550, processors=8)
```

```
mothur>     filter.seqs(fasta=all.good.unique.
good.align, processors=8)
```

```
mothur> unique.seqs(fasta=all.good.unique.good.
filter.fasta, count=all.good.good.count_table)
```

4. Remove sequences that occur only once among all samples (singletons) (*see* **Note 16**):

```
mothur>     split.abund(fasta=all.good.unique.
good.filter.unique.fasta, count=all.good.unique.
good.filter.count_table, cutoff=1)
```

5. Remove potential chimeric sequences using UCHIME [19] de novo mode:

```
mothur> chimera.uchime(fasta=all.good.unique.
good.filter.unique.abund.fasta, count=all.good.
unique.good.filter.abund.count_table,
processors=8)
```

```
mothur>   remove.seqs(accnos=all.good.unique.
good.filter.unique.abund.uchime.accnos,
fasta=all.good.unique.good.filter.unique.
abund.fasta,   count=all.good.unique.good.fil-
ter.abund.count_table)
```

6. Assign taxonomy to the sequences using the Wang approach [20]. Taxonomic assignments are done using the aligned reference database and the reference taxonomy file created in Subheading 3.3:

```
mothur>     classify.seqs(fasta=all.good.unique.
good.filter.unique.abund.pick.fasta, count= all.
good.unique.good.filter.abund.pick.count_table,
template=BOLDrefdb.fasta, taxonomy=BOLDreftax.
txt, cutoff=90, method=wang, processors=8)
```

7. Cluster sequences into "Operational Taxonomic Units" (OTUs) based on the previous taxonomic classification. Count the number of times an OTU is observed in order to have information about the incidence of the OTUs in the different samples.

```
mothur>   phylotype(taxonomy=all.good.unique.
good.filter.unique.abund.pick.BOLDreftax.
wang.taxonomy)
```

```
mothur>     make.shared(list=all.good.unique.
good.filter.unique.abund.pick.BOLDreftax.
```

```
wang.tx.list, count=all.good.unique.good.fil-
ter.abund.pick.count_table)
```

This will create a file with the count of the number of reads in each OTU, for each sample.

8. Assign taxonomy to each OTU:

```
mothur>    classify.otu(list=all.good.unique.
good.filter.unique.abund.pick.BOLDreftax.
wang.tx.list, count=all.good.unique.good.fil-
ter.abund.pick.count_table,    taxonomy=all.
good.unique.good.filter.unique.abund.pick.
BOLDreftax.wang.taxonomy)
```

9. Combine the files obtained in **steps 7** and **8** into a single table to generate the OTU table that contains the count of the number of sequences in each OTU, for each sample, and the taxonomy of that OTU.

The OTU table is the final output obtained using this protocol, which can be used as an input file for diversity metrics estimations (i.e., alpha and beta diversity). *See* also Chapters 1 by Lehmann and 15 by Leray and Knowlton on the calculation of diversity indices using the OTU table. The OTU table can also be used for the calculation of biotic indices, biodiversity monitoring programs, and other biodiversity studies that are based on sample taxonomic composition.

3.5 Calculation of Benthic Indices from Sequence Data

The biotic index calculation procedure described here is based on presence/absence data obtained from the taxonomic analysis of amplicon reads performed in Subheading 3.4 and carried out according to the "Instructions for the use of the AMBI index" protocol [21]. Detailed information about each step can be found in the manual.

We assume that we start with the OTU table, for which taxonomic assignment of the reads has been performed.

1. Import the OTU table into a spreadsheet and open it in R, Excel, or any other program to manipulate data.

2. Transform relative abundance of the retained taxa into presence/absence data. Simply change the number of reads to 1 if they represent more than 0.01% of the total taxa and keep the rest of the cells blank.

3. Open the AMBI software, import the spreadsheet, and calculate the AMBI index. The result will show the ecological quality of the stations under study (Fig. 2b), allowing the monitoring of a site after an impact or the detection of gradients from the source of a certain impact. In addition, detailed information on the percentage of taxa assigned to each ecological group for each station can be displayed (Fig. 2a).

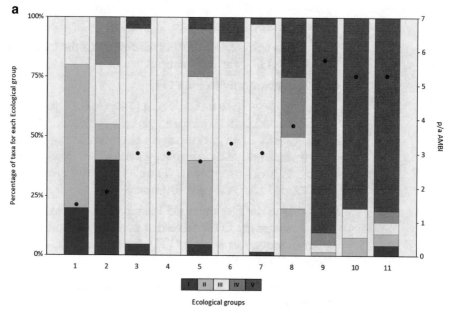

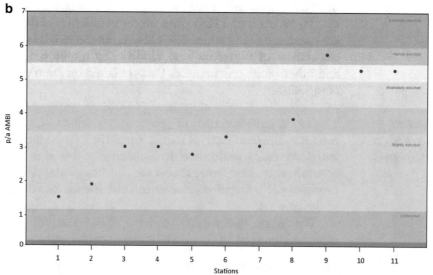

Fig. 2 (**a**) Percentage of taxa from each ecological group and derived presence/absence AMBI (p/a AMBI) values for 11 arbitrary stations used as an illustrating example. (**b**) Ecological quality for 11 arbitrary stations used as an illustrating example

4   Notes

1. A new BOLD account can be created at http://www.boldsys-tems.org/index.php/MAS_Management_NewUserApp.

2. Minimum required fields in the record search are Taxonomy, Marker and select to include public records. Note that record search can be performed by taxonomic level (e.g., phylum), although some groups need to be split into lower levels

(e.g., Chordata has to be split into classes) due to download limitations of 50,000 records in a unique search. If that is the case, you will need to concatenate the resulting files to create a single file.

3. Subheadings 3.1 and 3.2 describe the steps needed to process one sample (named here "S1") for which two raw data files (S1_R1.fastq.gz and S1_R2.fastq.gz), corresponding to 300 bp long forward and reverse reads, have been provided. Processing the hundreds of files usually generated in one MiSeq run would require the use of scripts including loops, which is not covered in this chapter.

4. mothur can be executed using an interactive mode, batch mode, and command line mode; see the mothur webpage for more explanations on how to use each mode.

5. It is expected that quality drops toward the end of the reads. For the analysis of the "short region," this is not an issue because the large overlapping region allows the poor quality bases at the ends of the forward reads to be compensated by the good quality ones of the beginning of the reverse reads and vice versa.

6. If different primers are used, these values need to be adjusted to the appropriate primer length.

7. We found that using a minimum and a maximum overlap of, respectively, minus and plus 20 bases from the expected overlap (237 bp in the case of the "short region") provides good results.

8. Quality score thresholds are somewhat arbitrary. We found that 25 is not too strict, neither too loose, but other values are equally appropriate.

9. It is expected that the quality of the read drops toward the end; for the analysis of the "long region," this is an issue because there is no overlap.

10. The taxonomy file downloaded from BOLD also includes taxa for which no barcode is available. Because the database must contain the same identifiers in both alignment and taxonomy files, these additional taxa need to be removed.

11. Removing the 249 bp gap fragment in the database facilitates the alignment of the query sequences to the reference alignment. We found that even changing the alignment parameters, mothur is not able to correctly aligning the CO1 "long region" sequences to the complete reference database.

12. Discarding all reads that contain at least one ambiguous base may lead to too few reads remaining; in such cases, it is possible to exclude only those reads with more than a certain number of ambiguous bases.

13. The unique.seqs commands is applied several times in order to reduce the number of reads analyzed by returning only the

unique sequences found; it has no effect on the output as it is not a filtering step.

14. Before aligning sequences to the reference alignment, verify the start and end positions on the alignment—this will facilitate following filtering steps. For the CO1 "short region," we retained sequences that start at or before position 420 and end at or after position 550; for the CO1 "long region" these positions are 60 and 300, respectively.

15. We used 200 bp for the CO1 "short region" and 300 bp for the CO1 "long region."

16. It is assumed that reads that occur only once (singletons) are most likely to be due to PCR or sequencing errors than to be real data.

Acknowledgements

This work was funded by the European Union (7th Framework Program 'The Ocean of Tomorrow' Theme, grant agreement no. 308392) through the DEVOTES (DEVelopment Of innovative Tools for understanding marine biodiversity and assessing good Environmental Status—http://www.devotes-project.eu) project and by the Basque Water Agency (URA) through a Convention with AZTI. E. Aylagas was supported by a doctoral grant from Fundación Centros Tecnológicos—Iñaki Goenaga. This is contribution number 742 from the Marine Research Division (AZTI).

References

1. Zepeda Mendoza ML, Sicheritz-Ponten T, Gilbert MT (2015) Environmental genes and genomes: understanding the differences and challenges in the approaches and software for their analyses. Brief Bioinform. doi:10.1093/bib/bbv001

2. Aylagas E, Borja A, Rodriguez-Ezpeleta N (2014) Environmental status assessment using DNA metabarcoding: towards a genetics based Marine Biotic Index (gAMBI). PLoS One 9(3), e90529. doi:10.1371/journal.pone.0090529

3. Tedersoo L, Ramirez KS, Nilsson RH, Kaljuvee A, Koljalg U, Abarenkov K (2015) Standardizing metadata and taxonomic identification in metabarcoding studies. GigaScience 4:34. doi:10.1186/s13742-015-0074-5

4. Hebert PD, Ratnasingham S, deWaard JR (2003) Barcoding animal life: cytochrome c oxidase subunit 1 divergences among closely related species. Proc Biol Sci 270(Suppl 1):S96–S99. doi:10.1098/rsbl.2003.0025

5. Folmer O, Black M, Hoeh W, Lutz R, Vrijenhoek R (1994) DNA primers for amplification of mitochondrial cytochrome c oxidase subunit I from diverse metazoan invertebrates. Mol Mar Biol Biotechnol 3(5):294–299

6. Meyer PC (2003) Molecular systematics of cowries (Gastropoda: Cypraeidae) and diversification patterns in the tropics. Biol J Linn Soc 79:401–459

7. Geller J, Meyer C, Parker M, Hawk H (2013) Redesign of PCR primers for mitochondrial cytochromecoxidase subunit I for marine invertebrates and application in all-taxa biotic surveys. Mol Ecol Resour 13(5):851–861. doi:10.1111/1755-0998.12138

8. Leray M, Yang YJ, Meyer PC, Mills CS, Agudelo N, Ranwez V, Boehm TJ, Machida JR (2013) New versatile primer set targeting a short fragment of the mitochondrial COI region for metabarcoding metazoan diversity: application for characterizing coral reef fish gut contents. Front Zool 10(34)

9. Borja A, Franco J, Perez V (2000) A marine biotic index to establish the ecological quality of soft-bottom benthos within european estuarine and coastal environments. Mar Pollut Bull 40:12

10. Yu DW, Ji Y, Emerson BC, Wang X, Ye C, Yang C, Ding Z (2012) Biodiversity soup: metabarcoding of arthropods for rapid biodiversity assessment and biomonitoring. Meth Ecol Evol 3(4):613–623. doi:10.1111/j.2041-210X.2012.00198.x

11. Elbrecht V, Leese F (2015) Can DNA-based ecosystem assessments quantify species abundance? Testing primer bias and biomass--sequence relationships with an innovative metabarcoding protocol. PLoS One 10(7), e0130324. doi:10.1371/journal.pone.0130324

12. Andrews S (2010) FastQC: a quality control tool for high throughput sequence data. http://www.bioinformatics.babraham.ac.uk/projects/fastqc

13. Bolger AM, Lohse M, Usadel B (2014) Trimmomatic: a flexible trimmer for Illumina Sequence Data. Bioinformatics 30:2114–2120

14. Magoč T, Salzberg S (2011) FLASH: fast length adjustment of short reads to improve genome assemblies. Bioinformatics 27(21):2957–2963

15. Schloss PD (2009) Introducing mothur: open-source, platform-independent, community-supported software for describing and comparing microbial communities. Appl Environ Microbiol 75(23):7537–7541

16. Li W, Godzik A (2006) Cd-hit: a fast program for clustering and comparing large sets of protein or nucleotide sequences. Bioinformatics 22(13):1658–1659. doi:10.1093/bioinformatics/btl158

17. Kozich JJ, Westcott SL, Baxter NT, Highlander SK, Schloss PD (2013) Development of a dual-index sequencing strategy and curation pipeline for analyzing amplicon sequence data on the MiSeq Illumina sequencing platform. Appl Environ Microbiol 79(17):5112–5120. doi:10.1128/AEM.01043-13

18. Hall TA (1999) BioEdit: a user-friendly biological sequence alignment editor and analysis program for Windows 95/98/NT. Nucleic Acids Symp Ser 41:4

19. Edgar RC, Haas BJ, Clemente JC, Quince C, Knight R (2011) UCHIME improves sensitivity and speed of chimera detection. Bioinformatics 27(16):2194–2200. doi:10.1093/bioinformatics/btr381

20. Wang Q, Garrity GM, Tiedje JM, Cole JR (2007) Naive Bayesian classifier for rapid assignment of rRNA sequences into the new bacterial taxonomy. Appl Environ Microbiol 73(16):5261–5267. doi:10.1128/AEM.00062-07

21. Borja A, Muxika I, Mader J (2012) Instructions for the use of the AMBI index software (Version 50). Rev Invest Mar 19(3):11

INDEX

Sarah J. Bourlat (ed.), *Marine Genomics: Methods and Protocols*, Methods in Molecular Biology, vol. 1452,
DOI 10.1007/978-1-4939-3774-5, © Springer Science+Business Media New York 2016

Printed in the United States
By Bookmasters